Study Guide for

The Practice of Nursing Research: Appraisal, Synthesis, and Generation of Evidence

Sixth Edition

Susan K. Grove, PhD, RN, ANP-BC, GNP-BC
Professor
School of Nursing
The University of Texas at Arlington
Arlington, Texas
Adult Nurse Practitioner
Family Practice
Grand Prairie, Texas

Susanne Mohnkern, PhD, RN
Professor and Chairperson, Division of Nursing
Director, Graduate Program
Roberts Wesleyan College
Rochester, New York

Nancy Burns, PhD, RN, FCN, FAAN
Professor Emeritus
School of Nursing
The University of Texas at Arlington
Arlington, Texas
Faith Community Nurse
St. Matthew Cumberland Presbyterian Church
Burleson, Texas

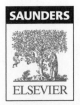

SAUNDERS

ELSEVIER

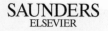

11830 Westline Industrial Drive
St. Louis, Missouri 63146

STUDY GUIDE FOR THE PRACTICE OF NURSING RESEARCH: ISBN: 978-1-4160-6108-3
APPRAISAL, SYNTHESIS, AND GENERATION OF EVIDENCE,
SIXTH EDITION
Copyright © 2009, 2005, 1997 by Saunders, an imprint of Elsevier Inc.

Notice

ISBN: 978-1-4160-6108-3

Senior Editor: Lee Henderson
Developmental Editor: Rae Robertson
Publishing Services Manager: Hemamalini Rajendrababu
Project Manager: Srikumar Narayanan
Cover Design Direction: Paula Catalano

Working together to grow
libraries in developing countries

www.elsevier.com | www.bookaid.org | www.sabre.org

ELSEVIER   BOOK AID International   Sabre Foundation

Printed in the United States of America

Last digit is the print number: 9 8 7 6 5 4 3 2

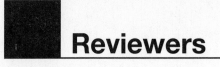

Reviewers

Maureen C. Creegan, EdD, RN
Department of Nursing
Dominican College of Blauvelt
Orangeburg, New York

Teresa Tarnowski Goodell, PhD, RN, CNS, CCRN, APRN-BC
Assistant Professor
School of Nursing
Oregon Health & Science University
Portland, Oregon

Cynthia Parkman, MSN, RN, MA
Assistant Professor
Nursing Division
California State University, Sacramento
Sacramento, California

Preface

The amount of knowledge generated through research is rapidly escalating in the nursing field. This knowledge is critical to the promotion of quality, cost-effective, evidence-based nursing care. We recognize that learning research terminology and reading and critically appraising research reports are complex and sometimes overwhelming activities. Therefore we have developed this study guide to assist you in clarifying, comprehending, analyzing, synthesizing, and applying the content presented in your textbook, *The Practice of Nursing Research: Appraisal, Synthesis, and Generation of Evidence*.

Your study guide is organized into 29 chapters, consistent with the chapters of your textbook. Each chapter of the study guide presents you with learning exercises that require various levels of cognitive skills. These exercises are organized into the following sections: Relevant Terms, Key Ideas, Making Connections, Puzzles, Exercises in Critical Appraisal, and Going Beyond. After completing the exercises for each chapter, you can review the answers in Appendix A and assess your knowledge of each chapter's content. Since your learning is enhanced by exposure to a variety of visual and written experiences, we have supplemented this study guide with an Evolve website to facilitate your comprehension of the research process.

The **Evolve Learning Resources,** http://evolve.elsevier.com/Burns/practice, include an Author Index, an alphabetical list of authors that are referenced in the textbook. Also included are approximately 400 Interactive Review Questions, references appendices, sample research proposals, data sets that provide practice in working with actual qualitative and quantitative data, and free access to **Mosby's Nursing Index,** a robust search tool for seeking articles on evidence-based practice.

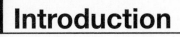

Introduction

This study guide was developed to accompany your textbook, *The Practice of Nursing Research: Appraisal, Synthesis, and Generation of Evidence*. The exercises included have been designed to assist you in comprehending the content of your textbook, conducting critical appraisals of nursing studies, using research findings to promote an evidence-based practice, and writing an initial proposal for research. It is important that you read each chapter in your text *before* completing the chapters in this study guide. First, scan the entire chapter to get an overall view of the content. Then reread the chapter with the intent of increasing your comprehension of each section. As you examine each section, pay careful attention to any terms that are defined. Underline or highlight definitions of terms in the text. If the meaning of a term is not clear to you, look up its definition in the glossary at the back of your text or in a dictionary. Highlight key ideas in each section. Examine tables and figures as they are mentioned in the text. Mark any sections that you do not fully understand. Reread these sections one sentence at a time to increase your understanding. Jot down questions to ask your instructor in class or privately.

After carefully reading a chapter in the text, use the study guide to further enhance your understanding. (Note: Each chapter in the study guide corresponds to its related chapter in your textbook.) There are six main sections to each study guide chapter: Relevant Terms, Key Ideas, Making Connections, Puzzles, Exercises in Critical Appraisal, and Going Beyond.

Relevant Terms have been identified to help you become more familiar with the terms necessary to comprehend the chapter content. Knowing these terms before you attend a class lecture on the content will give you an edge in grasping the lecture ideas and doing well on course exams. To improve your understanding of the research process, do not skip over terms in the chapter that are unfamiliar to you. Get in the habit of marking unfamiliar words as you read and looking up their definitions.

The **Key Ideas** section identifies information in the chapter important for you to note. The fill-in-the-blank questions will assist you in identifying important content that you might have missed in your first reading of the chapter. You may need to refer to specific sections of the text to complete some of these questions.

Making Connections between important ideas is critical to comprehending and synthesizing content. This section assists you in the process. Matching questions are frequently used for this purpose, although other strategies relevant to particular content may be used.

Puzzles, including Word Scrambles, Secret Messages, and Crossword Puzzles, are designed to help you have fun while learning. Each Word Scramble contains an important idea expressed in the chapter. The letters in each word have been rearranged. For example, "study" might be scrambled to read "tysud." Unscramble the words to decipher the message. (Hint: You may find it easier to start with the short words. Also, remember that the most commonly used letter in the English language is "e.") The Secret Message puzzles are similar to the Word Scrambles, but instead of rearranging letters, you will translate each message by substituting one letter for another, thus unravelling the secret code. Finally, Crossword Puzzles have been included to help you increase your familiarity with the terms and ideas expressed in the chapter.

Exercises in Critical Appraisal are provided to give you experience in critically appraising published studies. In some cases, brief quotes are provided with questions addressing information specific to the chapter content. Other questions will refer to Appendix B of the study guide, which includes three published studies, two quantitative and one qualitative. Critical appraisal questions related to these studies are posed in each chapter of the study guide. On completing the study guide, you can combine the critique information you have gathered to perform an overall critical appraisal of these three studies.

The **Going Beyond** section provides suggestions for further study. You might use these exercises to test your new knowledge. If the content of a particular chapter interests you, this section might direct you in learning more.

Appendix A provides the answers to the exercises in this study guide. However, we recommend that you not refer to these answers except to check your own responses to questions. You will learn more by searching for the answers on your own.

Appendix B provides reprints of the three published studies critically appraised in this study guide.

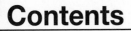

Contents

1 Discovering the World of Nursing Research

INTRODUCTION

Read Chapter 1, and then complete the following exercises. These exercises will help you to learn relevant terms, understand the framework that links nursing research with the world of nursing, and determine the significance of research in building an evidence-based practice for nursing. The answers to these exercises are in Appendix A.

RELEVANT TERMS

Framework for Nursing Research

Directions: Match each term with its correct definition.

Terms

a. Abstract thinking
b. Authority
c. Best research evidence
d. Concrete thinking
e. Empirical world

f. Evidence-based practice
g. Introspection
h. Intuition
i. Knowledge
j. Nursing research

k. Philosophy
l. Research
m. Theory
n. Science

Definitions

_____ 1. Information acquired in a variety of ways that is expected to be an accurate reflection of reality.

_____ 2. Scientific process that validates and refines existing knowledge and generates new knowledge that directly and indirectly influences nursing practice.

_____ 3. A person with expertise and power who is able to influence the opinions of others.

_____ 4. Integrative set of defined concepts and relational statements that present a way of explaining some segment of the empirical world and can be used to describe, explain, predict, or control that segment of the world.

_____ 5. Insight or understanding of a situation or event as a whole that usually cannot be logically explained.

_____ 6. Diligent, systematic inquiry to validate and refine existing knowledge and generate new knowledge.

_____ 7. A coherent body of knowledge composed of research findings, tested theories, principles, and laws for a specific discipline.

_____ 8. Thinking oriented toward and limited by tangible things or events that are observed and experienced in reality.

1

_____ 9. The world experienced through our senses; the concrete portion of our existence; often called *reality*.

_____ 10. Thinking oriented toward the development of an idea without application to, or association with, a particular instance.

_____ 11. The conscientious integration of best research evidence with clinical expertise and patient values and needs in the delivery of quality, cost-effective health care.

_____ 12. The process of turning your attention inward toward your own thoughts to increase your awareness of the flow and interplay of feelings and ideas that occur.

_____ 13. Belief system that provides a broad, global explanation of the world.

_____ 14. Extremely strong empirical knowledge generated from the synthesis of quality study findings that provides the basis for the best management of a practice problem.

Types of Reasoning

Directions: Match each term with its correct definition.

Terms

a. Deductive reasoning
b. Dialectic reasoning
c. Inductive reasoning
d. Logistic reasoning
e. Operational reasoning
f. Problematic reasoning

Definitions

_____ 1. Reasoning from the specific to the general.

_____ 2. Reasoning that involves the identification and discrimination among many alternatives and viewpoints and that focuses on the process of debating alternatives.

_____ 3. Reasoning from the general to the specific or from a general premise to a particular situation.

_____ 4. Reasoning that involves identifying a problem and the factors influencing the problem, selecting solutions to the problem, and resolving the problem.

_____ 5. Reasoning that is used to break the whole into parts that can be carefully examined, as can the relationships among the parts.

_____ 6. Reasoning from a holistic perspective that involves examining factors that are opposites and making sense of them by merging them into a single unit or idea.

KEY IDEAS

Directions: The research evidence generated for nursing needs to focus on the description, explanation, prediction, and control of phenomena important to nursing practice. Write a definition of these four types of research evidence, and provide an example of each.

1. Description:

   Example:

2. Explanation:

   Example:

3. Prediction:

   Example:

4. Control:

   Example:

MAKING CONNECTIONS

Directions: Fill in the blanks, or provide the appropriate responses.

1. List five ways of acquiring knowledge in nursing, and provide an example of each.

   a.

   b.

   c.

   d.

   e.

2. Benner's (1984) book *From Novice to Expert: Excellence and Power in Clinical Practice* describes the importance of

   _____ _____ in acquiring nursing knowledge.

3. Identify Benner's five levels of experience in the development of clinical knowledge and expertise.

   a.

   b.

   c.

   d.

   e.

3

4. Nurses _____ knowledge from other disciplines such as medicine, psychology, and sociology to provide care to patients.

5. _____ knowledge provides a scientific basis for the description, explanation, prediction, and control of nursing practice.

6. Nurses often have a "gut feeling" or "just know" when patients' conditions become serious. This is an example of

_____.

7. _____ provide knowledge based on customs and trends, such as giving a bath to hospitalized patients every morning.

8. New graduates sometimes enter internships provided by clinical agencies and are guided, supported, and educated

by experienced nurses, who act as _____ to the novice nurse.

9. In internships, new graduates are encouraged to _____ or imitate the behaviors of expert nurses.

10. Two types of logical reasoning are _____ and _____.

11. What type of reasoning is represented below? _____.

Human beings experience pain.
Babies are human beings.
Therefore, babies experience pain.

12. Identify three interventions that you use frequently in your nursing practice. What types or type of knowledge (authority, traditions, borrowing, trial and error, personal experience, role modeling, intuition, reasoning or research) provide(s) a basis for each intervention?

a. Intervention:
   Type(s) of knowledge:

b. Intervention:
   Type(s) of knowledge:

c. Intervention:
   Type(s) of knowledge:

13. What types of knowledge provide the basis for the majority of your interventions in clinical practice?

14. Is your practice evidence based? Provide a rationale for your response.

15. Why is evidence-based practice important in health care?

16. Identify two areas that are essential to the body of knowledge needed for nursing practice (American Nurses Association, 2003).

   a.

   b.

17. Identify two types of research that could be conducted to generate a science for nursing.

   a.

   b.

18. Identify two philosophical beliefs or values that provide a basis for the nursing profession.

19. The Seventh Report of the Joint National Committee on the Prevention, Detection, Evaluation, and Treatment of High Blood Pressure (JNC 7 Report) (2003) is an example of a research-based national guideline that is implemented

   to promote _____ _____.

20. Evidence-based practice includes three major concepts or ideas, which are:

   a.

   b.

   c.

PUZZLES

Directions: Using the framework developed for this textbook, circle the concepts that are directly linked to nursing research.

   Philosophy

   Theory

   Nursing practice

   Science

Abstract thought processes

Knowledge

Ways of knowing

Word Scramble

Directions: Unscramble the following sentence by rearranging the letters to form actual words. Note: You will use all the letters in every word.

Nrusgin sereahcr si rtecidly kinled ot hte rlwod fo singurn.

GOING BEYOND

Develop a framework that links research and evidence-based practice to the profession of nursing. Use the ideas and the framework presented in Chapter 1 as a basis for generating your framework. Share this framework with your instructor and classmates.

Use the framework you developed to deliver evidence-based care to a particular patient and family.

2 The Evolution of Evidence-Based Practice in Nursing

INTRODUCTION

Read Chapter 2, and then complete the following exercises. These exercises will help you to learn relevant terms, understand the historical development of research in nursing, identify the methodologies for developing nursing research evidence, and determine the best research evidence for practice. The answers to these exercises are in Appendix A.

RELEVANT TERMS

Methodologies Used to Develop Research Evidence in Nursing

Directions: Match each term with its correct definition.

Terms

a. Correlational research
b. Critical social theory
c. Descriptive research
d. Ethnographic research
e. Experimental research

f. Grounded theory research
g. Historical research
h. Intervention research
i. Outcomes research
j. Phenomenological research

k. Philosophical inquiry
l. Qualitative research
m. Quantitative research
n. Quasi-experimental research
o. Scientific method

Definitions

_____ 1. A type of quantitative research that provides an accurate portrayal or account of characteristics of a particular individual, situation, or group; these studies are often conducted when little is known about a phenomenon.

_____ 2. Research that is considered the most objective, systematic, and controlled of the different types of quantitative research.

_____ 3. A type of qualitative research that involves describing an experience as the person lives it.

_____ 4. A formal, objective, systematic research process to describe, test relationships, or examine cause-and-effect interactions among variables.

_____ 5. Procedures that scientists have used, currently use, or may use in the future to pursue knowledge.

_____ 6. A type of quantitative research that involves the systematic investigation of relationships among two or more variables.

_____ 7. Inductive research technique initially described by Glaser and Strauss that is useful in discovering what problems exist in a social scene and the processes people use to handle them, with the result being the development of a theory.

_____ 8. Systematic, subjective research methodology used to describe life experiences and give them meaning.

_____ 9. A type of quantitative research that involves examining cause-and-effect relationships but has a lower level of control than experimental research.

_____ 10. Research that involves a narrative description or analysis of events that occurred in the remote or recent past.

7

_____ 11. A type of qualitative research that involves the use of intellectual analysis to clarify meanings, make values manifest, identify ethics, and study the nature of knowledge.

_____ 12. A type of research that was developed within the discipline of anthropology for investigating cultures through an in-depth study of the members of the culture.

_____ 13. A theory that provides the basis for research that focuses on understanding how people communicate and how they develop symbolic meanings in a society.

_____ 14. A type of research conducted to examine the end result of care or to measure the change in health status of a patient to determine if the care is cost-effective and of high quality.

_____ 15. Important new research methodology for examining the effectiveness of nursing interventions in achieving the desired outcomes in natural settings.

Processes for Synthesizing Research Evidence for Practice

Directions: Match each term below with its correct definition.

Terms
a. Integrative review
b. Meta-analysis
c. Metasummary
d. Metasynthesis
e. Systematic review

Definitions

_____ 1. A structured, comprehensive synthesis of quantitative studies in a particular health care area to determine the best research evidence available for expert clinicians to use to promote evidence-based practice.

_____ 2. The synthesis or summing of the findings across qualitative research reports to determine the current knowledge in an area.

_____ 3. A type of study that statistically pools the results from previous studies into a single quantitative analysis that provides one of the highest levels of evidence for an intervention's efficacy.

_____ 4. A research synthesis process that includes the identification, analysis, and synthesis of research findings from independent quantitative and qualitative studies to determine the current knowledge (what is known and not known) in a particular area.

_____ 5. A complex synthesis of qualitative research that provides a fully integrated, novel description or explanation of a target event or experience versus a summary view.

KEY IDEAS

Directions: Fill in the blanks, or provide the appropriate responses.

1. _____ is considered the first nurse researcher.

2. _Nursing Research,_ the first research journal in nursing, was first published in _____.

3. The American Nurses Association (ANA) Commission on Nursing Research established the

_____ in 1972.

4. Many national and international _____ conferences have been sponsored by Sigma Theta Tau, the international honor society for nursing since 1970 to communicate nursing studies.

5. _____ is a Scottish epidemiologist who promoted the idea of evidence-based practice through his book published in 1972.

6. The research journal first published in 1978 is _____.

7. Identify two other research journals that were first published in 1987 or 1988.

   a.

   b.

8. _____was the project directed by J. Horsley to promote the use of research findings in practice, the results of which were published in 1982 to 1983.

9. What does the *Annual Review of Nursing Research* include?

10. The National Center for Nursing Research (NCNR) was established in _____ by the National Institutes for Health.

11. The NCNR is now called the _____.

12. _____ is based on the logical empiricism or positivism philosophy and is the most common type of research conducted in nursing.

13. Identify two areas of emphasis presented in the NINR mission for 2007.

   a.

   b.

14. A new type of research was initiated in the late 1980s and early 1990s to determine the quality endpoints or results of care and was called _____ research.

15. David Sacket and his research team developed methodologies to determine the best _____ _____ for practice.

16. In 1989, the _____ was established to facilitate the conduct of outcomes research.

17. The development of a(n) _____ practice for nursing requires the conduct and synthesis of numerous high-quality studies to determine the current best research evidence available for implementation in practice.

18. In 1999, the Agency for Health Care Policy and Research (AHCPR) was reauthorized, and its name was changed to the _____.

19. Identify two goals of the Agency for Healthcare Research and Quality (AHRQ).

a.

b.

20. What are the two major foci of *Healthy People 2010,* published in 2000 by the Department of Health and Human Services?

a.

b.

21. _____ provide the best research evidence for making a change in clinical practice.

22. What is the weakest evidence for making a change in clinical practice?

23. In Figure 2-2, Levels of Research Evidence, what is the second best type of research evidence that might be used to promote evidence-based practice in nursing?

MAKING CONNECTIONS

Synthesis Processes

Directions: Match the research synthesis processes listed here with the ideas that follow.

Process

a. Integrative review
b. Meta-analysis
c. Metasummary
d. Metasynthesis
e. Systematic review

Steps

_____ 1. Statistical synthesis of study results.

_____ 2. Summary of qualitative studies to determine what is known about the concept of health.

_____ 3. Narrative integration of quantitative studies, qualitative studies, and theoretical literature to determine what is currently known about the adaptation to chronic pain.

_____ 4. Synthesis of qualitative studies to provide a new perspective or theory about caring in nursing.

_____ 5. Synthesis of randomized controlled trials to determine the best pharmacological agent to use in the management of hypertension in the elderly.

_____ 6. Synthesis of a variety of independent quantitative and qualitative studies to determine the differences between associate and baccalaureate prepared registered nurses.

_____ 7. Summary of qualitative studies to provide a basis for metasynthesis.

_____ 8. Statistical analysis of the results of quantitative studies to determine the most effective pain assessment scale to use to assess pain in school-age children.

_____ 9. A synthesis process that includes both a narrative and a statistical analysis of studies.

_____ 10. Synthesis of original qualitative studies and metasummaries.

Research Methods

Directions: Match the following research methods with the specific types of research.

Methods
a. Qualitative research method
b. Quantitative research method

Types

_____ 1. Correlational research

_____ 2. Descriptive research

_____ 3. Ethnographic research

_____ 4. Experimental research

_____ 5. Critical social theory

_____ 6. Grounded theory research

_____ 7. Historical research

_____ 8. Phenomenological research

_____ 9. Quasi-experimental research

_____ 10. Philosophical inquiry

Nurses' Educational Preparation

Directions: Match the levels of nurses' educational preparation with the research activities that each group of nurses is *primarily responsible for* according to the guidelines of the American Nurses Association (ANA).

Educational Level
a. Associate degree
b. Baccalaureate degree
c. Master's degree
d. Doctoral degree (PhD or DNS)
e. Postdoctorate

Research Activities

_____ 1. Uses research findings in practice with supervision

_____ 2. Develops and coordinates funded research programs

_____ 3. Critically appraises studies

_____ 4. Develops nursing knowledge through research and theory development

_____ 5. Uses research findings to promote evidence-based practice

_____ 6. Collaborates in conducting research projects

_____ 7. Conducts funded independent research projects

PUZZLES

Word Scramble

Directions: Unscramble the following sentence by rearranging the letters to form actual words. Note: You will use all the letters in every word.

Tobh tiqutaantive nad aliqutaivte sereacrh htdosem era esenstial to singnur ledkngeow.

Searerch nowkdegle si deende to tropome vieenecd-sdeba urinngs actripce.

EXERCISES IN CRITICAL APPRAISAL

Research Types

Directions: The three studies listed here are provided in Appendix B. Review the titles and abstracts of these articles. Match each study with the type of research conducted.

Methods

a. Qualitative research method
b. Quantitative research method

Studies

_____ 1. Bindler, Massey, Shultz, Mills, and Short (2007)

_____ 2. Sethares and Elliott (2004)

_____ 3. Wright (2003)

Introduction to Quantitative Research

INTRODUCTION

Read Chapter 3, and then complete the following exercises. These exercises will help you to learn the steps of the quantitative research process and to identify the different types of quantitative research (descriptive, correlational, quasi-experimental, and experimental). The answers to these exercises are in Appendix A.

RELEVANT TERMS

Steps of the Research Process

Directions: Match each term with its correct definition.

Terms

a. Assumptions
b. Communicating research findings
c. Control
d. Data analysis
e. Data collection
f. Design

g. Framework
h. Interpretations of research outcomes
i. Intervention
j. Measurement
k. Methodological limitations
l. Pilot study

m. Research problem
n. Research purpose
o. Review of literature
p. Sample
q. Setting
r. Theoretical limitations
s. Variables

Definitions

_Q_ 1. Location for conducting research that can be natural, partially controlled, or highly controlled by the investigator.

_C_ 2. Occurs when the researcher imposes rules to decrease the possibility of error and increase the probability that the study's findings are an accurate reflection of reality.

_L_ 3. Smaller version of a proposed study conducted to develop or refine the methodology, such as the treatment, instruments, or data collection process to be used in the larger study.

_G_ 4. The abstract, logical structure of meaning that guides the development of the study and enables the researcher to link the findings to the body of nursing knowledge.

_N_ 5. The step of the research process that is generated from the problem and identifies the specific goal or aim of the study.

_A_ 6. Statements that are taken for granted or are considered true, even though they have not been scientifically tested.

_F_ 7. A blueprint for conducting a study that maximizes control over factors that could interfere with the study's desired outcome.

_M_ 8. An area of concern in which there is a gap in the knowledge base needed for nursing practice.

_O_ 9. A review and synthesis of sources (studies and theories) conducted to generate a picture of what is known and not known about a particular situation or problem of concern.

10. Terms or concepts at various levels of abstraction that are measured, manipulated, or controlled in a study.

11. A subset of a population that is selected for a particular study, the members of which are called *subjects*.

12. The process of assigning numbers to objects, events, or situations in accord with some rule.

13. Involves examining the results from data analysis, forming conclusions, exploring the significance of the findings, generalizing the findings, considering the implications for nursing practice, and suggesting further studies. *Interpretation*

14. Involves the development and dissemination of a research report to appropriate audiences, including nurses, health professionals, health care consumers, and policy makers. *Communicating* *Research Findings*

15. Limitations that restrict the abstract generalization of the findings and are reflected in the study framework. *Theoretical limitations*

16. Mechanism used to reduce, organize, and give meaning to data. *Analyze (Data Analysis)*

17. Limitations that result from weaknesses in the development of the study design, such as a nonrepresentative sample, threats to design validity, a single setting, limited control over the treatment, instruments with limited reliability and validity, limited control over data collection, and improper use of statistical analyses. *Methodological research*

18. An independent variable that is manipulated to create an effect on the dependent variable. *intervention*

19. The precise, systematic gathering of information relevant to the research purpose or the specific objectives, questions, or hypotheses.

Types of Study Settings
Directions: Match each term with its correct definition or example study setting.

Terms
a. Highly controlled setting

b. Natural setting

c. Partially controlled setting

Definitions

1. A field setting that the researcher does not control; it includes real-life situations that might be examined in a study

2. A setting for a study in which the researcher manipulates or modifies the environment in some way

3. Artificially constructed environments that are developed for the sole purpose of conducting research

4. Neonatal intensive care research unit

5. Cardiac rehabilitation center with structured programs

6. Nursing home

KEY IDEAS

Control in Quantitative Research

Directions: Fill in the blanks in the following sentences.

1. An experimental study is conducted in a(n) __*highly*__ __*controlled*__ setting.

2. Extraneous variables need to be controlled in __*Quasi-Exp.*__ and __*Experimental*__ studies to ensure that the findings about the effect of the treatment or intervention are an accurate reflection of reality.

3. __*Descriptive*__ or __*Correlational*__ studies are usually uncontrolled by the researcher and conducted in natural settings.

4. __*Experimental*__ studies should have random selection of the sample.

5. Frequently a(n) __*non random*__ sampling method is used in descriptive and correlational studies; however, a(n) __*Random*__ sampling method might also be used.

6. __*Basic Research*__ refers to scientific investigations conducted for the pursuit of "knowledge for knowledge's sake" or for the pleasure of learning.

7. Laboratories or research centers are examples of __*Highly*__ __*controlled*__ settings.

8. Researcher control is greatest in __*Experimental*__ research.

9. Hospital units are __*Partially Controlled*__ settings that allow the researcher to control some of the extraneous variables.

10. __*Quasi-Experimental (non-random)*__ research is conducted to determine the effect of a treatment but often involves less control than experimental research.

Steps of the Research Process

Directions: Fill in the blanks or provide the appropriate responses.

1. The __*Quantitative Research Process*__ is the formal, objective, systematic process to describe, test relationships, and examine cause-and-effect interactions among variables.

2. List the steps of the quantitative research process in their order of occurrence.

Step 1: *Formulate a Research Problem & Purpose*

Step 2: *Review relevant Literature*

Step 3: *Develop a framework*

Step 4: *Formulate research objectives, questions, hypothesis*

Step 5: *Define research variables*

Step 6: *Make assumptions explicit*

Step 7: *Identify limitations*

Step 8: _Select Research Design_

Step 9:

Step 10:

Step 11:

Step 12:

Step 13:

3. Identify four common assumptions on which nursing studies have been based.

   a.

   b.

   c.

   d.

4. What are the two types of study limitations?

   a. _Theoretical_

   b. _Methodolgical_

5. Identify five possible methodological limitations that you might find in published studies.

   a.

   b.

   c.

   d.

   e.

6. A study with no clearly identified framework has a(n) _Theoretical_ _Limitations_

7. Identify five reasons for conducting a pilot study.

   a.

   b.

   c.

   d.

   e.

MAKING CONNECTIONS

Directions: Match the types of quantitative research listed here with the sample study titles that follow.

Research Types

a. Descriptive research   c. Quasi-experimental research

b. Correlational research   d. Experimental research

Sample Study Titles

C 1. Determining the Effect of a Relaxation Technique on Patients' Post-Operative Pain

A 2. Identifying the Incidence of HIV in Adolescents and Young Adults

B 3. Examining the Relationships among Age, Gender, Knowledge of AIDS, and Use of Condoms in College Students

A 4. Describing the Coping Strategies of Chronically Ill Men and Women

C 5. Determining the Effects of Position on Sacral and Heel Pressures in Hospitalized Elderly

D 6. Determining the Effect of Impaired Physical Mobility on Skeletal Muscle Atrophy in Laboratory Rats

A 7. Identifying Current Nursing Practice for Male and Female Nurses

B 8. Examining the Relationship among Intensive Care Unit (ICU) Stress, Anxiety, and Recovery Rate

C 9. Examining the Effects of a Preadmission Self-Instruction Program on Patients' Postoperative Exercise Performance, Mood State, and Recovery Rate

D 10. Examining the Effects of Thermal Applications on the Abdominal Temperature of Laboratory Dogs

B 11. Examining the Relationships among Hardiness, Depression, and Coping in Institutionalized Elderly

A 12. Determining the Incidence of Drug Abuse in Registered Nurses in Community and Hospital Settings

☆ C 13. Examining the Effect of Warm and Cold Applications on the Resolution of IV Infiltrations in Hospitalized Patients

A 14. Determining the Stress Levels and Needs of Family Caregivers of Elderly Adults with Alzheimer's Disease

☆ C 15. Examining the Effectiveness of a Breast Cancer Screening Program for Women Residing in Rural Areas

A 16. Identifying the Types of Care Provider (Nurse Practitioner, Physician, and Physician Assistant) Who Are Responsible for Patient Care in Primary Care Settings

C 17. Determining the Effectiveness of Three Wound Dressings in Patients Undergoing Heart Surgery

★ C 18. Examining the Effectiveness of Home Health Visits in Promoting Recovery from Stroke

A 19. Determining the Differences between Associate and Baccalaureate Prepared Nurses in Their Use of Evidence-Based Protocols in Practice

C 20. Examining the Effectiveness of Two Types of Pain Medication for Abdominal Surgery Patients

Chapter **3** **Introduction to Quantitative Research**

Word Scramble

Directions: Unscramble the following sentence by rearranging the letters to form actual words. Note: You will use all the letters in every word.

Taquntiatiev sereacrh thodmes duclein cridpseitve, rrelacotiaonl, saiqu-perexienmtal,

dna eperxmiealnt udiests.

Crossword Puzzle

Directions: Complete the crossword puzzle. Note: If the answer is more than one word, there are no blank spaces left between the words.

Across

2. Study blueprint.
4. Research method.
8. Nursing concern.
9. Null _____.
10. Type of research that seeks knowledge for knowledge's sake.
12. _____ of dependent variables in research.
14. Becker's Health Belief model could be a study _____.
16. Location of research.
17. Strict adherence to the research plan.
18. This is composed of subjects.
19. Directs a study.

Down

1. Research finding.
2. What is collected in a study?
3. Research project.
5. Known truths.
6. Study treatment is an independent _____.
7. What is reviewed before conducting a study?
11. Researchers _____ extraneous variables.
13. Nursing _____ directs nursing care.
15. Practice-related studies are _____ research.

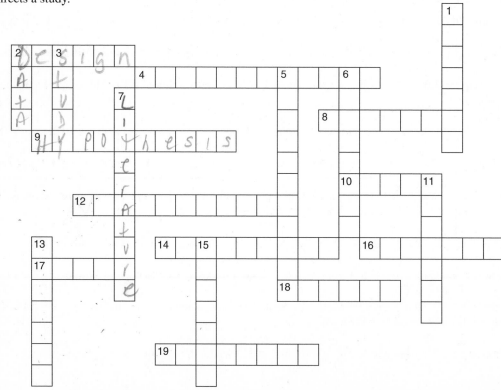

Directions: Read the research articles in Appendix B. Then identify the type of quantitative research conducted in each of the articles, choosing from the types of research listed here.

Research Types

a. Descriptive research
b. Correlational research
c. Quasi-experimental research

d. Experimental research
e. Qualitative research

Studies

_____ 1. Bindler, Massey, Shultz, Mills, and Short (2007)

_____ 2. Sethares and Elliott (2004)

_____ 3. Wright (2003)

Directions: Now indicate whether each of the studies in Appendix B is applied or basic nursing research.

Research Types

a. Applied nursing research
b. Basic nursing research

Studies

_____ 4. Bindler et al. (2007)

_____ 5. Sethares and Elliott (2004)

_____ 6. Wright (2003)

GOING BEYOND

Describe two quantitative studies that you would like to conduct. Have your instructor critically appraise the potential of conducting these studies.

4 Introduction to Qualitative Research

INTRODUCTION

Read Chapter 4, and then complete the following exercises. These exercises will help you to learn relevant terms and to read and comprehend published qualitative studies. The answers to these exercises are in Appendix A.

RELEVANT TERMS

Directions: Match each term with its correct definition.

Terms

a. Ascendance to an open context
b. Being-in-time
c. Deconstructing sedimented views
d. Embodied

e. Gestalt
f. Reconstructing new views
g. Sedimented view
h. Situated

Definitions

_____ 1. Ability to see depth and complexity within the phenomenon examined and a greater capacity for insight than with the sedimented view.

_____ 2. Person experiences being within the framework of time.

_____ 3. Seeing things from the perspective of a specific frame of reference, worldview, or theory that gives a sense of certainty, security, and control.

_____ 4. Organization of knowledge about a particular phenomenon into a cluster of linked ideas. The clustering and interrelatedness enhances the meaning of the ideas.

_____ 5. Rigorous qualitative research process that requires the researcher to ascend to an open context and to be willing to let go of sedimented views, which involves being open to new views.

_____ 6. Forming new views after examining many dimensions of the area being studied.

_____ 7. Heideggarian belief that a person is self within a body and the body makes concrete actions possible.

_____ 8. A person is shaped by his or her world.

KEY IDEAS

Directions: Fill in the blanks with the appropriate responses.

1. Qualitative research is a way to gain insights through _____ meanings.

2. The reasoning process used in qualitative research involves perpetually putting pieces together to make

   _____.

3. To form new gestalts, the researcher must get _____ of existing theories or gestalts that explain

   the _____ of interest.

4. In qualitative research, rather than using frameworks, the study is guided by a particular _____.

5. The purpose of phenomenological research is to describe or capture experiences as they are _____.

6. Symbolic interaction theory, on which grounded theory is based, explores how people define

   _____ and how their beliefs are related to their actions.

7. According to symbolic interaction theory, reality is _____ by people by attaching meanings

   to _____.

8. The word *ethnographic* means _____.

9. The purpose of anthropological research is to describe a(n) _____ by examining various
   characteristics of a group.

10. The primary questions of history are where _____, who _____, and

    where _____.

11. Foundational inquiry studies analyze the _____ of a science and the process of thinking about

    and _____ certain phenomena held in common by the science.

12. In ethical inquiry, the researcher identifies _____ to guide conduct based on

    _____ theory.

13. According to Stevens (1989), the purpose of _____
    is to uncover the distortions and constraints that impede free, equal, and uncoerced actions in society.

14. Identify the six types of qualitative research that are presented in this textbook.

    a.

    b.

    c.

    d.

    e.

    f.

15. List the three types of philosophical inquiry.

    a.

    b.

    c.

MAKING CONNECTIONS

List three characteristics of rigor in qualitative studies.

a.

b.

c.

Understanding Qualitative Research Methods
Directions: Match the type of qualitative research with the following characteristics.

Research Type
a. Phenomenological research
b. Grounded theory research
c. Ethnographic research
d. Historical research

Characteristics

_____ 1. Studies of ways of life within a give culture or group.

_____ 2. Nine elders were interviewed regarding the meaning of their day-to-day experiences with receiving family care.

_____ 3. A study of individuals' response to grief to develop a grief theory.

_____ 4. A study of Pakistani men's and women's views of crying.

_____ 5. Studies of the meaning of a lived experience.

_____ 6. Promotes culturally specific care.

_____ 7. Used to study the development and changes in Parse's theory over time.

_____ 8. A study of the social, economic, and legal influences on side rail use in the twentieth century.

_____ 9. Studies of the past nursing interventions.

_____ 10. Leininger's theory directs this type of qualitative research.

_____ 11. Theory has roots in the data.

_____ 12. Prefers primary source documents.

_____ 13. Considers an experience unique to the individual.

_____ 14. A model and theory emerged from a study of persons with HIV disease.

_____ 15. A study of the treatment of terminally ill patients over the past 100 years.

Linking Qualitative Philosophies and Methods with Types of Qualitative Research
Directions: Place the appropriate qualitative research approach/method in the center of each Venn diagram.

Critical social theory

Ethnographic research

Grounded theory research

Historical research

Phenomenological research

Philosophical inquiry

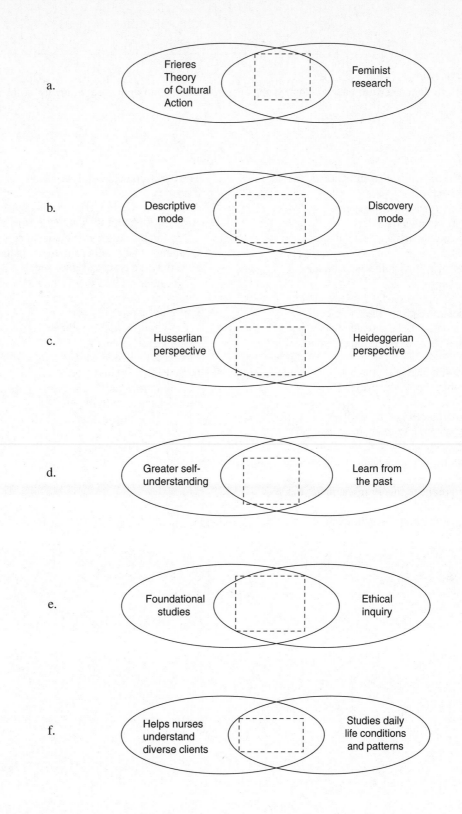

a.

Frieres Theory of Cultural Action

Feminist research

b.

Descriptive mode

Discovery mode

c.

Husserlian perspective

Heideggerian perspective

d.

Greater self-understanding

Learn from the past

e.

Foundational studies

Ethical inquiry

f.

Helps nurses understand diverse clients

Studies daily life conditions and patterns

Chapter **4**   **Introduction to Qualitative Research**

Crossword Puzzle

Directions: Complete the crossword puzzle. Note: If the answer is more than one word, there are no blank spaces left between the words.

Across

1. _____ mode: a strategy used to refine substantive theory.
3. _____ research: a strategy of research emerging from Leininger's theory.
5. Letting go of sedimented views to be open to new views.
6. _____ culture: man-made objects associated with a particular group.
7. _____ research: an approach to research in which representatives from the group being studied are included in the research team.
8. Theory that has its roots in the data from which it was derived.
10. Striving for excellence in research.
14. A branch of philosophy that deals with morality.
16. Describes experiences as they are lived.
18. Experiencing within a framework of time.
20. _____ ethnography: research focused on the ideas, beliefs, and knowledge that a group holds.
21. _____ mode: grounded theory research approach that provides rich detail.
22. _____ view: seeing things from a specific frame of reference.
23. A self within a body.
24. Being shaped by your world, which constrains your ability to establish meanings.

Down

2. The philosophical bases, concepts, and theories of a science.
4. A way of life belonging to a designated people.
9. A way of organizing data that forms new ideas.
11. _____ inquiry: uses intellectual analyses to clarify meanings, make values manifest, identify ethics, and study the nature of knowledge.
12. _____ mode—Used to test the relationships of a substantive theory.
13. Portrait of a people.
15. _____ anthropology: studies patterns of behavior, customs, and ways of life.
17. Elements unique to each person within which that person can be understood.
19. _____ mode: identifies patterns in the life experiences of individuals.

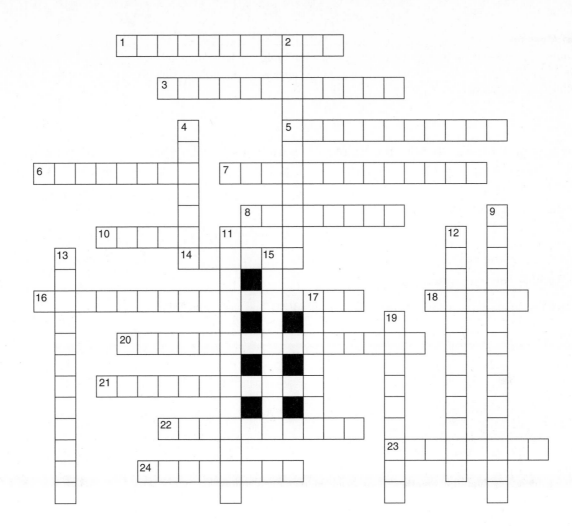

Word Scramble

Directions: Unscramble the following sentence by rearranging the letters to form actual words. Note: You will use all the letters in every word.

Cnoe oyu vaeh scadnede ot het noep txencot, ouy oancnt og kabc ot eth edai hatt het

mohennopne uoy veha revsobed nac eb nese olny noe yaw.

Secret Message

Directions: Translate the following secret message by substituting one letter for another. For example, if you decide that "b" should really be "d," then "b" will be "d" every time it appears in this puzzle. Hint: Try to translate short words first to establish vowel patterns.

Gr gq apgrgayj rm slbcpqrylb rfl cnfgjmqmnfw ml ufgaf lyaf osyjgryrgtc crfmb gq zyqcb.

EXERCISES IN CRITICAL APPRAISAL

Directions: Examine the study by Wright (2003) in Appendix B, and answer the following questions.

1. What is the philosophical base for Wright's study?

2. What evidence can you find that the author ascended to an open context?

3. Whose method did Wright select for her study?

4. What strategies did Wright use to achieve rigor in her study?

Seek out a variety of published qualitative studies. Identify the philosophy on which each study is based. Does the researcher explain the philosophical base? What is the research question? How was a sample acquired? Identify the data collection and analysis strategies used. What is the outcome of the analysis process? For each study, write a paragraph summarizing information you have gathered in answering these questions.

5 Research Problem and Purpose

INTRODUCTION

Read Chapter 5, and then complete the following exercises. These exercises will help you to critically appraise problems and purposes in published studies and formulate a problem and purpose for conducting a study. The answers to these exercises are in Appendix A.

RELEVANT TERMS

Directions: Match each term with its correct definition.

Terms

a. Approximate replication
b. Concurrent replication
c. Exact replication
d. Feasibility of study

e. Landmark study
f. Replication
g. Research problem

h. Research purpose
i. Research topic
j. Systematic replication

Definitions

_____ 1. Internal replication that involves collecting data for the original study and simultaneously replicating it to check the reliability of the original study.

_____ 2. Clear, concise statement of the specific goal or aim of the study that is generated from the problem.

_____ 3. An area of concern in which there is a gap in the knowledge base needed for nursing practice.

_____ 4. Operational replication that involves repeating the original study under similar conditions, following the original methods as closely as possible.

_____ 5. Reproducing or repeating a study to determine whether similar findings are obtained.

_____ 6. Concept or broad problem area that provides the basis for generating numerous research problems.

_____ 7. Precise, identical duplication of the initial researcher's study to confirm the original findings.

_____ 8. Constructive replication performed under distinctly new conditions in which the researchers conducting the replication do not follow the design or methods of the original researcher; rather, the second investigative team begins with a similar problem statement but formulates new means to verify the first investigator's findings.

_____ 9. A determination made by examining the time and money commitment; the researcher's expertise; the availability of subjects, facility, and equipment; the cooperation of others; and the study's ethical considerations.

_____ 10. Major study generating knowledge that influences a discipline and sometimes society in general.

KEY IDEAS

Directions: Fill in the blanks, or provide the appropriate responses.

1. A clearly stated research purpose includes:

   a.

   b.

   c.

   d.

2. Research problems and purposes are significant if they have the potential to generate and refine relevant knowledge that:

   a.

   b.

   c.

   d.

3. Williams's (1972) study, conducted to examine factors that contribute to skin breakdown, is considered a(n)

   _____ study in the area of pressure ulcer prevention. Williams's study and many other studies of pressure ulcers are summarized in the document "Pressure Ulcers in Adults: Prediction and Prevention," published

   by the _____.

4. Studies need to be _____ to determine whether the findings are consistent from one study to another and whether they provide strong evidence for use in practice.

5. Researchers are conducting a(n) _____ replication of a study if they are repeating the study but are using different subjects and measuring the variables with improved methods of measurement.

6. The feasibility of a research problem and purpose is determined by examining the following:

   a.

   b.

   c.

   d.

32

Chapter **5** **Research Problem and Purpose**

7. Three ways to determine researchers' expertise are by examining the _____ preparation,

   conduct of previous _____, and _____ experience in nursing.

8. Identify four sources of research problems.

   a.

   b.

   c.

   d.

9. Identify four goals of outcomes research.

   a.

   b.

   c.

   d.

10. Coping patterns, pain management, health promotion, and social support are examples of _____

    _____ that have directed the generation of research in nursing.

11. Numerous research problems can be generated from a research topic, and a research problem can be used to generate

    numerous _____ _____.

MAKING CONNECTIONS

Directions: Match the types of research listed here with the specific purpose statements that follow.

Research Types
a. Correlational research
b. Critical social theory
c. Descriptive research
d. Ethnography
e. Experimental research
f. Grounded theory research
g. Historical research
h. Phenomenological research
i. Philosophical analysis
j. Quasi-experimental research

Purpose Statements

_____ 1. To examine the evolution of the American Nurses Association's position on health care for the aged from 1935 to 1990.

_____ 2. To determine how the employment, income, and coping patterns of parents changed following the birth of a low-birth-weight infant.

_____ 3. To describe the lived experience of being in an intensive care unit.

_____ 4. To develop a theory to describe the suffering of people with dementia of the Alzheimer type (DAT).

_____ 5. To examine the relationships among spirituality, perceived social support, and income of adult children caring for their elderly parents.

_____ 6. To examine the effect of a relaxation technique on perceived anxiety in working adults in high-stress jobs.

_____ 7. To examine the effect of heat application on the healing rate of abdominal incisions in dogs.

_____ 8. To determine the essential elements of caring, a significant concept in nursing, with the use of a concept analysis.

_____ 9. To examine the health practices of Hispanic women and the impact of these practices on their families.

_____ 10. To determine the smoking status, alcohol dependence, and bone mineral density in postmenopausal women.

_____ 11. To describe the experience of sleeplessness in depressed women.

_____ 12. To determine whether social support, employment, and marital status are predictive of coping with the loss of a child.

_____ 13. To examine the impact of an exercise program on muscle mass and bone mineral density in premenopausal women.

_____ 14. To describe the implementation of skin care by nurses from 1850 to 1950.

_____ 15. To explore the childbirth practices of Asian women.

EXERCISES IN CRITICAL APPRAISAL

Bindler, Massey, Shultz, Mills, and Short Study

Directions: Review the Bindler et al. (2007) research article in Appendix B, and answer the following questions.

1. Identify the following parts of the problem for this study.

   a. Significance of the problem:

   b. Background of the problem:

   c. Problem statement:

2. State the purpose of this study.

3. Are the problem and the purpose significant? Provide a rationale.

4. Does the purpose identify the concept(s) of interest, population, and setting for this study?

   a. Identify the research concept(s):

   b. Identify the population:

   c. Identify the setting:

5. Are the problem and purpose feasible for the researchers to study? Provide a rationale.

Sethares and Elliott Study

Directions: Review the Sethares and Elliott (2004) research article in Appendix B, and answer the following questions.

1. Identify the following parts of the problem for this study.

   a. Significance of the problem:

   b. Background of the problem:

   c. Problem statement:

2. State the purpose of this study.

3. Are the problem and the purpose significant? Provide a rationale.

4. Does the purpose identify the variables, population, and setting for this study?

   a. Identify the variables:

   b. Identify the population:

   c. Identify the setting:

5. Are the problem and purpose feasible for the researchers to study? Provide a rationale.

Wright Study

Directions: Review the Wright (2003) research article in Appendix B, and answer the following questions.

1. Identify the following parts of the problem for this study.

   a. Significance of the problem:

   b. Background of the problem:

   c. Problem statement:

2. State the purpose of this study.

3. Are the problem and the purpose significant? Provide a rationale.

4. Does the purpose identify the concept(s) of interest, population, and setting for this study?

   a. Identify the research concept(s):

   b. Identify the population:

   c. Identify the setting:

5. Are the problem and purpose feasible for the researchers to study? Provide a rationale.

GOING BEYOND

1. Following the steps outlined in Figure 5-2 in your textbook, identify a research topic and formulate a research problem and purpose for a study of interest to you.

2. Seek feedback from your classmates and instructor in clarifying the problem and purpose you have identified.

3. Analyze whether the purpose is feasible to direct the conduct of your study by examining the time and money commitment; your expertise as a researcher; the availability of subjects, facility, and equipment; the cooperation of others; and the study's ethical considerations.

6 Review of Relevant Literature

INTRODUCTION

Read Chapter 6, and then complete the following exercises. These exercises will help you to read and critically appraise research reports and summarize the findings for use in practice or for conducting research. The answers to these exercises are in Appendix A.

RELEVANT TERMS

Directions: Match each term with its correct definition.

Terms

a. Bibliographic database
b. Complex search
c. Dissertation
d. Empirical knowledge
e. Empirical literature

f. Landmark study
g. Literature review
h. Periodicals
i. Primary source
j. Secondary source

k. Seminal study
l. Serial
m. Synonym
n. Theoretical literature
o. Thesis

Definitions

_____ 1. An organized, written presentation of what scholars have published on a topic.

_____ 2. The first study that prompted the initiation of a field of research.

_____ 3. A major project that generates knowledge that influences a discipline and sometimes society in general and marks an important stage of development in a field of research.

_____ 4. Includes concept analyses, maps, theories, and conceptual frameworks that support a selected research problem and purpose.

_____ 5. Literature published over time or in multiple volumes; they do not necessarily have a predictable publication date.

_____ 6. Subsets of serials with predictable publication dates, such as journals, which are published over time and are numbered sequentially for the years published.

_____ 7. Includes relevant studies published in journals, in books, and online, as well as unpublished studies such as master's theses and doctoral dissertations.

_____ 8. Research project completed by a master's student as part of the requirements for a master's degree.

_____ 9. An extensive, usually original, research project that is completed as the final requirement for a doctoral degree.

_____ 10. Knowledge derived from research.

_____ 11. A source that is written by the person who originated or is responsible for generating the ideas published.

_____ 12. A source that summarizes or quotes content from primary sources.

_____ 13. Database that consists of citations relevant to a specific discipline or may be a broad collection of citations from a variety of disciplines.

_____ 14. Alternative terms that authors might use to search for concepts or variables.

_____ 15. The combination of two or more concepts or synonyms in one search.

KEY IDEAS

Directions: Fill in the blanks, or provide the appropriate responses.

1. Provide five correct ways to complete the following statement: As a researcher, your goal is to develop a literature search strategy designed to:

   a.

   b.

   c.

   d.

   e.

2. List three advantages of using a library that provides access to large numbers of electronic databases.

   a. Provides a large scope of available literature nationally and _____.

   b. Identifies relevant sources _____.

   c. Allows the researcher to print _____ versions of sources immediately.

3. Identify three reasons for keeping a written search plan.

   a. It helps you from going back _____.

   b. It helps you _____ your steps if need be.

   c. It helps you select _____ paths to search.

4. The two main types of information cited in the review of literature for research are _____ and _____ sources.

5. Predominately _____ sources, not secondary sources, are used in developing a research proposal.

6. Sources for developing a literature review for a proposal can be identified through _____ and

_____ searches.

7. Number the steps below in the correct order for reviewing the literature.

_____ Locate relevant sources

_____ Develop a search strategy

_____ Systematically record references

_____ Synthesize sources

_____ Select keywords

_____ Analyze sources

8. Manual search of the literature involves examining the following:

a.

b.

c.

d.

9. What is the name of the original index for nursing literature?

10. Identify two databases commonly used by nurses to locate relevant sources.

a.

b.

11. The _____ is a good source of integrative reviews of research relevant to nursing practice.

12. Reviewing the literature requires a _____ of research sources to determine what is known and not known about a clinical problem.

13. What is the purpose of reference management software?

14. Identify the four common headings or content areas covered in a literature review.

   a.

   b.

   c.

   d.

15. Consider the following research problem: "Women's delay in seeking treatment for acute myocardial infarction symptoms results in higher rates of mortality and morbidity for women" (Rosenfeld, A. G. [2004]. Treatment-seeking delay among women with acute myocardial infarction. *Nursing Research,* 53[4], p. 225). What key terms would you use to direct your review of literature for this research problem?

16. Consider the following research problem: "The southern Appalachian states show a high prevalence of smoking, with associated high rates of both heart disease and cancer; yet cultural differences raise questions concerning the applicability of the most frequently used model for smoking cessation, the transtheoretical model, for smokers from this region of the county" (Macnee, C. L., & McCabe, S. [2004]. The transtheoretical model of behavior change and smokers in southern Appalachia. *Nursing Research,* 453[4], p. 243). What key terms would you use to direct your review of literature for this research problem?

17. Consider the following research problem: "Cancer-related pain often is undertreated despite the availability of effective interventions." (Vallerand, A. H., Riley-Doucet, C., Hasenau, S. M., & Templin, T. [2004]. Improving cancer pain management by homecare nurses. *Oncology Nursing Forum,* 31[4], p. 809). What key terms would you use to direct your review of literature for this research problem?

18. List three steps for limiting your search if you get too many hits.

   a.

   b.

   c.

19. The most common sources for nursing research reports are professional journals. Identify four nursing research journals.

   a.

   b.

   c.

   d.

20. Identify the four major sections of a research report.

a.

b.

c.

d.

21. Summarizing sources to develop a literature review section for a research proposal involves _____,

_____, _____, and _____.

22. When writing the literature review section for a research proposal, it is better to _____ the content of your sources than to use long direct quotes.

MAKING CONNECTIONS

Purpose of the Literature Review

Directions: Match each type of qualitative research listed below with the appropriate purpose of the literature review.

Research Types

a. Ethnographic research
b. Grounded theory research
c. Historical research
d. Phenomenological research

Literature Review Purpose

_____ 1. Compare and combine findings from the study with the literature to determine current knowledge of a phenomenon.

_____ 2. Review literature to develop study questions; the literature is a source of data in the study.

_____ 3. Review the literature to provide a background for conducting the study, as in quantitative research.

_____ 4. Use the literature to explain, support, and extend the theory generated in the study.

Theoretical and Empirical Literature

Directions: Theoretical and empirical literature sections are included in the literature review of a published study. Consider the following sources; then place a "T" next to the theoretical sources and an "E" next to those sources that are empirical.

_____ 1. Lazarus and Folkman's *Theory of Coping*.

_____ 2. Abstracts from a research conference.

_____ 3. Theses.

_____ 4. Watson's *Philosophy of Human Caring*.

_____ 5. Orem, D. E. (2001). *Nursing: Concepts of practice* (6th ed.). St. Louis: Mosby.

_____ 6. Bakitas, M. A. (2007). Background noise: The experience of chemotherapy-induced peripheral neuropathy. *Nursing Research, 56*(5), 323-331.

_____ 7. Cricco-Lizza, R. (2007). Ethnography and the generation of trust in breastfeeding disparities research. *Applied Nursing Research, 20*(4), 200-204.

_____ 8. Dissertations.

_____ 9. von Bertalanffy, L. (1968). *General systems theory*. New York: Braziller.

_____ 10. Lewin's change theory.

_____ 11. Tullmann, D. F., Haugh, K. H., Dracup, K. A., & Bourguignon, C. (2007). A randomized controlled trial to reduce delay in older adults seeking help for symptoms of acute myocardial infarction. *Research in Nursing & Health, 30*(5), 485-497.

Primary and Secondary Sources

Directions: A literature review includes mainly primary sources rather than secondary ones. Label the following sources with a "P" if they are primary or an "S" if they are secondary.

_____ 1. Integrated review of research

_____ 2. Dissertations

_____ 3. Theses

_____ 4. Textbooks

_____ 5. Summary of theoretical and empirical sources

_____ 6. Study published in *Applied Nursing Research*

EXERCISES IN CRITICAL APPRAISAL

Directions: Review the three articles in Appendix B, then answer the following questions.

1. In the nursing field, the most common way to cite a reference is by using the format of the American Psychological Association (APA). Knowing the different parts of a reference citation will assist you in locating and recording sources for a formal paper. The following source is presented in APA format:

Sethares, K. A., & Elliott, K. (2004). The effect of a tailored message intervention on heart failure readmission rates, quality of life, and benefit and barrier beliefs in persons with heart failure. *Heart & Lung, 33*(4), 249-260.

Chapter **6**   **Review of Relevant Literature**

a. What is *Heart & Lung* in this reference?

b. What is "2004" in this reference?

c. What is "33" in this reference?

d. What is "249-260" in this reference?

e. What is "(4)" in this reference?

f. Who are the authors of this article?

2. Write a proper reference citation for the Bindler et al.'s (2007) article using APA format.

3. Carefully review the three reference citations listed below. Are they complete? If not, indicate what elements are missing.

a. Wright, V. L. (1994). *Archives of Psychiatric Nursing, 17*(4).

b. Macnee, C. L., & McCabe, S. (2004). The transtheoretical model of behavior change and smokers in southern Appalachia. *Nursing Research,* (4).

c. Rosenfeld, A. G. Treatment-seeking delay among women with acute myocardial infarction: Decision trajectories and their predictors. *Nursing Research,* 225-236.

4. What are the titles of the literature review sections of the three articles in Appendix B?

   a. Sethares and Elliott (2004):

   b. Wright (2004):

   c. Bindler et al. (2007):

5. Are relevant studies identified and described in Bindler et al.'s study? Give examples of two studies that are cited in the study's literature review.

6. Are relevant theories identified and described in the Bindler et al. (2007) study? Identify a theoretical source that is cited in the study's literature review.

7. In Bindler et al.'s (2007) references, is the source by Williams et al. (2002) a primary or secondary source?

8. Are the references in Bindler et al.'s (2007) study current? Provide a rationale.

9. Does the literature review in the Sethares and Elliott (2004) study present the current knowledge base for the research problem? Provide a rationale.

10. Are relevant studies identified and described in the Sethares and Elliott (2004) study? Give examples of two studies that are cited in the literature review of the article.

11. Are relevant theories identified and described in the following:

   a. Sethares and Elliott (2004) study? Identify one theoretical source that is cited in the study's literature review.

   b. Bindler et al. (2007) study?

12. In the Sethares and Elliott (2004) study, is the source by Hunt et al. (2003) a primary or secondary source?

13. Are the references in the Sethares and Elliott (2004) study current? Provide a rationale.

14. Does the literature review of Bindler et al.'s (2007) study provide the current knowledge base of the problem examined in this study? Provide a rationale.

15. Are relevant studies identified and described in the Wright (2003) study? Give examples of two studies that are cited in the study's literature review.

16. Are relevant theories identified and described in the Wright (2003) study? Identify two theoretical sources that are cited in the study's literature review.

17. a. In Wright's (2003) study, is the source by Davis (1997) a primary or secondary source?

   b. In Wright's (2003) study, is the source by Giorgi (1985) a primary or secondary source?

Chapter **6**   **Review of Relevant Literature**

18. Are the references in Wright's (2003) study current? Provide a rationale.

19. Does the literature review in Wright's (2003) study provide a current knowledge base for the research problem examined in the study? Explain your answer.

GOING BEYOND

1. Identify a problem in clinical practice, and conduct a summary of the research literature on this topic.

2. Search the literature for relevant research sources for the problem you identified.

3. Locate relevant studies via your university library.

4. Read each study, and identify the steps of the research process.

5. Outline key information from each study, including the study purpose, framework, sample size, design, results, and findings.

6. Critically appraise the quality of each study.

7. Write a description of each research report, and critically appraise the quality of the report.

8. Write a summary paragraph that indicates what is known and not known about your clinical problem.

7 Frameworks

INTRODUCTION

Read Chapter 7, and then complete the following exercises. These exercises will help you to learn relevant terms and to identify and critically appraise frameworks in published studies. The answers to these exercises are in Appendix A.

RELEVANT TERMS

Terms Related to Theory

Directions: Match each term with its correct definition.

Terms

a. Abstract thinking
b. Asymmetrical relationship
c. Concept
d. Concept analysis

e. Concept derivation
f. Concept synthesis
g. Conceptual definition
h. Conceptual map

i. Conceptual model
j. Concrete thinking

Definitions

_____ 1. A process of extracting and defining concepts from theories in other disciplines.

_____ 2. If A occurs, then B will occur, but there may be no indication that if B occurs, A will occur.

_____ 3. A set of highly abstract, related constructs that broadly explains phenomena of interest, expresses assumptions, and reflects a philosophical stance.

_____ 4. A strategy for expressing a framework of a study that diagrammatically shows the interrelationship of the concepts and statements.

_____ 5. Oriented toward the development of an idea without application to or association with a particular instance; independent of time and space.

_____ 6. A process of describing and naming a previously unrecognized concept.

_____ 7. Provides a variable or concept with connotative (abstract, comprehensive, theoretical) meaning and is established through concept analysis, concept derivation, or concept synthesis.

_____ 8. Thinking that is oriented toward and limited by tangible things or events observed and experienced in reality.

_____ 9. A strategy through which a set of attributes or characteristics essential to the connotative meaning or conceptual definition of a concept are identified.

_____ 10. A term that abstractly describes and names an object or phenomenon.

Terms Related to Relational Statements

Directions: Match each term with its correct definition.

Terms

a. Concurrent relationship
b. Construct
c. Contingent relationship
d. Curvilinear relationship
e. Denotative definition
f. Deterministic relationship
g. Direction of a proposition
h. Effect size

i. Existence statement
j. Framework
k. General proposition
l. Hierarchical statement
m. Hypothesis
n. Intervening variable
o. Linear relationship
p. Mediator variable

q. Necessary relationship
r. Negative relationship
s. Positive relationship
t. Probability statement
u. Proposition
v. Relational statement
w. Research tradition

Definitions

_____ 1. May be positive, negative, or unknown.

_____ 2. Occurs only if a third variable or concept is present.

_____ 3. A program of research that is important for building a body of knowledge related to the phenomena explained by a particular conceptual model.

_____ 4. Formal statement of the expected relationship(s) between two or more variables in a specified population.

_____ 5. Dictionary definition.

_____ 6. Expresses the likelihood that something will happen in a given situation and addresses relative rather than absolute causality.

_____ 7. A relationship in which both variables and concepts occur simultaneously.

_____ 8. The degree to which the phenomenon is present in the population or to which the null hypothesis is false.

_____ 9. Variables that bring about the effects of the intervention after it has occurred and thus influence the outcomes of the study.

_____ 10. The abstract, logical structure of meaning that guides development of the study and enables the researcher to link the findings to nursing's body of knowledge.

_____ 11. The relationship between two variables or concepts will remain consistent regardless of the values of each of the variables or concepts.

_____ 12. Composed of a specific proposition and a hypothesis or research question.

_____ 13. Indicates that as one variable or concept changes, the other variable or concept changes in the opposite direction.

_____ 14. Can affect the occurrence, strength, or direction of a relationship.

_____ 15. A highly abstract statement of the relationship between two or more concepts that is found in a conceptual model.

_____ 16. Declares that a given concept exists or that a given relationship occurs.

50

_____ 17. One variable or concept must occur for the second variable or concept to occur.

_____ 18. The relationship between two variables varies depending on the relative values of the variables.

_____ 19. Indicates that as one variable changes, the second variable will also change in the same direction.

_____ 20. Statements of what always occurs in a particular situation, such as a scientific law.

_____ 21. Declares that a relationship of some kind exists between two or more concepts.

_____ 22. Concept at a very high level of abstraction that has general meaning.

_____ 23. An abstract statement that further clarifies the relationship between two concepts.

More Terms Related to Statements and Theory

Directions: Match each term with its correct definition.

Terms

a. Scientific theory
b. Sequential relationship
c. Specific proposition
d. Strength of relationship
e. Substitutable relationship
f. substantive theory
g. Substruction
h. Sufficient relationship
i. Symmetrical relationship
j. Tendency statement
k. Tentative theory
l. Theoretical substruction
m. Theory
n. Variable

Definitions

_____ 1. The amount of variation explained by the relationship.

_____ 2. Qualities, properties, or characteristics of persons, things, or situations that change or vary and are manipulated, measured, or controlled in research.

_____ 3. A relationship in which one concept occurs later than the other.

_____ 4. A theory with valid and reliable methods of measuring each concept and relationship statements that have been tested repeatedly.

_____ 5. A theory recognized within the discipline as useful for explaining important phenomena.

_____ 6. A relationship in which a similar concept can be substituted for the first concept and the second concept will occur.

_____ 7. The opposite of construction; to take apart.

_____ 8. A deterministic relationship that describes what always happens in the absence of interfering conditions.

_____ 9. If A occurs, B will occur and if B occurs, A will occur.

_____ 10. States that when the first variable or concept occurs, the second will occur regardless of the presence or absence of other factors.

_____ 11. A statement found in theories that are at a moderate level of abstraction and provide the basis for the generation of hypotheses to guide a study.

_____ 12. Consists of an integrated set of defined concepts, existence statements, and relational statements that present a view of a phenomenon and can be used to describe, explain, predict, or control that phenomenon.

_____ 13. A process in which the framework of a published study is separated into component parts to evaluate the logical consistency of the theoretical system and the interaction of the framework with the study methodology.

_____ 14. A theory that is newly proposed, has had minimal exposure to critical appraisal by the discipline, and has had little testing.

KEY IDEAS

Directions: Fill in the blanks, or provide appropriate responses.

1. We use _____ to organize what we know about phenomenon.

2. Testing theory involves determining the _____ of each relational statement in the theory.

3. _____ are not generally considered testable.

4. A research framework is based on _____.

5. The strength of a relationship is sometimes referred to as the _____.

6. Research findings are interpreted in terms of the study _____.

7. In a framework, all _____ should be defined.

8. Concepts in conceptual models are referred to as _____.

9. A _____ is more specific than a concept and is defined so that it is measurable in a study.

10. The _____ of a theory are tested through research.

11. Statements at the lowest level of abstraction are referred to as _____.

12. The purpose of a conceptual map is to explain which concepts _____ to or partially _____ an outcome.

13. A conceptual map includes all the major _____ in a theory or framework linked together by _____ expressing the _____ proposed between the concepts.

14. An organized program of research designed to build a body of knowledge related to a particular conceptual model is referred to as a _____.

MAKING CONNECTIONS

Directions: Match each term with its definition.

Terms

a. Theory
b. Concept
c. Conceptual model

d. Variable
e. Statement
f. Conceptual map

g. Framework
h. Construct
i. Hypothesis

Definitions

_____ 1. Broadly explains phenomena of interest.

_____ 2. The basic element of a theory.

_____ 3. Expresses a claim important to a theory.

_____ 4. Graphically shows interrelations among concepts.

_____ 5. Integrated set of defined concepts and statements.

_____ 6. Statement expressed at low level of abstraction.

_____ 7. Provides general meanings of terms.

_____ 8. Defines a term so that it is measurable.

_____ 9. Presents portions of a theory to be tested in a study.

Levels of Abstraction

Directions: Place the following terms in order from the highest level of abstraction to the lowest level of abstraction.

Variable	Construct	Operational definition	Concept

_____ (Highest level of abstraction)

_____

_____

_____ (Lowest level of abstraction)

PUZZLES

Word Scramble

Directions: Unscramble the following sentence by rearranging the letters to form actual words. Note: You will use all the letters in every word.

Amyn tusidse rea duirqere ot diatvelat lal fo eht tesnamtets ni a yrehto.

Secret Message

Directions: Translate the following secret message by substituting one letter for another. For example, if you decide that "i" should really be "g," then "i" will be "g" every time it appears in this puzzle. Hint: Try to translate short words first to establish vowel patterns.

Aqw pggf vq fgvgtokpg nkpmu coqpi vjg eqpegrvwcn fghkpkvkqpu, vjg xctkcdngu kp vjg

uvwfa, cpf vjg tgncvgf ogcuwtgogpv ogvjqfu.

Crossword Puzzle

Directions: Complete the crossword puzzle. Note: If the answer is more than one word, there are no blank spaces left between the words.

Across

1. Not considered testable through research.
4. Framework with ideas not fully developed.
6. Portion of a theory to be tested in a study.
7. Specific statement expressed at lowest level of abstraction.
11. Focus of Orem's model.
12. Expression of an idea apart from any specific instance.
13. Term in which numerical values vary from one instance to another.
14. An organized program of research designed to build a body of knowledge related to a particular conceptual model.

Down

1. Ideas concerned with realities or actual instances.
2. Process of determining the truth of a relational statement.
3. Developed to illustrate which concepts contribute to or partially cause an outcome.
5. Used to describe, explain, predict, or control a phenomenon.
8. Statement found in theories.
9. Clarifies the type of relationship that exists between or among concepts.
10. Focus of Roy's model.

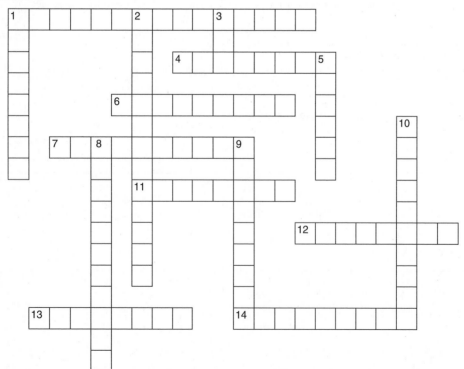

Directions: Examine the framework of Bindler et al.'s (2007) study provided in Appendix B.

1. List the concepts in the study.

2. State the definition of each concept as defined by the author(s). Are the definitions clear and adequate? If not, identify the inadequacies.

3. List the variables used in the study.

4. Identify the concept(s) with which each study variable is associated.

5. Complete the following table by listing each concept, the related variable(s), and the measurement method(s).

Concepts	Variables	Measurement Methods

55

6. Compare the measurement method for each variable with its associated concept and conceptual definition. Is each measurement method consistent with its associated concept and conceptual definition? If not, what are the inconsistencies?

7. List the statements expressed within the Bindler et al. (2007) study. Then underline the concepts included in each statement. Are all of the study concepts included within each statement? Provide a map of each statement.

8. State the propositions being tested in the study and the related hypotheses or research questions.

9. Are the statements tested by the study design? How?

10. Is the framework expressed as a conceptual map? Are all of the concepts in the study included in the map? Are all of the statements you identified included in the map? If there is no map, develop one and draw it here.

11. Does the author provide statements for each linkage between concepts shown on the map? Does the author provide references from the literature to support the linkages? If so, list the references for each linkage.

12. Develop a short summary paragraph describing the strengths and weaknesses of the framework of the Bindler et al. (2007) study.

GOING BEYOND

Critique the framework of the Sethares and Elliott (2004) study in Appendix B by doing the following:

a. Drawing a model of the conceptual framework described in the article

b. Diagramming the relationship posited in each of the three hypotheses of the study

c. Completing the following table:

Concept(s)	Variable(s)	Measurement Method(s)

8 Objectives, Questions, and Hypotheses

INTRODUCTION

Read Chapter 8, and then complete the following exercises. These exercises will help you to critically appraise objectives, questions, hypotheses, and variables in published studies. The content will also help you to develop research objectives, questions, or hypotheses for a study and conceptually and operationally define the variables to be studied. The answers to these exercises are in Appendix A.

RELEVANT TERMS

General Concepts

Directions: Match each term with its correct definition.

Terms
a. Hypothesis
b. Research objective
c. Research question
d. Variables

Definitions

_____ 1. Clear, concise, declarative statement that is expressed in the present tense and are used to direct the conduct of a study.

_____ 2. Concepts at various levels of abstraction that are measured, manipulated, or controlled in a study.

_____ 3. A formal statement of the expected relationship(s) between two or more variables in a specified population.

_____ 4. Concise interrogative statement developed to direct a study; focuses on description of variables, examination of relationships among variables, and determination of differences between two or more groups.

Types of Hypotheses

Directions: Match each type of hypothesis with its correct definition.

Terms
a. Associative hypothesis
b. Causal hypothesis
c. Complex hypothesis
d. Directional hypothesis
e. Nondirectional hypothesis
f. Null hypothesis
g. Research hypothesis
h. Simple hypothesis

Definitions

_____ 1. Hypothesis stating the relationship (associative or causal) between two variables.

_____ 2. Alternative hypothesis to the null hypothesis, which states that a relationship exists between two or more variables.

_____ 3. Hypothesis stating a relationship between two variables where one variable (independent variable) is thought to cause or determine the presence of the other variable (dependent variable).

_____ 4. Hypothesis stating that a relationship exists but does not predict its exact nature.

_____ 5. Hypothesis predicting the relationships (associative or causal) among three or more variables.

_____ 6. Hypothesis stating a relationship in which variables or concepts that occur or exist together in the real world are identified; when one variable changes, the other variable changes.

_____ 7. Hypothesis stating the specific nature of the interaction or relationship between two or more variables.

_____ 8. Hypothesis stating that no relationship exists between the variables being studied.

Types of Variables

Directions: The following terms are related to variables. Match each term with its correct definition.

Terms

a. Conceptual definition
b. Demographic variables
c. Dependent variable

d. Extraneous variable
e. Independent variable
f. Operational definition

g. Research concept
h. Research variables

Definitions

_____ 1. Definition that provides a variable or concept with a connotative (abstract, comprehensive, theoretical) meaning.

_____ 2. Variable that exists in all studies and can affect the measurement of study variables and the relationships among these variables.

_____ 3. Definition that describes how variables or concepts will be measured or manipulated in a study.

_____ 4. Response, behavior, or outcome that is predicted or explained in research; changes in this variable are presumed to be caused by the independent variable.

_____ 5. Treatment or experimental activity that is manipulated or varied by the researcher to create an effect on the dependent variable.

_____ 6. Characteristics or attributes of subjects that are collected to describe the sample.

_____ 7. Specific qualities, properties, or characteristics that are identified in the study purpose and objectives or questions that are observed or measured in quantitative studies.

_____ 8. An abstract idea, such as caring, that is described in a qualitative study.

KEY IDEAS

Directions: Fill in the blanks, or provide the appropriate responses.

1. The research problem and purpose provide a basis for the formulation of specific _____,

_____, or _____ to direct the conduct of a study.

2. Causal relationships identify a cause-and-effect interaction between two or more variables, which are referred to as

_____ and _____ variables.

3. Terms such as *less, more, increase,* and *decrease* indicate the _____ of relationships in hypotheses.

4. H_0 is the symbol used to represent a(n) _____ _____.

5. A testable hypothesis is one that:

6. Other terms that are used for or mean independent variable include:

7. Other terms that are used for or mean dependent variable include:

8. Qualitative studies sometimes involve the investigation of _____ instead of variables.

9. Variables that are not recognized until the study is in process or are recognized before the study is initiated but cannot be controlled are referred to as _____ variables.

10. _____ variables are a type of extraneous variable that make up the setting where the study is conducted.

11. Three important demographic variables that need to be measured in all studies to describe the sample are

_____, _____, and _____.

MAKING CONNECTIONS

Directions: Types of hypotheses are listed. Following the list are 10 specific example hypotheses. Identify each specific hypothesis by indicating which terms apply to it. Hint: Four terms are needed to identify each hypothesis. The correct answer for hypothesis 1 is provided as an example.

Types of Hypotheses

a. Associative
b. Causal
c. Complex
d. Direction
e. Nondirectional
f. Null
g. Research
h. Simple

Sample Hypotheses

_____ 1. Relaxation therapy is more effective than standard care in decreasing pain perception and use of pain medications in adults with chronic arthritic pain.

_____ 2. Age, family support, and health status are related to the self-care abilities of nursing home residents.

_____ 3. Heparinized saline is no more effective than normal saline in maintaining the patency and comfort of a heparin lock.

_____ 4. Poor health status is related to decreasing self-care abilities in institutionalized elderly adults.

_____ 5. Low-back massage is more effective in decreasing one's perception of low-back pain than no massage in patients with chronic low-back pain.

_____ 6. Healthy adults involved in a diet and exercise program have lower low-density lipoprotein (LDL), higher high-density lipoprotein (HDL), and lower cardiovascular risk levels than adults not involved in the program.

_____ 7. Time on the operating table, diastolic blood pressure, age, and preoperative albumin levels are related to development of pressure ulcers in hospitalized elderly adults.

_____ 8. There are no differences in complications or incidence of phlebitis in heparin locks changed every 72 hours and those locks left in place up to 168 hours.

_____ 9. Nurses' perceived work stress, internal locus of control, and social support are related to their psychological symptoms.

_____10. Cancer patients with chronic pain who listen to music with positive suggestion of pain reduction have less pain than those who do not listen to music.

11. Rewrite hypothesis 2 as a directional hypothesis.

12. Rewrite hypothesis 5 as a null hypothesis.

Directions: Match the types of variables with the sample variables that follow.

Types of Variables
a. Demographic variable

b. Dependent variable

c. Independent variable

Sample Variables

_____ 1. Age

_____ 2. Perception of pain

_____ 3. Exercise program

_____ 4. Gender

_____ 5. Length of hospital stay

_____ 6. Incidence of phlebitis

_____ 7. Relaxation therapy

_____ 8. Low-back massage

_____ 9. Educational level

_____ 10. Postoperative pain

_____ 11. Ethnic background

_____ 12. Marital status

EXERCISES IN CRITICAL APPRAISAL

Bindler, Massey, Shultz, Mills, and Short Study

Directions: Read the Bindler et al. (2007) research article in Appendix B and answer the following questions.

1. Are objectives, questions, or hypotheses stated in the study? Identify them.

2. Are objectives, questions, or hypotheses appropriate and clearly stated? Provide a rationale.

3. List the variables in this article, and identify the type of each variable (independent, dependent, or research).

4. Identify the conceptual and operational definitions for the dependent variable: fasting serum insulin levels.

5. Identify the demographic variables in this study.

Sethares and Elliott Study

Directions: Review the Sethares and Elliott (2004) research article in Appendix B, and answer the following questions.

1. Are objectives, questions, or hypotheses stated in the study? Identify them.

2. Are objectives, questions, and hypotheses appropriate and clearly stated? Provide a rationale.

Chapter **8**   **Objectives, Questions, and Hypotheses**

3. List the concept(s) or variables in this article and identify the type of each variable (independent, dependent, or research).

4. Identify the conceptual and operational definitions for the independent variable: tailored message for patients with heart failure.

5. Identify the demographic variables in this study.

Wright Study

Directions: Review the Wright (2003) research article in Appendix B, and answer the following questions.

1. Are objectives, questions, or hypotheses stated in the study? Identify them.

2. Are objectives, questions, or hypotheses appropriate and clearly stated? Provide a rationale.

3. List the concepts or variable(s) in this article, and identify the type of each variable (independent variable, dependent variable, or research variable or concept).

4. Identify the conceptual and operational definitions for the research concept: lived experience of spirituality of recovery from substance abuse.

5. Identify the demographic variables in this study.

GOING BEYOND

1. Develop specific objectives, questions, or hypotheses to direct a proposed study.

2. Link the objectives, questions, or hypotheses developed to the study purpose and framework.

3. Identify the variables to be studied, and develop conceptual and operational definitions for each variable.

9 | Ethics in Research

INTRODUCTION

Read Chapter 9, and then complete the following exercises. These exercises will help you to understand the historical events affecting the development of ethical codes and regulations, protect the rights of research subjects, balance benefits and risks for a study, obtain informed consent from subjects, and participate in institutional reviews of research. The answers for these exercises are in Appendix A.

RELEVANT TERMS

Directions: Match each term with its correct definition

Terms

a. Anonymity
b. Benefit-risk ratio
c. Breach of confidentiality
d. Confidentiality
e. Covert data collection
f. Declaration of Helsinki
g. Deception
h. Department of Health and Human Services Protection of Human Subjects Regulations
i. Ethical principles
j. Food and Drug Administration Protection of Human Subjects Regulations
k. Health Insurance Portability and Accountability Act (HIPAA)
l. Human rights
m. Informed consent
n. Institutional review
o. Nontherapeutic research
p. Nuremberg Code
q. Privacy
r. Research or scientific misconduct
s. Therapeutic research
t. Voluntary consent

Definitions

_____ 1. Claims and demands that have been justified in the eyes of an individual or by the consensus of a group of individuals and are protected in research.

_____ 2. Condition in which a subject's identity cannot be linked, even by the researcher, with his or her individual responses.

_____ 3. Agreement by a prospective subject to voluntarily participate in a study after he or she has assimilated essential information about the study.

_____ 4. Research conducted to generate knowledge for a discipline; the results might benefit future patients but will probably not benefit the research subjects.

_____ 5. Occurs when subjects are unaware that research data are being collected.

_____ 6. Process of examining studies for ethical concerns by a committee of peers.

_____ 7. Ethical document that was adopted in 1964 and recently revised in 2000 by the World Medical Assembly to differentiate therapeutic research from nontherapeutic research.

_____ 8. Ratio considered by researchers and reviewers of research as they weigh potential benefits and risks in a study to promote the conduct of ethical research.

67

_____ 9. Principles of respect for persons, beneficence, and justice, which are relevant to the conduct of research.

_____ 10. Management of private data in research in such a way that subjects' identities are not linked with their responses.

_____ 11. Ethical code of conduct developed in 1949 that contains rules to guide the investigators in conducting research ethically.

_____ 12. Freedom of an individual to determine the time, extent, and general circumstances under which private information will be shared with or withheld from others.

_____ 13. Occurs when the subject is actually misinformed about a study for the purposes of the research; the classic example is the Milgram (1963) study.

_____ 14. Occurs when a researcher, by accident or direct action, allows an unauthorized person to gain access to raw data of a study.

_____ 15. This means that the prospective subject has decided to take part in a study of his or her own volition without coercion or any undue influence.

_____ 16. Research that provides a patient with an opportunity to receive an experimental treatment that may have beneficial results.

_____ 17. The governmental act that established the category of protective health information, which allows covered entities—such as health plans, health care clearinghouses, and health care providers—to transmit health information to others in only certain situations.

_____ 18. Involves such practices as fabrication, falsification, or forging of data; dishonest manipulation of the study design or methods; and plagiarism.

_____ 19. Government regulations developed to protect the rights and welfare of human subjects involved in research conducted or supported by the U.S. Department of Health and Human Services.

_____ 20. Government regulations developed to protect the rights, safety, and welfare of subjects involved in clinical investigations regulated by the Food and Drug Administration (FDA).

Human Rights Based on Ethical Principles

Directions: Match each human right with its correct definition and ethical principle.

Terms
a. Right to fair treatment
b. Right to protection from discomfort and harm
c. Right to self-determination

Definitions

_____ 1. A human right, based on the principle of beneficence, which states subjects should be protected from physical, emotional, social, and economic discomfort and harm.

_____ 2. A human right, based on the principle of justice, which states the selection of subjects and their treatment during the course of a study should be fair.

_____ 3. A human right, based on the ethical principle of respect for persons, which states that humans are capable of controlling their own destinies.

Types of Institutional Review of Research

Directions: Match each type of institutional review of research with its correct definition.

Terms

a. Complete institutional review
b. Exempt from institutional review
c. Expedited institutional review

Definitions

_____ 1. Studies that have some risks, viewed as minimal, require this type of institutional review.

_____ 2. Studies that have no apparent risks for the research subjects require this type of institutional review.

_____ 3. Studies that have greater than minimal risks must receive this type of review.

KEY IDEAS

Directions: Fill in the blanks, or provide the appropriate responses.

1. You randomly selected subjects for your study, to ensure that the ethical principle of _____ was respected in the study.

2. List three examples of legally or mentally incompetent subjects.

   a.

   b.

   c.

3. Children 7 years of age and older are relatively _____ (*competent* or *incompetent*) to give permission to be part of a study.

4. Children must be given the opportunity to _____ to participation in research.

5. Levine (1986) identified two approaches that families, guardians, researchers, or institutional review boards (IRBs) may use when making decisions on behalf of legally and mentally incompetent individuals, such as those with senile dementia of the Alzheimer type (SDAT): (1) best interest standard and (2) substituted judgment standard. Describe what these approaches involve.

   a. Best interest standard

   b. Substituted judgment standard

6. Maintaining confidentiality is more difficult in _____ (*quantitative* or *qualitative*) research.

7. Identify the elements of informed consent.

    a.

    b.

    c.

    d.

8. Identify five types of information that must be included on the consent form.

    a.

    b.

    c.

    d.

    e.

9. _____ consent means that the prospective subject with hypertension has decided, based on his or her own volition without coercion or any undue influence, to take part in a study focused on a new medication to treat high blood pressure.

10. In hospitals, before a study is conducted, it must be reviewed by a committee of peers called a(n)

    _____ _____ _____.

11. Identify mechanisms by which consent may be documented.

    a.

    b.

    c.

12. Fabrication of data in a study is an example of _____ _____.

13. The Office of Research Integrity (ORI) is responsible for:

14. Identify four issues that are relevant in addressing the problem of research misconduct.

    a.

    b.

c.

d.

15. Identify the three levels of institutional review of research.

   a.

   b.

   c.

16. Identify two important questions that need to be addressed related to the use of animals in research.

   a.

   b.

17. More than 700 institutions conducting health-related research with animals have sought accreditation by the

   _____ to ensure the humane treatment of animals in research.

18. How do you assess the benefit-risk ratio of a published study?

19. You are using school-age children in your study to implement a treatment to promote weight management. What type of consent must you obtain and from whom?

20. Social Security numbers are an example of _____ _____

   _____ under HIPAA.

MAKING CONNECTIONS

Levels of Discomfort or Harm
Directions: Match the levels of discomfort or harm listed here with the examples that follow.

Levels
a. No anticipated effects
b. Temporary discomfort
c. Unusual levels of temporary discomfort
d. Risk of permanent damage
e. Certainty of permanent damage

Examples

_____ 1. Collecting an additional blood sugar sample from a diabetic patient.

_____ 2. Reviewing patient records for medical diagnoses, complications, and length of hospital stay.

_____ 3. Confining a patient to bed for 10 days to determine the impact on muscle strength, joint mobility, and bone density.

_____ 4. Collecting data on a person's child abuse and drug use behavior.

_____ 5. Data collected during the Nazi medical experiments.

_____ 6. Involving sedentary females over 45 years of age in an exercise program with slow progressive increases in the strenuousness of the exercises.

_____ 7. Completing an anonymous survey on satisfaction with a health care agency's services.

_____ 8. Examining the effect of new drugs that may have some serious side effects.

_____ 9. The conduct of the Tuskegee syphilis study and the continuation of the study for several years after the treatment for syphilis was identified.

_____ 10. Studying the emotional impact of experiencing a rape.

Unethical Studies

Directions: Match the unethical studies listed here with the correct descriptions.

Studies
a. Jewish chronic disease hospital study
b. Nazi medical experiments
c. Tuskegee syphilis study
d. Willowbrook study

Descriptions

_____ 1. Subjects were exposed to freezing temperatures, high altitudes, poisons, untested drugs, and experimental operations.

_____ 2. Study was conducted to determine the natural course of syphilis in the adult black male.

_____ 3. Subjects were deliberately infected with the hepatitis virus.

_____ 4. Subjects were frequently killed or sustained permanent physical, mental, or social damage during these studies.

_____ 5. Subjects did not receive penicillin, even after it was identified as an effective treatment for their disease.

_____ 6. The purpose of this study was to determine the patients' rejection responses to live cancer cells.

_____ 7. The subjects in this study were institutionalized mentally retarded children.

_____ 8. These experiments resulted in the development of the Nuremberg Code.

_____ 9. The subjects were injected with live cancer cells without their knowledge.

_____ 10. This study continued until 1972, when an account of the study appeared in the *Washington Star* and public outrage demanded the study be stopped.

PUZZLES

Crossword Puzzle

Directions: Complete the crossword puzzle. Note: If the answer is more than one word, there are no blank spaces left between the words.

Across

1. Keeping data private.
4. Agency evaluation of a study to protect potential subjects.
6. Subjects who can legally choose whether or not to participate in a study are _____.
7. Code developed after World War II.
10. Controlling your own fate.
11. Focuses on human rights of research.
13. Child's agreement to be in a study.
14. _____ act of 1974.
15. Subjects whose identities are unknown are _____.

Down

2. Subjects should receive _____ during a study.
3. Opposite of benefit; a factor that must be examined to determine whether a study is ethical.
5. Institutional review board.
8. Misinforming subjects.
9. Subject's permission to be in a study.
12. _____ are considered incompetent to give consent.

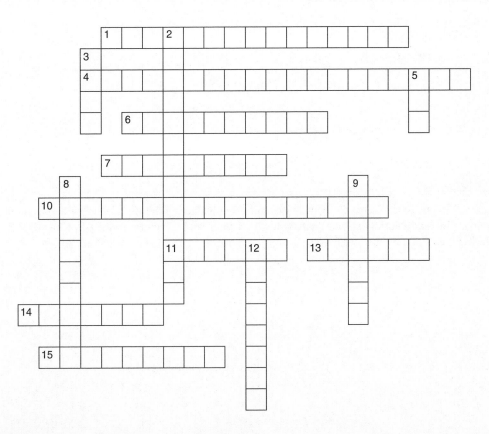

EXERCISES IN CRITICAL APPRAISAL

Directions: Review the research articles in Appendix B, and answer the following questions.

1. Is the Bindler, Massey, Shultz, Mills, and Short (2007) study ethical? What information in the study indicates that the subjects' rights were protected and that institutional review was obtained?

2. Is the Sethares and Elliott (2004) study ethical? What information in the study indicates that the subjects' rights were protected and that institutional review was obtained?

3. Is the Wright (2003) study ethical? What information in the study indicates that the subjects' rights were protected and that institutional review was obtained?

GOING BEYOND

Develop a proposal for a study. Discuss the benefit-risk ratio for conducting the study, develop a consent form, and complete a preliminary institutional review board (IRB) form for your study. Use the content in Chapter 9 to direct you in developing these aspects of a research proposal.

10 Understanding Quantitative Research Design

INTRODUCTION

Read Chapter 10, and then complete the following exercises. These exercises will help you to learn relevant terms and identify and critically appraise designs in published studies. The answers to these exercises are in Appendix A.

RELEVANT TERMS

Terms Related to Triangulation

Directions: Match each term with its correct definition or description.

Terms

a. Analysis triangulation
b. Between method triangulation
c. Data triangulation
d. Investigator triangulation
e. Methodological triangulation
f. Multiple triangulation
g. Theoretical triangulation
h. Triangulation
i. Within method triangulation

Definitions

_____ 1. Exists when two or more research-trained investigators with divergent backgrounds explore the same phenomenon.

_____ 2. The use of both quantitative and qualitative research strategies in conducting a study but within one method (i.e., only data triangulation).

_____ 3. Combining research methods or strategies from two or more research traditions in the same study.

_____ 4. Collection of data from multiple sources in the same study.

_____ 5. Using two or more analysis techniques to analyze the same set of data for the purpose of validation.

_____ 6. The use of two or more frameworks or theoretical perspectives in the same study, with development of hypotheses based on the different theoretical perspectives and tested on the same data set.

_____ 7. The use of two or more theories, methods, data sources, investigators, or analysis methods in a study; it usually involves combining qualitative and quantitative research methodologies.

_____ 8. The use of two or more research methods or procedures in a study, such as different designs, instruments, and data collection procedures, usually from both quantitative and qualitative research.

_____ 9. The use of two or more types of triangulation (theoretical, data, methodological, investigator, or analysis) in a study.

Concepts Important to Design

Directions: Match each term with its correct definition or description.

Terms

a. Bias
b. Causality
c. Control
d. Control group

e. Intermediate mediation
f. Micromediation
g. Molar

h. Multicausality
i. Manipulation
j. Probability

Definitions

_____ 1. The controlled implementation of a treatment or an independent variable in a study to determine its effect on the study dependent variable.

_____ 2. Any influence or action in a study that distorts the findings or slants them away from the true or expected.

_____ 3. Causal laws that relate to large and complex objects.

_____ 4. Imposing of rules by the researcher to decrease the possibility of error and increase the probability that the study's findings are an accurate reflection of reality.

_____ 5. Examines causal connections at the level of small particles, such as atoms.

_____ 6. The recognition that a number of interrelating variables can be involved in causing a particular effect.

_____ 7. Addresses relative rather than absolute causality.

_____ 8. Includes three conditions: (a) there must be a strong relationship between the proposed cause and effect, (b) the proposed cause must have preceded the effect in time, and (c) the cause has to be present whenever the effect occurs.

_____ 9. The group of elements or subjects not exposed to the experimental treatment; used in studies with random sampling methods.

_____ 10. Considers causal factors operating between molar and micro levels.

Terms Important to Design Validity

Directions: Match each term with its correct definition or description.

Terms

a. Construct validity
b. Threats to validity
c. External validity
d. Fishing
e. History

f. Internal validity
g. Matching
h. Maturation
i. Selection

j. Statistical conclusion validity
k. Statistical regression
l. Study validity
m. Threats to statistical conclusion validity

Definitions

_____ 1. Reasons why false conclusions can be drawn about the presence or absence of a statistically significant relationship or difference between groups.

_____ 2. A measure of the truth or accuracy of a claim that is an important concern throughout the research process.

_____ 3. Issues within a study that could provide alternate explanations about the relationships identified during the study.

_____ 4. The process by which subjects are chosen to take part in a study and how subjects are grouped within a study.

_____ 5. An event that is not related to the planned study but occurs during the time of the study and could influence the responses of subjects to the treatment.

_____ 6. Increasing the risk of a type I error by conducting multiple statistical analyses of relationships or differences looking for a significant relationship or difference.

_____ 7. The movement or regression of extreme scores toward the mean in studies using a pretest-posttest design.

_____ 8. This technique is used when an experimental subject is randomly selected and a subject similar in relation to important extraneous variables is randomly selected for inclusion in the control or comparison group.

_____ 9. The extent to which the effects detected in the study are a true reflection of reality rather than being the result of the effects of extraneous variables.

_____ 10. Concerned with whether the conclusions about relationships and differences drawn from statistical analyses are an accurate reflection or reality.

_____ 11. Examines the fit between conceptual and operational definitions of variables and determines whether the instrument actually measures the theoretical construct that it purports to measure.

_____ 12. Unplanned and unrecognized changes experienced during a study—such as subjects growing older, wiser, stronger, or hungrier—that can influence the findings of a study.

_____ 13. The extent to which the study findings can be generalized beyond the sample used in the study.

Controlling Extraneous Variables

Directions: Match each term with its correct definition or description.

Terms

a. Blocking
b. Design
c. Extraneous variable
d. Heterogeneity
e. Homogeneity
f. Monomethod bias
g. Mono-operation bias
h. Randomized block design
i. Rival hypothesis
j. Stratification

Definitions

_____ 1. The researcher's attempt to obtain subjects with a wide variety of characteristics to reduce the risk of bias in studies not using random sampling.

_____ 2. Design in which the researcher includes subjects with various levels of an extraneous variable in the sample but controls the number of subjects at each level of the variable and their random assignment to groups within the study.

_____ 3. Used in a design so that subjects are distributed throughout the sample by using sampling techniques similar to those used in blocking, but the purpose of the procedure is even distribution throughout the sample.

_____ 4. The possibility of an alternative explanation of cause.

Chapter **10** **Understanding Quantitative Research Design**

_____ 5. The degree to which objects are similar or a form of equivalence, such as limiting subjects to only one level of an extraneous variable to reduce its impact on the study findings.

_____ 6. The blueprint for conducting the study that maximizes control over factors that could interfere with the validity of the findings.

_____ 7. Occurs when only one method of measurement is used to measure a construct, such as the use of one paper-and-pencil scale to measure chronic pain.

_____ 8. More than one measure of a variable is used in a study, but all measures use the same method of recording.

_____ 9. Exists in all studies and can affect the measurement of study variables and the relationships among these variables.

_____ 10. Designs using blocking where the extraneous variable is used as an independent variable in the data analysis.

KEY IDEAS

Directions: Fill in the blanks in the following sentences.

1. According to causality theory, things have causes, and causes lead to _____.

2. From the perspective of probability, a(n) _____ may not produce a specific _____ each time that particular _____ occurs.

3. Designs are developed to reduce the possibilities and effects of _____.

4. The purpose of research designs is to maximize _____ of factors that can interfere with the validity of the findings.

5. The most commonly used manipulation in a study is the _____.

6. Critical analysis of research involves being able to think through the _____ to _____ that have occurred and make judgments about how seriously these affect the integrity of the findings.

7. Quasi-experimental and experimental studies are designed to examine _____ and _____.

8. Threats to external validity consist of interactions with _____, _____, and _____.

9. Designs are developed to reduce threats to the validity of the _____ made in the study.

Chapter **10** **Understanding Quantitative Research Design**

MAKING CONNECTIONS

Directions: Match the methods of design control listed here with the following statements describing the research design of a study. You might identify more than one design control method for each statement. Note: Not all design control methods will be used, and some might be used more than once.

Design Control Methods

a. Controlling the environment
b. Controlling subject and group equivalence
c. Control groups
d. Controlling the treatment
e. Counterbalancing

f. Controlling measurement
g. Controlling extraneous variables
h. Random sampling
i. Random assignment
j. Homogeneity

k. Heterogeneity
l. Blocking
m. Stratification
n. Matching
o. Statistical control

Statements

_____ 1. "Patients who met the inclusion criteria on admission to labor and delivery were approached to be in the study using a random table of numbers. Participants receiving an even number were included in the study (total of 75 patients)" (Radzyminski, 2005, p. 336).

_____ 2. "Chi-square demonstrated no significant differences between success and failure groups in gender, admitting diagnosis, type of surgery, cardiac rhythm, and weaning technique" (Hanneman, 1994, p. 5).

_____ 3. "All data were obtained by the principal investigator who stayed with the mother-infant dyads during the data collection sessions and recorded and timed all observed behaviors. The principal investigator was blind to whether the mother received an epidural or not." (Radzyminski, 2005, p. 337).

_____ 4. "First, census block groups were selected using age, income, and ethnicity to facilitate the selection of a sample of menstruating women between the ages of 18 and 45 with a wide range of incomes. The ethnic mix was representative of the northwestern metropolitan area that was sampled" (Mitchell, Woods, & Lentz, 1994, p. 25).

_____ 5. "This correlational descriptive study included a convenience sample of 50 women who had resided for at least 21 days in one of four battered women's shelters in the San Francisco Bay Area." (Humphreys, 2000, p. 274).

_____ 6. "17 [mother-infant dyads] were eliminated from the analysis for failure of the labor and delivery nurse to follow the protocol of placing the newborn immediately on the mother's chest postdelivery" (Radzyminski, 2005, p. 336).

_____ 7. "A separate preadmission testing area was used to provide privacy and confidentiality during interactions with patients who participated in the study" (Wagner, Byrne & Kolcaba, 2006, p. 427).

_____ 8. "To obtain sufficient power for analyses, data collection was designed to continue until at least 300 blue-collar, 200 skilled trades, and 100 white-collar subjects volunteered" (Lusk, Ronis, Kerr, & Atwood, 1994, p. 152).

_____ 9. "Data collectors alternated the order of mothers and fathers completing the instruments and doing the parent-infant interaction tasks. Different teaching tasks were alternately assigned to each parent" (Broom, 1994, p. 140).

_____ 10. "The researcher used a two-group independent sample experimental design. A randomized block design controlled for gender" (Treloar, 1994, p. 54).

Chapter **10**   **Understanding Quantitative Research Design**

PUZZLES

Word Scramble

Directions: Unscramble the following sentence by rearranging the letters to form actual words. Note: You will use all the letters in every word.

Sjut sa hte libunetpr rof a usheo tmus eb vidnuizliddaie ot eth fseccipi esuho giben itlub,

os tsum eht anedig eb daem piseccif ot a yudst.

Secret Message

Directions: Translate the following secret message by substituting one letter for another. For example, if you decide that "c" should really be "x," then "c" will be "x" every time it appears in this puzzle. Hint: Try to translate short words first to establish vowel patterns.

Ymj uzwutxj tk f ijxnls nx yt xjy zu f xnyzfynts ymfy rfcnrnejx ymj txxngnqnynjx tk tgyfnsnsl

fhhzwfyj fsxajwx yt tgojhynajx, vzjxynts, tw mdutymjxjx.

Crossword Puzzle

Directions: Complete the crossword puzzle. Note: If the answer is more than one word, there are no blank spaces left between the words.

Across

1. Selection of a control group subject who has similar characteristics to an experimental group subject.
. Good design reduces threats to the validity of _____.
   A cause leads to an _____.
   Administration of multiple treatments in random order.
   The purpose of sampling criteria is to establish ____ among subjects.
   dependent variable.
   examination of whether the study provides nvincing test of the framework propositions.
   nger to the integrity of the findings.
   ive, rather than absolute, causality.
   rint for conducting a study.
   strategy used to ensure even distribution of nt variables throughout the sample.
   that provide greatest control in examining

Down

2. A design strategy in which subjects with a wide variety of characteristics are obtained for the sample.
3. A visual depiction of the design.
5. Treatment or study intervention.
6. Group of subjects selected for a study.
8. Imposition of rules by the researcher to decrease the possibility of errors.
9. Controls the number of subjects at various levels of an extraneous variable in a sample.
11. Designs used to examine relationships between two or among more than two variables in a single group.
13. Strategy used to increase the probability that the sample is equivalent to the population.
14. Deviation of findings from the true.
15. Design used to provide a picture of situations as they naturally happen.
17. A design in which the patterns of responses of various samples are examined over time.

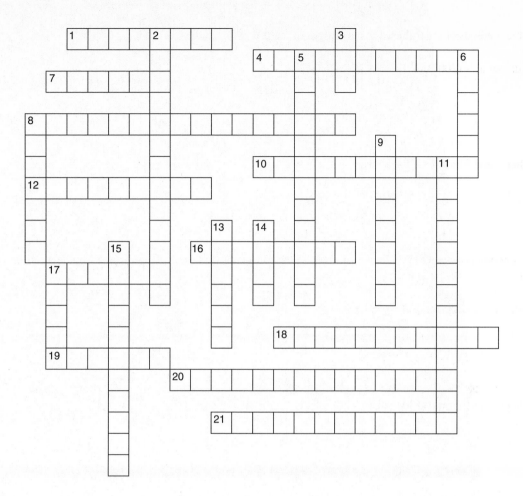

Directions: Review the research articles in Appendix B, and answer the following questions.

1. Identify three sources of potential bias in the designs of the following studies.

   a. Bindler et al.'s (2007) study

   b. Sethares and Elliott's (2004) study

2. List three methods of control used in the designs of the following studies.

   a. Bindler et al.'s (2007) study

   b. Sethares and Elliott's (2004) study

3. To what populations can the findings from each of the following studies be generalized? Provide a rationale for your answer.

   a. Bindler et al.'s (2007) study

   b. Sethares and Elliott's (2004) study

4. What are the threats to external validity in each of the following studies?

   a. Bindler et al.'s (2007) study

   b. Sethares and Elliott's (2004) study

GOING BEYOND

Select a recently published study with a clearly stated framework. Examine the relationships among the study framework; the research objectives, questions, or hypotheses; and the design. Does the design allow an adequate test of the research objectives, questions, or hypotheses? Does the design facilitate application of the findings to the framework in the two quantitative studies presented in Appendix B?

11 Selecting a Quantitative Research Design

INTRODUCTION

Read Chapter 11, and then complete the following exercises. These exercises will help you to understand and select a design for a study. The answers to these exercises are in Appendix A.

RELEVANT TERMS

Types of Design (A)

Directions: Match each term with its correct definition.

Terms

a. Carryover effect
b. Case study design
c. Classic experimental design
d. Clinical trial
e. Cohort

f. Comparative descriptive design
g. Comparative experimental design
h. Comparison group
i. Correlational study
j. Cross-sectional design

k. Crossover
l. Dependent variable
m. Descriptive design
n. Double-blinding

Definitions

_____ 1. Less rigorous experimental design in which random sampling is difficult if not impossible so convenience sample is used with random assignment to groups.

_____ 2. Means of examining the effects of various treatments where the effects of a treatment are examined by comparing the treatment group with the no-treatment group.

_____ 3. The sample in the time-dimensional studies in the field of epidemiology.

_____ 4. A systematic investigation of relationships between two or more variables to explain the nature of relationships in the world and not to examine cause and effect.

_____ 5. The response, behavior, or outcomes that is predicted and measured in research; changes are presumed to be caused by the independent variable.

_____ 6. The application of one treatment can influence the response to following treatments.

_____ 7. Used to describe differences in variables in two or more groups in a natural setting.

_____ 8. The original, most commonly used design with two randomized groups, one receiving the experimental treatment and one receiving no treatment.

_____ 9. Includes the administration of more than one treatment to each subject, and the treatments are provided sequentially rather than concurrently.

_____ 10. Neither the patient nor the caregivers are aware of the group assignment of the patient.

_____ 11. Used to examine groups of subjects in various stages of development simultaneously with the intent of inferring trends over time.

_____ 12. Intensive exploration of a single unit of study, such as a person, family, group, community, or institution.

_____ 13. Used to describe variables that exist in a study situation.

_____ 14. This group is not selected using random sampling and usually does not receive a treatment.

Types of Variables and Designs

Directions: Match each term with its correct definition.

Terms

a. Endogenous variables
b. Event-partitioning design
c. Experimental design
d. Fatigue effect
e. Independent variable

f. Indicator
g. Inferred causality
h. Interventions
i. Longitudinal design
j. Matching

k. Methodological design
l. Model-testing design
m. Nested variables

Definitions

_____ 1. Variables found only at certain levels of the independent variable, such as gender, race, socioeconomic status, and education.

_____ 2. This technique is used when an experimental subject is randomly selected and a subject similar in relation to an important extraneous variable is randomly selected for inclusion in the control or comparison group.

_____ 3. Merger of the longitudinal and trend designs to increase sample size and avoid the effects of history on the validity of findings.

_____ 4. A cause-and-effect relationship is identified from numerous studies conducted over time to determine risk factors or causal factors in selected situations.

_____ 5. When a subject becomes tired or bored with a study, which can affect the findings from the study.

_____ 6. Panel designs used to examine changes in the same subjects over an extended period of time.

_____ 7. Those variables whose variations are explained within the theoretical model as part of a study with a model-testing design.

_____ 8. A design that provides the greatest amount of control possible to examine causality more closely.

_____ 9. Treatments, therapies, procedures, or actions implemented by health care professionals to and with patients, in a particular situation, to move the patients' conditions toward desired health outcomes that are beneficial to them.

_____ 10. Used to test the accuracy of a hypothesized causal model or map.

_____ 11. The treatment, intervention, or experimental activity that is manipulated or varied by the researcher to create an effect on the dependent variable.

_____ 12. Used to develop the validity and reliability of instruments to measure research concepts and variables.

_____ 13. Variables in primary prevention studies in which changes in the community are examined to assess the effectiveness of a primary prevention program.

Types of Designs (B)

Directions: Match each term with its correct definition.

Terms

a. One-group posttest-only design
b. One-group pretest-posttest design
c. Phase I clinical trial
d. Phase II clinical trial
e. Phase III clinical trial
f. Phase IV clinical trial

g. Posttest only design with comparison group
h. Predictive design
i. Preexperimental
j. Pretest sensitization
k. Primary prevention design
l. Prospective study

m. Quasi-experimental design
n. Random assignment to groups
o. Randomized block design
p. Residual variable
q. Retrospective study
r. Survey
s. Treatment

Definitions

_____ 1. Subjects' responses to the posttest can be due, in part, to learning from or subjective reaction to the pretest.

_____ 2. A preexperimental design in which there is usually no attempt to select the subjects who receive the treatment, and the group is not pretested.

_____ 3. A preexperimental design in which the convenience sample is pretested in an attempt to assess the effects of the treatment.

_____ 4. The independent variable that is manipulated in a study to produce an effect on the dependent variable.

_____ 5. Developed to predict the value of the dependent variable based on values obtained from the independent variables.

_____ 6. The initial testing of a new drug; focuses on determining the best drug dose and identifying safety effects.

_____ 7. A trial that seeks preliminary evidence of efficacy and side effects of the drug dose determined by the phase I trial.

_____ 8. These trials are comparative definitive studies in which the new drug's effects are compared with those of the drug considered standard therapy.

_____ 9. These trials occur after regulatory approval of the drug and are designed to follow patients over time to identify uncommon side effects and test marketing strategies.

_____ 10. A data collection technique in which questionnaires or personal interviews are used to gather data about an identified population.

_____ 11. An epidemiological study that identifies a group composed of people who are at risk for experiencing a particular event.

_____ 12. A weak experimental design with many threats to validity, no randomization, and usually no attempt at control.

Chapter **11** **Selecting a Quantitative Research Design**

_____ 13. Variables that indicate the effect of unmeasured variables not included in the model in a model-testing design.

_____ 14. This preexperimental design includes a nonequivalent comparison group in an attempt to strengthen the findings.

_____ 15. A design that attempts to control for a confounding variable by rank-ordering the subjects in relation to the blocking variable.

_____ 16. A design with limited control that was developed to provide alternative means for examining causality in situations not conducive to experimental controls.

_____ 17. A procedure used to assign subjects to treatment or comparison groups in which the subjects have an equal opportunity to be assigned to either group.

_____ 18. An epidemiological study that identifies a group composed of people who have experienced a particular event.

_____ 19. A study that attempts to measure things that do not happen. One cannot select a sample to study, apply a treatment, and then measure an effect, therefore changes in the community are examined.

KEY IDEAS

Directions: Fill in the blanks, or provide the appropriate responses.

1. What is the purpose of a design?

2. Designs created to meet nursing needs need to be congruent with _____.

3. In epidemiological studies, _____ is an important dimension of the design.

4. Surveys are a means of gathering _____ data.

5. With a correlational design, it is important that the sample reflect:

6. The researcher cannot establish _____ using a correlational study.

7. In predictive correlational designs, independent variables most effective in prediction are

_____ correlated with the dependent variable but _____ correlated with other independent variables.

8. Interventions designed for use in quasi-experimental and experimental studies are expected to result in:

9. The power of quasi-experimental or experimental designs to examine causality is determined by the degree to which:

10. The method of randomization typically used in randomized clinical trials is _____.

11. Variables found only at certain levels of the independent variable are _____

   _____.

12. The research design organizes all the components of the study in a way that is most likely to lead to:

MAKING CONNECTIONS

Study Designs

Directions: Match the study designs listed here to the study descriptions that follow. Note: Some descriptions may match more than one design. Not all designs will be used.

Designs
a. Typical descriptive design
b. Comparative descriptive design
c. Longitudinal design
d. Trend design
e. Case study
f. Descriptive correlational design
g. Predictive correlational design
h. Model testing design
i. Pretest-posttest quasi-experimental design
j. Experimental or quasi-experimental design

Study Descriptions

_____ 1. The purpose of the present study was to investigate the predictive relationships among attachment, selected demographic variables, and quality of life (Rickelman, Gallman, & Parra, 1994, p. 68).

_____ 2. The purpose of this study was to explore the dimensions of disturbing behaviors in institutionalized elders and to identify the related environmental and personal characteristics. A model comparison approach was used to examine the effectiveness of the Kaiser-Jones model in explaining agitated psychomotor behavior (Kolanowski, Hurwitz, Taylor, Evans, & Strumpf, 1994, p. 73).

_____ 3. The purpose of this study was to determine whether men whose partners had experienced a low-risk pregnancy and men whose partners had been hospitalized during pregnancy for an obstetrical risk differed in paternal role competence from the time of their partners' early postpartum hospitalization to 1, 4, and 8 months after birth. Each subjects was recruited during the 24th to 34th week of his partner's pregnancy and followed until 8 months after the child was born (Ferketich & Mercer, 1994, p. 82).

_____ 4. The aim of this study was to assess elementary school nurses' perceptions of student bullying, actions when they encounter bullies or victims, and perceived level of preparation for dealing with this problem (Hendershot, Dake, Price, & Lartey, 2006, p. 229).

_____ 5. The aim of this study was to determine the feasibility of "Girls on the Move," an individually tailored computerized physical activity (PA) program plus nurse counseling intervention, in increasing PA using a pretest-posttest control group design (Robbins, Gretebeck, Kaxanis, & Pender, 2006, p. 206).

_____ 6. The aim of this study was to evaluate the short-and-long term effects of smoking cessation strategies tailored to help the pregnant adolescent to attain and maintain abstinence. The specific aim was to examine differences in short-and long-term smoking behaviors among three groups: Teen FreshStart, Teen FreshStart Plus Buddy, and Usual Care control. A randomized controlled intervention design was used (Albrecht et al., 2006, p. 402).

_____ 7. This study examined the relationship of less restrictive restraints with Seclusion/Restraint Usage, average years of psychiatric experience of nursing staff, and staff mix (Williams & Myers, 2001, p. 139).

MAPPING THE DESIGN

Directions: Map the design for each of the following quasi-experimental studies.

1. "Transcutaneous oxygen and behavioral state data were collected before, during, and after a prescribed diagnostic heelstick. … The 5-minute period immediately preceding heelstick was the precry episode (baseline); the 5-minute period commencing with the heelstick was the cry episode; and the final 2-minute period was the postcry episode. … For the NNS infants, the pacifier was inserted immediately after heelstick. The ONNS infants did not receive the pacifier after heelstick and were allowed to cry without interference for the 5-minute crying episode" (Treloar, 1994, p. 52).

2. "All consenting patients admitted to the SICU had their admitting core temperature recorded. Patients with admitting core temperatures of less than 36°C were entered into the study. Their temperatures were recorded and shivering assessed every 15 minutes until they reached a core temperature of 36°C and remained at that temperature for 30 minutes. Patients were randomly assigned to one of three treatment groups (radiant heat, forced warm air, and warm blankets)" (Giuffre, Heidenreich, & Pruitt, 1994, p. 176).

EXERCISES IN CRITICAL APPRAISAL

Directions: Review the research articles in Appendix B, and answer the following questions.

1. Identify the designs used in the following studies.

   a. Bindler et al.'s (2007) study

b. Sethares and Elliott's (2004) study

2. What group comparisons were made in the following studies?

a. Bindler et al.'s (2007) study

b. Sethares and Elliott's (2004) study

3. Identify three strengths in the designs used in each of the following studies.

a. Bindler et al.'s (2007) study

b. Sethares and Elliott's (2004) study

Chapter **11** **Selecting a Quantitative Research Design**

Identify a quasi-experimental study in a recent nursing journal. Identify the intervention or treatment. Was the intervention described in sufficient detail for you to provide the same intervention? Was the intervention provided consistently to all subjects? In your opinion, was the intervention sufficiently powerful to cause a difference in effect between the experimental and control groups? Write a brief paragraph judging the adequacy of the intervention.

12 Outcomes Research

INTRODUCTION

Read Chapter 12, and then complete the following exercises. These exercises will help you to learn relevant terms and to read and comprehend published outcomes studies. The answers for these exercises are in Appendix A.

RELEVANT TERMS

Outcomes Research Terms (A)

Directions: Match the terms with their definitions.

Terms

a. Aggregate
b. Clinical decision analysis
c. Consensus knowledge building
d. Cost-benefit analysis
e. Cost-effectiveness analysis
f. Donabedian's primordial cell

g. Efficiency
h. Geographic analysis
i. Health (as defined by Donabedian)
j. Individual
k. Interdisciplinary team

l. Intermediate end point
m. Latent transition analysis
n. Measurement error
o. Multicomponent treatment
p. Multilevel analysis
q. Opportunity costs

Definitions

_____ 1. The least expensive method of achieving a desired end while obtaining the maximum benefit from available resources.

_____ 2. A systematic method of describing clinical problems, identifying possible diagnostic and management courses of action, assessing the probability and value of the various outcomes, and then calculating the optimal course of action.

_____ 3. Analysis technique used in outcomes research that examines the costs and benefits of alternative ways of using resources assessed in monetary terms and the use that produces the greatest net benefit.

_____ 4. Type of outcomes research in which costs and benefits are compared for different ways of accomplishing a clinical goal, such as diagnosing a condition, treating an illness, or providing a service. The goal is to identify the strategy that provides the most value for the money.

_____ 5. Small area analysis used to examine variations in health status, health services, patterns of care, or patterns of use by a geographical area.

_____ 6. Events or markers that act as precursors to the final outcome and are sometimes used in place of the final outcome of care when it may not occur for weeks of months.

_____ 7. The difference between what exists in reality and what a research instrument measures.

_____ 8. A group of patients or persons considered with reference to the individual.

_____ 9. A single person or patient.

_____ 10. Used in epidemiology to study how environmental factors and individual attributes and behavior interact to influence individual-level health behavior and disease risk.

_____ 11. Outcomes design that requires the critique and synthesis of an extensive international search of literature on the topic of concern, including unpublished studies, studies in progress, dissertations, and theses.

_____ 12. Individuals from multiple health disciplines use their diversity of knowledge and skills to care for the same patients. The plan of care reflects an integrated set of goals shared by the providers of care, and the team members share information and coordinate their services through a systematic communication process.

_____ 13. The basic unit of Donabedian's framework—the physical-physiological function of the individual patient being cared for by the individual practitioner.

_____ 14. Occurs when a set of treatments are combined to manage a patient problem. Outcomes research designs have been developed to examine the effects of these treatment programs.

_____ 15. Lost opportunities that the patient, family members, or others experience. For example, a family member might have been able to earn more money if he or she had not had to stay home to care for the patient.

_____ 16. Outcomes research strategy used in situations in which stages or categories of recovery have been defined and transitions across stages can be identified. To use this analysis method, each member of the population is placed in a single category or stage for a given point of time.

_____ 17. Defined by the subject of care, not by the provider of care, and based on what the consumer expects, wants, or is willing to accept.

Outcomes Research Terms (B)

Directions: Match the terms with their definitions.

Terms

a. Out-of-pocket
b. Patient
c. Patient Outcomes Research Team (PORT) projects
d. Person
e. Population-based study
f. Practice pattern profiling

g. Prospective cohort study
h. Providers of care (as defined by Donabedian)
i. Research tradition
j. Retrospective cohort study
k. Sampling error
l. Standard of care

m. Standardized mortality ratio
n. Structures of care
o. Subject of care (as defined by Donabedian)
p. Variance analysis

Definitions

_____ 1. The difference between a sample statistic used to estimate a population parameter and the actual but unknown value of the parameter.

_____ 2. Important type of outcomes research that involves studying health conditions in the context of the community rather than the context of the medical system.

_____ 3. The elements of organization and administration that guide the processes of care.

_____ 4. A norm on which quality of care is judged. Clinical guidelines, critical paths, and care maps define quality care.

_____ 5. Those expenses incurred by the patient or family or both that are not reimbursable by the insurance company.

_____ 6. Include several practitioners, who might be of the same profession or different professions and "who may be providing care concurrently, as individuals, or jointly, as a team" (Donabedian, 1987, p. 5).

_____ 7. An individual who may or may not have gained access to care.

_____ 8. Outcomes research strategy to track individual and group variance from a specific critical pathway with the goal of decreasing preventable variance in process.

_____ 9. A measure of the relative risk of the studied group to die of a particular condition.

_____ 10. An epidemiological study in which a group of people are identified who have experienced a particular event to determine cause-and-effect relationships.

_____ 11. Someone who has already gained access to some care.

_____ 12. An epidemiological study in which a group is identified that is made up of people who are at risk for experiencing a particular event.

_____ 13. Large-scale, multifaceted, and multidisciplinary projects initiated by the Agency for Healthcare Research and Quality (AHRQ) that were designed to examine the outcomes and cost of current practice patterns, identify the best treatment strategy, and test methods for reducing inappropriate variations.

_____ 14. A program of research that is important for building a body of knowledge related to the phenomena explained by a particular conceptual model; defines acceptable research methodologies.

_____ 15. Either a patient or a person who has already or may in the future gain access to care.

_____ 16. An epidemiological technique used in outcomes research that focuses on patterns of care rather than individual occurrences of care.

KEY IDEAS

Directions: Fill in the blanks, or provide the appropriate responses.

1. What does outcomes research focus on?

2. The meeting of which two National Institutes of Health study sections ultimately led to the development of the Agency for Health Services Research (AHSR)?

   a.

   b.

3. What was the first large-scale study to examine factors influencing patient outcomes?

4. The Medical Outcomes Study (MOS) was flawed because it failed to control for the following three elements:

   a.

   b.

   c.

5. The MOS considered the following three components, commonly performed by nurses, to be components of medical practice:

   a.

   b.

   c.

6. Identify three questions that might be addressed by PORTs.

   a.

   b.

   c.

7. Clinical guideline panels were developed to:

8. Examining the impact of nursing on overall hospital outcomes will require:

9. To evaluate an outcome, the outcome must be _____ _____ to the

   _____ that _____ the outcome.

10. In outcomes research, the_____ _____ _____
    must clarify what outcomes are desirable.

11. List three examples of standards of care.

    a.

    b.

    c.

12. _____ _____ samples are preferred in outcome studies.

13. To allow evaluation or monitoring of individual patient care, the following information must be available in large databases:

    a.

    b.

    c.

    d.

14. Decision analysis is based on the following four assumptions:

a.

b.

c.

d.

15. From an outcomes research perspective, three questions that might be asked about interventions are:

a.

b.

c.

16. Outcomes selected for nursing studies should be those that are:

17. Instruments for outcomes studies should be selected for their sensitivity to:

18. The Nursing Care Report Card for acute care was developed by:

19. According to Gottman and Rushe (1993), what five fallacies do researchers hold related to the analysis of change?

a.

b.

c.

d.

e.

20. In analyzing improvement of patients' treatment with a particular intervention, the following parameters should be reported:

a.

b.

c.

d.

e.

21. In performing variance analysis, it is important to track:

a.

b.

c.

MAKING CONNECTIONS

Directions: Match the researchers with their contributions to outcomes research.

Researchers

a. Louis
b. Hinshaw
c. Wennberg
d. Donabedian
e. Sir William Petty

f. Chaput de Saintonge and colleagues
g. Lange and Jacox
h. Earnest A. Codman
i. Maynard

j. Florence Nightingale
k. Schmitt, Farrell, and Heinemann
l. Semmelweiss
m. Kelly and colleagues

Research Contributions

_____ 1. Proposed a method evaluating the effectiveness of care based on an examination of the patient 1 year after surgery or discharge from a hospital.

_____ 2. The first physician to question the effectiveness of medical care.

_____ 3. One of the first nurses to conduct outcome studies.

_____ 4. Examined small area variations in medical practice.

_____ 5. As director of the National Institute for Nursing Research, sponsored the Conference on Patient Outcomes Research: Examining the Effectiveness of Nursing Practice.

_____ 6. Viennese physician who used hospital records to show that women in labor who were assisted by midwives had lower mortality rates than those attended by physicians in hospital wards.

_____ 7. Criticized the MOS for not considering the influence of nursing actions while studying medical practice outcomes.

_____ 8. Recommended elements necessary to the description of interventions.

_____ 9. Developed a strategy for analyzing clinical decisions using "paper patients."

_____ 10. The first to use statistical methods to examine the effectiveness of medical interventions.

_____ 11. Proposed a theory of quality health care and the process of evaluating it.

_____ 12. Identified important health policy questions related to nursing that should be examined using large databases.

_____ 13. Identified the characteristics of interdisciplinary teams.

PUZZLES

Word Scramble
Directions: Unscramble the following sentence by rearranging the letters to form actual words. Note: You will use all the letters in every word.

Het tomrnenum rollpengip scemouto sharcere si mongic morf ployci karnrse, rinsures,

dan eht plibuc.

Secret Message
Directions: Translate the following secret message by substituting one letter for another. For example, if you decide that "c" should really be "x," then "c" will be "x" every time it appears in this puzzle. Hint: Try to translate short words first to establish vowel patterns.

Csy wcpxcynzyw kwyr zo jkcmjiy pywyxpms xpy, cj wniy ydcyoy, x rybxpcqpy gpji csy

xmmybcyr wmzyoczgzm iycsjr.

Crossword Puzzle

Directions: Complete the crossword puzzle. Note: If the answer is more than one word, there are no blank spaces left between the words.

Across

1. A norm on which quality of care is judged.
4. _____ analysis—technique used to determine alternate ways of using resources to produce the greatest net benefit.
6. Someone who has already gained access to care.
8. Someone who may or may not have gained access to care.
11. A group of people identified at a point of time as being at risk for or experiencing a health condition.
16. Very early statistical procedures developed by Louis.
20. _____ (economic)—the least costly method of achieving a desired end with the maximum benefit to be obtained from available resources.
21. _____ analysis—used to track individual and group variance from a specific critical pathway.
22. Single person or patient.
23. Defines acceptable research methodologies for a particular research focus.

Down

2. Those expenses incurred by the patient or family that are not reimbursable by the insurance company.
3. Difference between what exists in reality and what is measured.
5. Elements of organization and administration that guide the processes of care.
7. _____ analysis—Used to examine variations in patterns of care by geographic area
9. Proximate outcomes.
10. Individual practitioners, who might be of the same profession or different professions, working concurrently, as individuals or as a team.
12. Lost prospects that the patient, family member, or others experience as a consequence of illness.
13. The difference between a sample statistic used to estimate a population parameter and the actual but unknown value.
14. A patient, a person, a caseload, a community.
15. The physical-physiological function of the individual patient being cared for by the individual practitioner.
17. _____ analysis—studies how environmental factors, individual attributes, and behavior interact to influence health.
18. A caseload, target population, or community.
19. _____ analysis—examination of patterns of use by geographical area.

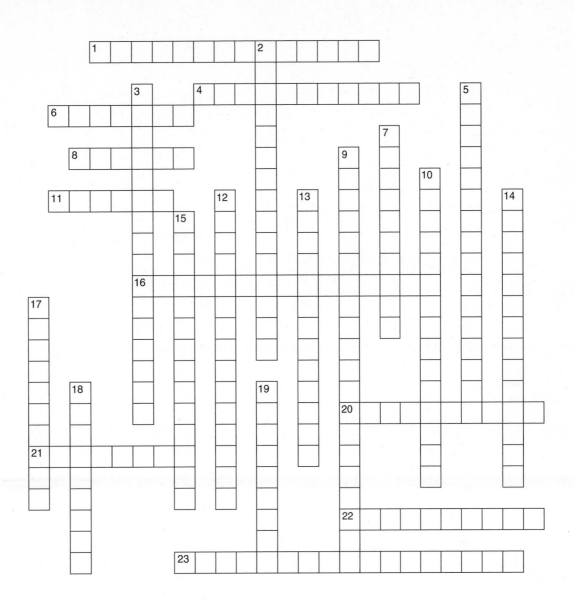

GOING BEYOND

Identify three nursing outcome studies published in the last year. Identify the design, sampling process, measurement methods, and treatments (if applicable) in these studies. Discuss how these outcome studies contribute to the empirical knowledge needed for providing evidence-based nursing practice.

13 Intervention Research

INTRODUCTION

Read Chapter 13, and then complete the following exercises. These exercises will help you to understand and critically appraise intervention studies. The answers to these exercises are in Appendix A.

RELEVANT TERMS

Intervention Studies (A)

Directions: Match each term with its correct definition.

Terms

a. Adaptation of intervention
b. Advanced testing
c. Analogue testing
d. Causal connection

e. Causal explanation
f. Complex intervention
g. Confounding variable
h. Constructive strategy

i. Creating a demand
j. Critical pathway
k. Descriptive theory
l. Disadvantaged group

Definitions

_____ 1. Theory-based scientific evidence to explain why the intervention causes changes in outcomes, how it does so, or both.

_____ 2. Some intervention prototypes are tested before pilot testing using actors to play roles in the intervention.

_____ 3. A variable that is recognized before the study is initiated but that cannot be controlled or a variable not recognized until the study is in process.

_____ 4. Interventions that have multiple elements that may act independently, interactively, or have additive effects.

_____ 5. Involves marketing the intervention to persuade potential purchasers that they will actually benefit from the intervention.

_____ 6. Describes the causal processes occurring.

_____ 7. Involves changing the intervention to fit local conditions and is sometimes referred to as reinvention.

_____ 8. Strategy used to test the effectiveness of complex interventions in which theoretical rationale is used to select interventions one at a time to add to the base intervention.

_____ 9. Recommended as stakeholders in interventions that would or should affect members of that group.

_____ 10. Clinical pathways that define expected or standard care activities and expected outcomes. These pathways are based on an extensive review of the literature focused on findings from previous studies.

_____ 11. The focus of a study is to provide evidence that the intervention causes the outcome.

_____ 12. Occurs after sufficient evidence is available to determine that the intervention is effective in achieving the desired outcomes.

Intervention Studies (B)

Terms

a. Dismantling strategy (substruction design)
b. Duration of intervention
c. Extraneous factors
d. Factorial ANOVA designs
e. Field test
f. Fractional factorial design
g. Integrity of intervention
h. Intermediate outcomes
i. Intervener
j. Interventions
k. Intervention complexity
l. Intervention doses

Definitions

_____ 1. Sometimes referred to as confounding variables, these elements of the environment or characteristics of the patient significantly affect the problem, the treatment process, or the outcomes; tend not to be well understood and often are unidentifiable before initiation of a study.

_____ 2. Simplification of the factorial design where the researcher systematically selects a portion of all possible intervention component combinations to implement. Such a design requires the researcher to be willing to assume that the effects of higher-order interactions (multiple combination effects) are negligible.

_____ 3. The full version of the program is compared with a reduced version in which one or more components have been removed.

_____ 4. The intensity of the intervention, the length of time of a single treatment, frequency of an intervention, or the span of time over which the intervention is continued or repeatedly given.

_____ 5. The extent to which the intervention is implemented as it was designed.

_____ 6. Outcomes that can be measured in a reasonable period of time when the end outcomes will not occur for some time. It is assumed these outcomes represent the end outcomes.

_____ 7. Determined by the type and number of activities to be performed for the intervention.

_____ 8. Commonly used in psychology, these designs are potentially the most powerful way to examine all possible combinations of an intervention.

_____ 9. Treatments, therapies, procedures, or actions implemented by health care professional to and with patients, in a particular situation, to move the patients' conditions toward desired health outcomes that are beneficial to them.

_____ 10. Conducted in clinical settings in which the intervention will typically be implemented; evaluates the effectiveness of the intervention when implemented in uncontrolled situations.

_____ 11. Individuals who are involved in the delivery of the study intervention. They are usually health care professionals functioning in the role of clinicians or researchers.

_____ 12. The total length of time the intervention is to be implemented (e.g., the number of days the intervention was implemented).

Intervention Studies (C)

Terms

a. Intervention effectiveness
b. Intervention research
c. Intervention strength
d. Intervention taxonomy
e. Intervention theory
f. Key informant
g. Lack of intervention integrity
h. Logical positivism
i. Mediating process
j. Mediator variables
k. Modeling the intervention
l. Moderator variable
m. Natural leader
n. Nursing interventions
o. Observation system
p. Participatory research
q. Pilot test
r. Potential market
s. Preference clinical trial

Definitions

_____ 1. Amount, frequency, and duration of the intervention.

_____ 2. A discrepancy between what was planned and what was actually delivered.

_____ 3. Involves showing experts, celebrities, or others who are easily identifiable by the market segment using the intervention and benefiting from its use.

_____ 4. One of the typical key informants who is a leader in a stakeholder group.

_____ 5. In complex studies, this research program is carried out to determine whether all or just some of the elements of an intervention are causing the outcome.

_____ 6. Alters the causal relationship between the intervention and the outcomes; occurs simultaneously with the intervention effect.

_____ 7. A strategy that includes representatives from all groups that will be affected by the change (stakeholders) as collaborators.

_____ 8. This theory includes a careful description of the problem to be addressed by the intervention, the intervening actions that must be implemented to address the problem, moderating variables, and expected outcomes.

_____ 9. An individual who can furnish information useful for determining and addressing the concerns or needs of stakeholder groups as the intervention project is being planned.

_____ 10. The series of changes that occur in participants and mediator variables after the initiation of the intervention; explains exactly how the intervention causes the outcome.

_____ 11. A test conducted before the initiation of the study to determine the behavior of the interventionist in relation to the administration of the intervention.

_____ 12. An organized categorization of all interventions performed by nurses.

_____ 13. Developed for use throughout the design and development process. This system allows the researchers to observe events related to the intervention naturalistically and to analyze these observations.

_____ 14. Identified by analyzing which people might benefit from the intervention, whether the goal is broad-based or restricted adoption, and which market segments are most likely to adopt the intervention.

_____ 15. A branch of philosophy that operates on strict rules of logic, truth, laws, axioms, and predictions and from which quantitative research emerged.

_____ 16. Rather than being randomized to subject groups, patients choose among all treatments available; patient preference is considered an important variable.

_____ 17. New methodology for investigating the effectiveness of a nursing intervention in achieving the desired outcome or outcomes in a natural setting.

_____ 18. "Deliberative cognitive, physical, or verbal activities performed [by nurses] with, or on behalf of, individuals and their families [that] are directed toward accomplishing particular therapeutic objectives relative to individuals' health and well-being" (Grobe, 1996, p. 50).

_____ 19. Variables that might alter the effect of the intervention.

Interventions Studies (D)

Terms

a. Prescriptive theory
b. Product sampling
c. Project team
d. Prototype
e. Reinvention

f. Response surface methodology
g. Stakeholders
h. Structural equation analysis
i. Technical support
j. Timing

k. Type II error
l. Type III error
m. Use standards
n. Validity of the cause

Definitions

_____ 1. Potential purchasers are allowed to try out portions of the product. This process might consist of demonstrations of the intervention and opportunities to review materials at regional and national professional conferences.

_____ 2. A methodology in which the dose response can be applied to more than one dimension of a treatment; used to determine which combination of components produces the optimum outcome.

_____ 3. Researchers and their staff who are the primary experts on an intervention are available to assist with adopting the intervention.

_____ 4. A primitive design that has evolved to the point that it can be tested clinically; includes establishing and selecting a mode of delivery of the intervention.

_____ 5. A type of error where there is a risk of asking the wrong question—a question that does not address the problem of concern.

_____ 6. All groups that will be affected by the change.

_____ 7. Used to examine the contribution of each component to the outcome.

_____ 8. A type of error that occurs when the researcher concludes that there is no significant difference between the samples examined when, in fact, a difference exists.

_____ 9. Involves changing the intervention to fit local conditions. Elements of the intervention may be modified or deleted, or new elements may be added.

_____ 10. Guidelines for using the intervention correctly that adopters must agree to before they receive it.

_____ 11. Specifies what must be done to achieve the desired effects, including the (1) components, intensity, and duration required; (2) human and material resources needed; and (3) procedures to be followed to produce the desired outcomes.

_____ 12. Established via the "true experiment."

_____ 13. A multidisciplinary team that facilitates distribution of the work and a broader generation of ideas.

_____ 14. The point in time after the intervention that a change is expected to occur.

KEY IDEAS

Directions: Fill in the blanks, or provide the appropriate responses.

1. Intervention research in nursing holds great promise for:

2. The _____ is being seriously questioned by a growing number of scholars because modifications in the original design have decreased its validity.

3. A nursing intervention can be defined in what four ways?

   a.

   b.

   c.

   d.

4. In medical and nursing research, the "true experiment" is commonly referred to as a _____.

5. In causal explanation, required in intervention theory research, in addition to demonstrating that the intervention causes the outcome, the researcher must provide scientific evidence to:

6. A participatory research strategy involves including representatives from _____ as collaborators.

7. An intervention theory includes a descriptive theory, which describes the causal processes, and a prescriptive theory, which specifies what must be done to achieve the desired results. The prescriptive theory includes:

   a.

   b.

   c.

8. Strength of the intervention is defined in terms of the _____, _____,

   and _____.

9. A moderator is a separate _____ variable affecting outcomes.

10. Extraneous variables, sometimes referred to as _____ _____, are elements of the environment or characteristics of the patient that significantly affect the problem, the treatment process, or the outcomes.

MAKING CONNECTIONS

Designing an Intervention

Directions: Match each term with its appropriate description.

Terms

a. Pilot testing
b. Analogue testing
c. Testing variations in effectiveness
d. Formal testing

e. Developing a prototype
f. Treatment matching
g. Field test

h. Preference clinical trial
i. Path analysis
j. Component testing

Descriptions

_____ 1. A primitive design to develop the elements of the intervention.

_____ 2. Using actors to play roles in the intervention.

_____ 3. Using small studies to determine whether the prototype will work.

_____ 4. Rigorous test of the intervention.

_____ 5. Advanced testing.

_____ 6. Analysis to examine the causal processes through which every component of the intervention has its effect.

_____ 7. Testing the effect on outcomes of active choice of subjects for the intervention on its outcomes.

_____ 8. Comparison of the relative effectiveness of various treatments.

_____ 9. Testing differential effects of aspects of complex interventions.

_____ 10. Testing an intervention in an uncontrolled clinical setting.

PUZZLES

Word Scramble

Directions: Unscramble the following sentence by rearranging the letters to form actual words. Note: You will use all the letters in every word.

Revittenspinon stum eb seddirebe roem lordaby sa lal fo het catoisn quireder ot sadreds a

cultrapira moplemb.

Secret Message

Directions: Translate the following secret message by substituting one letter for another. For example, if you decide that "g" should really be "f," then "g" will be "f" every time it appears in this puzzle. Hint: Try to translate short words first to establish vowel patterns.

Sehuh dt jruuhysan adssah jxytdtshyjn dy seh whugxuzlyjh xg ly dyshuqhysdxy.

Crossword Puzzle

Directions: Complete the crossword puzzle. Note: If the answer is more than one word, there are no blank spaces left between the words.

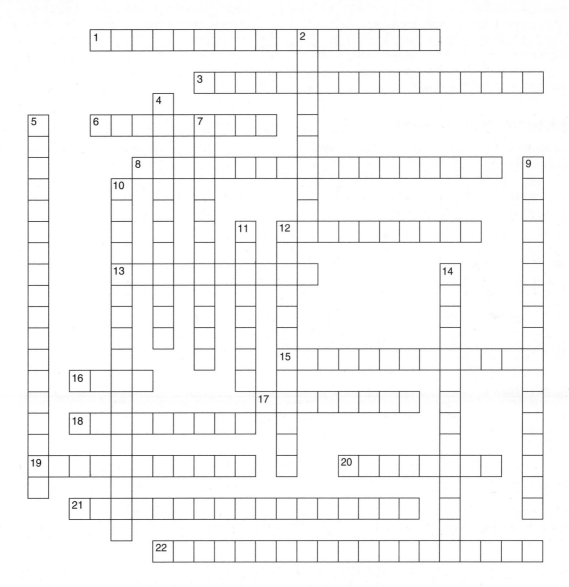

Across

1. Performed to compare the relative effectiveness of various treatments
3. Variable in intervention research that alters the causal relationship between the intervention and the outcomes.
6. Force, power, or amount of an intervention.
8. Minorities, the poor, the elderly, and so on.
12. The person providing the intervention.
13. Level of difficulty in understanding or using.
15. _____ (intervention)—extent to which treatment is successful.
16. _____ (intervention)—amount of the intervention at a specific point in time.

Down

2. Modification to meet the agency's need.
4. Important provider of information.
5. Prescribes actions to be taken by caregivers in a given situation.
7. All groups affected by the change resulting from the intervention.
9. Variables external to the phenomenon described.
10. A researcher who adheres to an atheoretical research strategy that focuses on discovering laws through the accumulation of facts.
11. Organized categorization of all interventions.
12. Deliberative activity directed toward accomplishing particular therapeutic objectives.

Chapter **13** Intervention Research

Across

17. Potency of the intervention.
18. _____ (of intervention)—intervention administered exactly as directed.
19. Changing the intervention to fit existing conditions.
20. Length of time the treatment must be provided.
21. Allows researchers to observe events related to the intervention naturalistically.
22. Occurs prior to the final result.

Down

14. Requires rigid adherence to design rules, including random sampling, equivalence of groups, complete control of the treatment, a control group that receives no treatment, control of the environment, and precise measurement of variables.

EXERCISES IN CRITICAL APPRAISAL

Directions: Review the intervention described in Sethares and Elliott's (2004) study in Appendix B, and answer the following questions.

1. Is the intervention described in sufficient detail for you to provide the intervention?

2. Is the intervention theory based?

GOING BEYOND

1. If you were to use Sethares and Elliott's (2004) intervention for a research program following intervention theory strategies, how would you plan the program of research?

2. Search the nursing literature for a nursing study using intervention theory methodology. Identify the process used to develop the intervention. Describe the method of observation used during the process. Was the intervention theory clearly presented? Was the intervention described in sufficient detail for you to provide the same intervention? Was the intervention provided consistently to all subjects? In your opinion, was the intervention sufficiently powerful to cause a difference in effect between the experimental and control groups? Write a brief paragraph judging the adequacy of the intervention.

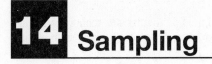 **Sampling**

INTRODUCTION

Read Chapter 14, and then complete the following exercises. These exercises will help you to understand the sampling process for critically appraising published studies and conducting research. The answers to these exercises are in Appendix A.

RELEVANT TERMS

Directions: Match each term with its correct definition.

Terms
a. Accessible population
b. Cluster sampling
c. Convenience sampling
d. Network sampling
e. Nonprobability sampling

f. Probability sampling
g. Purposive sampling
h. Quota sampling
i. Random sampling
j. Sampling

k. Sample criteria
l. Stratified random sampling
m. Systematic sampling
n. Target population
o. Theoretical sampling

Definitions

_____ 1. Process of selecting a group of people, events, behaviors, or other elements that are representative of the population being studied.

_____ 2. Portion of the target population to which the researcher has reasonable access.

_____ 3. All elements (individuals, objects, events, or substances) that meet the sample criteria for inclusion in a study.

_____ 4. Judgmental sampling that involves the conscious selection by the researcher of certain subjects or elements to include in a study.

_____ 5. Characteristics essential for membership in the target population.

_____ 6. Random sampling technique in which every member (element) of the population has a probability higher than zero of being selected for the sample; examples include simple random sampling, stratified random sampling, cluster sampling, and systematic sampling.

_____ 7. Sampling technique selecting every *k*th individual from an ordered list of all members of a population, using a randomly selected starting point.

_____ 8. Random selection of elements from the sampling frame for inclusion in a study.

_____ 9. Sampling technique used when the researcher knows some of the variables in the population that are critical to achieving representativeness; the sample is divided into strata or groups using these identified variables.

_____ 10. Sampling technique in which a frame is developed that includes a list of all states, cities, institutions, or organizations (clusters) that could be used in a study; a randomized sample is drawn from this list.

_____ 11. "Snowballing" technique that takes advantage of social networks and the fact that friends tend to hold characteristics in common; subjects meeting sample criteria are asked to assist in locating others with similar characteristics.

_____ 12. Sampling in which not every element of the population has an opportunity for selection, such as convenience sampling, quota sampling, purposive sampling, and network sampling.

_____ 13. Convenience sampling technique with an added strategy to ensure the inclusion of subjects who are likely to be underrepresented in the convenience sample, such as women, minority groups, and uneducated persons.

_____ 14. Sampling technique that involves including subjects in a study because they happen to be in the right place at the right time.

_____ 15. Sampling method often used in grounded theory research to advance the development of a theory throughout the research process. The researcher gathers data from any individual or group that can provide relevant data for theory generation.

KEY IDEAS

Directions: Fill in the blanks, or provide the appropriate responses.

1. The individual units of a population are called _____, and if these units are people, they are

   called _____.

2. The researcher desires to obtain a sample from an accessible population and generalize to a _____.

3. Representativeness means that the _____, _____

   _____, and _____ _____ are alike in as
   many ways as possible.

4. Identify two ways you might evaluate the representativeness of a sample in a published study.

   a.

   b.

5. Random variation is:

6. A list of every member of a population is referred to as a _____, _____.

7. A sampling plan outlines the:

8. In critically appraising the sampling plan in a study, several elements are examined. List at least three questions you need to ask when evaluating a sampling plan.

   a.

   b.

   c.

9. When the sampling criteria are narrowly defined or very specific, the sample desired is _____.

10. When the sampling criteria are broadly defined to include a variety of subjects, the sample desired is

    _____.

11. Subjects must be over the age of 18, able to read and write English, newly diagnosed with cancer, and have no other

    major illnesses. These are examples of _____ _____.

12. The sample was 65% female, 40% African American, 30% Hispanic, and 30% Caucasian. These are examples of

    _____ _____.

13. When subjects die or withdraw from the study, this is referred to as _____

    _____.

14. The term *control group* is limited to only those studies using _____ sampling methods.

15. If _____ sampling methods are used for sample selection, the group not receiving the treatment is referred to as a comparison group.

16. Identify four types of probability sampling.

    a.

    b.

    c.

    d.

17. If the original group of subjects is selected randomly before random assignment to treatment or control groups, it is

    considered a _____ sample.

18. Identify four types of nonprobability sampling.

    a.

    b.

    c.

    d.

19. Currently, the majority of nursing studies use _____ (*probability or nonprobability*) sampling methods.

20. Convenience sampling is also called _____ _____.

21. Purposive sampling is referred to as _____ _____.

22. The adequacy of the sample size can be evaluated using _____ _____.

23. Power is the capacity to detect _____ or _____ that actually exist in the population.

24. The minimal acceptable level of power for a study is _____.

25. If the findings of a study are nonsignificant, the researcher should examine the adequacy of the sample size by

    running a _____ _____.

26. Effect size is the extent to which the _____ _____ is false.

27. Identify five factors that influence the adequacy of a quantitative study's sample size.

    a.

    b.

    c.

    d.

    e.

28. Identify three sampling methods that are commonly used in qualitative research.

    a.

    b.

    c.

29. A qualitative study that included subjects selected based on their history of substance abuse and their judged severity

    of abuse over the previous year used _____ sampling method.

30. List three factors that need to be considered in determining the sample size of a qualitative study.

    a.

    b.

    c.

31. Identify the types of research settings used in nursing studies.

a.

b.

c.

32. A(n)_____ setting is an uncontrolled, real-life situation or environment for the conduct of a study.

33. A(n) _____ _____ setting is an artificially constructed environment for the sole purpose of doing research.

34. A(n) _____ _____ setting is an environment that is manipulated or modified in some way by the researcher but usually in a limited way.

35. The two types of sampling criteria that might be used in a study are _____ and

_____ criteria.

MAKING CONNECTIONS

Sampling Methods
Directions: Match the sampling methods listed here with the examples of sampling methods from published studies. Note: Some sampling methods will be used more than once.

Methods
a. Cluster sampling
b. Convenience sampling
c. Network sampling

d. Purposive sampling
e. Quota sampling
f. Simple random sampling

g. Stratified random sampling
h. Systematic sampling
i. Theoretical sampling

Examples

_____ 1. Five hundred nurses were randomly selected from a list of all registered nurses in the state of Texas.

_____ 2. A sample of 50 patients with diabetes was obtained from patients who came to an outpatient clinic; those 5 patients were randomly placed in the comparison and experimental groups.

_____ 3. A sample of 10 HIV-positive subjects was obtained by asking 3 subjects to identify friends with HIV w might participate in the study.

_____ 4. A sample of 1000 critical care nurses was obtained by asking 100 critical care nurse managers in 50 rando selected, large hospitals to identify 10 staff nurses to complete a survey.

_____ 5. Subjects with a history of asthma, who effectively managed their disease over the previous year, were recr to provide relevant information to develop a theory of asthma management.

_____ 6. Gender was used to stratify a sample of 100 randomly selected subjects.

_____ 7. The researcher obtained a list of all certified nurse practitioners, picked a random starting point, an n selected every 25th individual to participate in the study.

_____ 8. Fifty hypertensive subjects were recruited in a clinic to participate in a study.

_____ 9. An equal number of patients with asthma, emphysema, and chronic bronchitis were recruited from the local Better Breathers chapter to participate in a study.

_____ 10. The sample included 50 patients; 25 were examples of strong self-care, and 25 were examples of poor self-care.

_____ 11. Five thousand military personnel were randomly selected to participate in a study.

_____ 12. A sample of drug-addicted nurses was obtained by asking five subjects to identify friends who were drug addicted.

_____ 13. Twenty-five home health patients were asked to participate in a study because they had a history of pressure ulcers that would not heal.

_____ 14. Ten subjects were selected because they could provide rich, relevant data for the generation of a theory of pain management and assessment.

_____ 15. Fifty surgery patients were randomly selected from a hospital and randomly placed in control and treatment groups.

Types of Settings

Directions: Match the types of settings listed here with the examples of settings from published studies. Note: Some types of settings will be used more than once.

Settings

a. Highly controlled setting
b. Natural setting
c. Partially controlled setting

Examples

_____ 1. Research unit in a pediatric hospital

_____ 2. Home of a patient who is on continuous oxygen

_____ 3. School for severely disabled children

_____ 4. A rehabilitation center that has a structured protocol for exercise activities

_____ 5. Rat research on new drugs done in a pharmaceutical lab

PUZZLES

Crossword Puzzle

Directions: Complete the crossword puzzle. Note: If the answer is more than one word, there are no blank spaces left between the words.

Across

2. Group in a study.
5. Equal opportunity to be a subject.
6. Used to determine sample size.
7. _____ make up the population.
9. Used to select subjects.
11. Slanted from truth.
12. Portion of the target population within the range of researcher.
13. Population designated by sample criteria.
14. Possible sampling method used when studying subjects with HIV.
15. Nonprobability sampling method.

Down

1. _____ determine who is in a sample.
3. Random sampling.
4. Number of subjects in a study.
5. Sample is _____ of population.
8. People in a quantitative study.
10. All members of a refined set of elements.

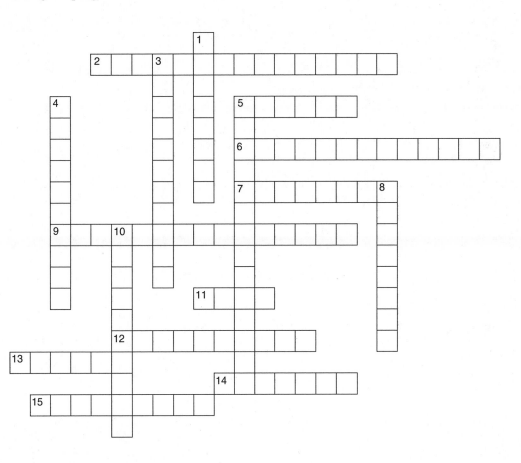

EXERCISES IN CRITICAL APPRAISAL

Bindler, Massey, Shultz, Mills, and Short Study

Directions: Review the Bindler et al. (2007) research article in Appendix B, and answer the following questions.

1. How would you identify the study population?

2. What sample criteria were used for this study?

3. How would you identify the sample characteristics for this study?

4. What is the sample size? Was a power analysis used to determine the sample size?

5. Was the sample size adequate? Provide a rationale.

6. What was the sample attrition or mortality for this study?

7. Was probability or nonprobability sampling used in this study? What specific type of sampling method was used in this study?

8. Was the sample in this study representative of the population studied? Provide a rationale.

9. Can the findings be generalized? Provide a rationale.

Sethares and Elliott Study

Directions: Review the Sethares and Elliott (2004) research article in Appendix B, and answer the following questions.

1. How would you identify the study population?

2. What sample criteria were used for this study?

3. What sample characteristics were used for this study?

4. What is the sample size? Was a power analysis used to determine the sample size?

5. Was the sample size adequate? Provide a rationale.

6. What was the sample attrition or mortality for this study?

7. Was probability or nonprobability sampling used in this study? What specific type of sampling method was used in this study?

8. Was the sample in this study representative of the target population? Provide a rationale.

9. Can the findings be generalized? Provide a rationale.

Wright Study

Directions: Review the Wright (2003) research article in Appendix B and answer the following questions.

1. How would you identify the study population?

2. What sample criteria were used for this study?

3. What sample characteristics were used for this study?

4. What is the sample size? Was a power analysis used to determine the sample size?

5. Was the sample size adequate? Provide a rationale.

6. What was the sample attrition or mortality for this study?

7. Was probability or nonprobability sampling used in this study? What specific type of sampling method was used in this study?

8. Was the sample in this study representative of the population studied? Provide a rationale.

9. Can the findings be generalized? Provide a rationale.

Study Settings

Directions: Identify the type of setting for each of the studies in Appendix B. Note: More than one type of setting may apply to each study.

Setting Types
a. Natural setting
b. Partially controlled setting
c. Highly controlled setting

Studies

_____   1. Bindler et al. (2007)

_____   2. Sethares and Elliott (2004)

_____   3. Wright (2003)

15 Measurement Concepts

INTRODUCTION

Read Chapter 15, and then complete the following exercises. These exercises will help you to learn the terms relevant to measurement and to critically appraise measurement methods in studies. The answers to these exercises are in Appendix A.

RELEVANT TERMS

Levels of Measurement
Directions: Match each term with its correct definition.

Terms
a. Absolute zero
b. Interval-level measurement
c. Levels of measurement
d. Measurement

e. Nominal-level measurement
f. Ordered metric scales
g. Ordinal-level measurement
h. Ratio-level measurement

Definitions

_____ 1. The lowest of the four measurement categories. It is used when data can be organized into categories, but the categories cannot be rank ordered.

_____ 2. The process of assigning numbers to objects, events, or situations in accord with some rule.

_____ 3. Scales with unequal intervals are sometimes referred to as this.

_____ 4. The point at which a value of zero indicates the absence of the property being measured.

_____ 5. The highest form of measurement that meets all the rules of the lower forms of measurement (mutually exclusive categories, exhaustive categories, rank ordering, equal spacing between intervals, and a continuum of values) and also has an absolute zero.

_____ 6. A level of measurement where data can be assigned to categories that can be ranked.

_____ 7. A categorization system for measurement.

_____ 8. A level of measurement in which the distances between intervals of the scale are numerically equal.

Types of Reliability and Validity for Measurement Methods
Directions: Match each type of reliability or validity with its correct definition.

Terms
a. Accuracy of physiological measure
b. Alternate forms reliability
c. Construct validity
d. Content-related validity
e. Errors in physiological measurement
f. Homogeneity
g. Precision of physiological measure

h. Interrater reliability
i. Interpretive reliability
j. Readability of an instrument
k. Reliability
l. Split-half reliability
m. Test-retest reliability
n. Validity

o. Validity from contrasting groups
p. Validity from examining convergence
q. Validity from examining divergence
r. Validity from factor analysis
s. Validity from prediction of future events
t. Validity from successive verification
u. Unitizing reliability

Definitions

_____ 1. Validity determined by comparison of an instrument's values with those of other instruments that measure the same concept.

_____ 2. Type of reliability obtained by splitting the instrument items in two halves (such as odd and even items) and performing correlational procedures between the two halves.

_____ 3. Considered comparable to validity and addresses the extent to which a physiological instrument measures the variable being studied.

_____ 4. Type of reliability that examines the consistency of measurement of two raters.

_____ 5. Instrument validity determined by identifying groups that are expected (or known) to have opposing scores on the instrument.

_____ 6. Environment, user, subject, machine, and interpretation problems that lead to inaccuracy in the measurements of physiological instruments.

_____ 7. Type of reliability that evaluates consistency of repeated measures.

_____ 8. Validity of an instrument determined by comparison of values with those of other instruments that measure opposite concepts.

_____ 9. Validity of an instrument is enhanced when the instrument values have the ability to predict future performance.

_____ 10. Degree of consistency or reproducibility of measurements made with physiological instruments.

_____ 11. Reliability of an instrument that is determined by correlation of the items within an instrument.

_____ 12. Comparison of the equivalence of two paper-and-pencil instruments and is also referred to as parallel forms reliability.

_____ 13. Type of validity that examines the extent to which an instrument includes all the major elements of the concept being measured.

_____ 14. Denotes the consistency of measures obtained in the use of a particular instrument and is an indication of the extent of random error in the measurement method.

_____ 15. In qualitative research, the extent to which each judge (data collector, coder, or researcher) consistently identifies the same units within the data as appropriate for coding.

_____ 16. In qualitative research, the extent to which each judge assigns the same category in which the overall rate of reliability is examined.

_____ 17. Validity is considered a single broad method of measurement evaluation, and this is referred to as what?

_____ 18. The extent to which an instrument actually reflects the abstract construct being examined. Thus, the instrument measures what it is supposed to measure.

_____ 19. Essential element of instrument validity and reliability that indicates the reading level of an instrument.

_____ 20. Type of validity determined by conducting analysis to examine relationships among the various items of the instrument to reveal the presence of the factors or subconcepts measured by an instrument.

_____ 21. Validity of an instrument is enhanced when other researchers use the instrument in unrelated studies.

KEY IDEAS

Directions: Fill in the blanks, or provide the appropriate responses.

1. The purpose of measurement is to produce _____ data.

2. The ideal, perfect measure is referred to as the _____ measure.

3. Measurement _____ is the difference between true measure and what, in reality, is measured.

4. Weight is an example of _____ measurement.

5. A coping scale is an example of _____ measurement.

6. A reliability value of _____ is considered the lowest acceptable coefficient for a well-developed measurement tool.

7. A reliability value of _____ is considered the lowest acceptable coefficient for a new measurement tool.

8. Describe three situations that might result in random error.

   a.

   b.

   c.

9. Describe three measurement situations that might result in systematic error.

   a.

   b.

   c.

10. The two types of testing involving referencing are:

   a.

   b.

MAKING CONNECTIONS

Error Types
Directions: Identify the type of measurement error likely to occur with each of the measurement methods.

Types
a. Random error   b. Systematic error

Methods

_____ 1. Community income was determined using a white, middle-class sample.

_____ 2. Severity of cancer at diagnosis in a community was determined using patients in a county hospital.

_____ 3. Average body weight was measured at work at noon.

_____ 4. Blood pressure was taken with an electric monitor that records pressures high.

_____ 5. Scores on drug calculation test were taken in the clinical setting anytime during the work shift.

Measurement Levels
Directions: Match the levels of measurement shown here with the specific types of measures that follow.

Levels
a. Nominal-level measurement
b. Ordinal-level measurement
c. Interval- or ratio-level measurement

Types

_____ 1. Temperature

_____ 2. Gender

_____ 3. Educational level

_____ 4. Final exam grade

_____ 5. Type of cancer

_____ 6. Severity of illness rank

_____ 7. Score from visual analogue scale

_____ 8. Level of fatigue measured as minimal, moderate, and severe

_____ 9. Systolic and diastolic blood pressures

_____ 10. Triglyceride level on lab report

Sensitivity and Specificity

Directions: Complete the other three cells in the following table.

1.

Diagnostic Test Results	Disease Present	Disease Not Present or Absent
Positive test	a (true positive)	
Negative test		

2. What is the formula for sensitivity?

3. What is the formula for specificity?

Sensitivity and Specificity of Colonoscopy Screening Tests		
Diagnostic Test Results	Disease Present	Disease Not Present or Absent
Positive test N = 200	180 (90%)	
Negative test N = 200		170 (85%)

4. What is the percentage of false positive for the colonoscopy screening test using the data in the table above?

5. What is the percentage of false negative for the colonoscopy screening test?

6. What is the sensitivity of the colonoscopy screening test?

7. What is the specificity of the colonoscopy screening test?

PUZZLES

Word Scramble

Directions: Unscramble the following sentence by rearranging the letters to form actual words. Note: You will use all the letters in every word.

Rethe si on fertpec semarue.

Secret Message

Directions: Translate the following secret message by substituting one letter for another. For example, if you decide that "y" should really be "p," then "y" will be "p" every time it appears in this puzzle. Hint: Try to translate short words first to establish vowel patterns.

Anurjkrurch cnbcrwp wnnmd cx kn ynaoxavnm xw njlq rwbcadvnwc dbnm rw j bcdmh.

Crossword Puzzle

Directions: Complete the crossword puzzle. Note: If the answer is more than one word, there are no blank spaces left between the words.

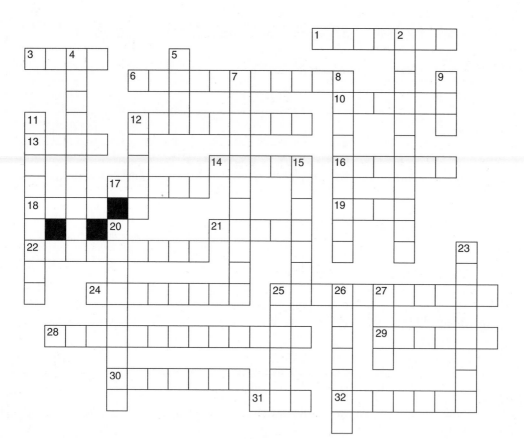

Across

1. Gather data.
3. Common method of obtaining questionnaire data.
6. Strategies used to assign numbers to a variable.
10. The crudest form of scale.
12. Concerned with the consistency of repeated measures.
13. Infrequent occurrence.
14. Highest level of measurement.

Down

2. Interrater reliability.
4. Measurement tool.
5. Information obtained through measurement.
7. Consistency of measurement.
8. Score obtained if there were no measurement error.
9. Commonly used demographic data.
11. Reproducibility of physiological measurements.
12. A measurement tool can be used to generate a _____ for each subject for a study variable.

Across

16. Self-report measures with summated scores.
17. The difference between true measure and what is measured.
18. Thought related to a creative way to measure a nursing phenomenon.
19. Unstructured.
21. Site of data collection.
22. Measurement strategy involving verbal communication between the researcher and the subject.
24. Evaluation of the adequacy of a physiological operational definition.
25. The amount of change in a physiological parameter that can be measured precisely.
28. A printed self-report form with individual items that are not summated.
29. Scale with options rated from negative to positive.
30. Level of measurement in which values must be ranked.
31. Common method of obtaining demographic data.
32. Lowest level of measurement.

Down

15. Measurement strategy used in qualitative research.
20. Approach to judging reliability of physiological measures.
23. Level of measurement with equal numerical distances.
25. Selye identified and measured the concept of _____ in his research.
26. Place in which data collection occurs.
27. Done by researchers and study participants to obtain interview data.

EXERCISES IN CRITICAL APPRAISAL

Directions: Review the Bindler, Massey, Shultz, Mills, and Short (2007) and Sethares and Elliott (2004) studies in Appendix B, and answer the following questions about measurement methods.

1. Using the following tables, identify the variables measured, the method of measurement, and the directness of measurement (D = direct, I = indirect).
   a. Bindler et al. study

Variable	Method of Measurement	Directness

b. Sethares and Elliott study

Variable	Method of Measurement	Directness

2. Bindler et al. (2007) study: Identify the precision and accuracy information for each of the physiological measures listed in question 1. Identify the reliability and validity information for each of the non-physiological measures listed in question 1. Indicate if the reliability and validity values are from previous studies or the current study.

a. Physiological measures:

Precision and Accuracy	Information Listed in Study

b. Questionnaires:

Type of Reliability or Validity	Values Previous Studies or Current Study?

3. Sethares and Elliott (2004) Study: Identify the specific types of reliability and validity for the scales listed in question 1. Indicate if the reliability and validity values are from previous studies or the current study.
   Scales:

Scale and Type of Reliability or Validity	Values & Indicate Previous Studies or Current Study?

4. Using the information gathered earlier, judge the adequacy of the measurement methods used in each study.
   a. Bindler et al. (2007) study:

   b. Sethares and Elliott (2004) study:

16 Measurement Methods Used in Developing Evidence for Practice

INTRODUCTION

Read Chapter 16, and then complete the following exercises. These exercises will help you to learn relevant terms and to identify and critically appraise measurement methods in published studies. The answers to these exercises are in Appendix A.

RELEVANT TERMS

Directions: Match each term with its correct description.

Measurement Methods

a. Delphi technique
b. Diary
c. Likert scale
d. Questionnaire

e. Physiological measures
f. Projective technique
g. Rating scale
h. Semantic differential

i. Structured interview
j. Structured observation
k. Visual analogue scale

Descriptions

_____ 1. Instruments used to measure physical characteristics of a subject, such as a laboratory test to determine hemoglobin level.

_____ 2. A printed self-report form designed to elicit information that can be obtained through subjects' written responses to closed-ended questions.

_____ 3. A recording of events over time by individuals to document experiences, feelings, or behavior patterns.

_____ 4. Specific verbal questions that the researcher will ask when collecting data. The questions are designed before data collection begins.

_____ 5. Another name for this scale is magnitude scaling technique.

_____ 6. The crudest form of scaling technique that lists an ordered series of categories of a variable that are assumed to be based on an underlying continuum.

_____ 7. Based on the assumption that the responses of individuals to unstructured or ambiguous situations reflect the attitudes, desires, personality characteristics, and motives of the individual. Most frequently used in psychology.

_____ 8. Designed to determine the opinion or attitude of a subject and contains a number of declarative statements with a scale after each statement.

_____ 9. Consists of two opposite adjectives with a 7-point scale between them.

Chapter **16** **Measurement Methods Used in Developing Evidence**

_____ 10. Used to measure the judgments of a group of experts for the purpose of making decisions, assessing priorities, or making forecasts. Provides a means of obtaining the opinions of a variety of experts nationally and internationally.

_____ 11. Observational data recorded using preestablished category systems.

KEY IDEAS

Directions: Fill in the blanks, or provide the appropriate responses.

1. Knowledge of measurement methods is important in nursing research and _____ practice.

2. For some variables, such as dizziness, _____ may be the only means of obtaining information needed for research.

3. _____ physiological measures are most valid.

4. One disadvantage of using sensors to measure physiological variables is that the presence of a transducer within the body can _____.

5. In observational measurement, as with any type of measurement, _____ is very important.

6. Structured interviews include strategies that provide increasing amounts of _____ by the researcher over the content of the interview.

7. There is a(n) _____ response rate to interviews than to questionnaires.

8. Compared with interviews, questionnaires tend to have less _____.

9. Scales are a more _____ means of measuring phenomena than are questionnaires.

10. What is the most commonly used scaling technique?

11. What type of scale has the finest discrimination of values?

12. What is the name (and common abbreviated name) of the computerized database for locating existing measurement methods?

13. What measurement method is often used to determine the research priorities for a professional organization so experts' opinions can be obtained across the nation?

14. List three main activities for selecting an existing instrument for a study?

   a.

   b.

   c.

15. As a novice researcher, we recommend that you not _____ a scale to be used in a study.

MAKING CONNECTIONS

Directions: Match each type of scale listed here with specific names of scales or characteristics of the scales.

Type of Scales
a. Likert scale
b. Rating scale
c. Semantic differential
d. Visual analogue scale

Specific Scales and Characteristics

_____ 1. Zung Depression Scale

_____ 2. Magnitude scaling technique used to measure pain, mood, or severity of clinical symptoms.

_____ 3. State and Trait Anxiety Scale

_____ 4. Developed by Osgood et al. (1957) to measure attitudes or beliefs.

_____ 5. Faces Pain Scale

_____ 6. This scale always has seven possible choices for response.

_____ 7. Response choices might include strongly disagree, disagree, uncertain, agree, and strongly agree.

_____ 8. Scale that produces ratio-level data.

_____ 9. "On a scale of 1 to 10, how would you rank your anxiety?" is an example of what type of scale?

_____ 10. Which is the more sensitive scale for measuring pain in the clinical setting: rating scale or visual analogue scale?

PUZZLES

Word Scramble

Directions: Unscramble the sentence by rearranging the letters to form actual words. Note: You will use all the letters in every word.

Ni slubiphgin eht stulers fo a slogiochipy dusty, eth steaumemen thinquece desen ot eb

brisedced ni bonedricales laited.

Secret Message

Directions: Translate the secret message by substituting one letter for another. For example, if you decide that "b" should really be "d," then "b" will be "d" every time it appears in this puzzle. Hint: Try to translate short words first to establish vowel patterns.

Ksgqilfhzkcfa nfhqwkizqg gxkjvu sq bjhjfaap qntajgzlq

EXERCISES IN CRITICAL APPRAISAL

Directions: Review the Bindler, Massey, Shultz, Mills, and Short (2007) and the Sethares and Elliott (2004) research articles in Appendix B. Critically appraise the quality of the measurement methods listed here for the Bindler et al. (2007) and Sethares and Elliott (2004) studies. In making this judgment, look for the following information about the measurement method: (a) developer of the method of measurement, (b) date measurement method was developed, (c) detailed description of method of measurement (e.g., number of items in scale or steps of performing a physiological measure), and (d) range of values possible using the measure.

1. Bindler et al. study:

   a. Physiological measure: Blood sample of fasting insulin—Critical appraisal:

   b. Physiological measure: Blood pressure—Critical appraisal:

c. Youth/Adolescent Question (YAQ) used to measure dietary variables—Critical appraisal:

d. Smoking History Questionnaire—Critical appraisal:

2. Sethares and Elliott study:

a. Heart failure readmission rates—Critical appraisal:

b. Ways of Coping Quality of Life Scale—Critical appraisal:

c. Benefits and Barriers Scale—Critical appraisal:

Chapter **16**   **Measurement Methods Used in Developing Evidence**

17 Collecting and Managing Data

INTRODUCTION

Read Chapter 17, and then complete the following exercises. These exercises will help you to learn relevant terms and to identify and critique measurement and data collection procedures in published studies. The answers to these exercises are in Appendix A.

RELEVANT TERMS

Directions: Match each term with its correct definition.

Terms

a. Code book
b. Coding
c. Computerized data collection
d. Data collection
e. Data collection form

f. Data collection plan
g. Data collection problems
h. Personal digital assistant (PDA)
i. Serendipity
j. Support systems

Definitions

_____ 1. Detailed plan of how the study will be implemented that is specific to the study being conducted and requires consideration of the commonplace elements of research.

_____ 2. Small hand-held computer that allows the researcher to enter data directly into the computer during the data collection process.

_____ 3. The actual process of selecting subjects and gathering data from these subjects.

_____ 4. Form that is developed or modified by the researcher, which is used for recording data.

_____ 5. Identifies and defines each variable in your study and includes an abbreviated variable name (often limited to six to eight characters), a descriptive variable label, and a range of possible numerical values of every variable entered in a computer file. Also often identifies the source of each datum, which provides a link to the data collection forms.

_____ 6. Process of transforming data into numerical symbols that can be entered easily into the computer. For example, gender has two categories, and male might be identified by a 1 and female by a 2.

_____ 7. Concerns or issues that develop as data are collected and might include concerns with people, researchers, institutions, and events.

_____ 8. The accidental discover of something useful or valuable during the conduct of a study.

_____ 9. Individuals and groups who can provide assistance, consultation, and clarification during the data collection process.

_____ 10. Use of the microcomputer to collect large amounts of data with few errors that can be readily analyzed with a variety of statistical software packages.

KEY IDEAS

Directions: Provide the appropriate responses.

1. List three decision points during the data collection phase of a study that involve the subjects.

   a.

   b.

   c.

2. Describe three situations that might affect consistency in data collection.

   a.

   b.

   c.

3. List four direct costs related to data collection and management.

   a.

   b.

   c.

   d.

4. List three indirect costs related to data collection and management.

   a.

   b.

   c.

5. List five tasks of the researcher during data collection.

   a.

   b.

   c.

d.

e.

MAKING CONNECTIONS

1. Identify three problems with the following planned method of coding data of ages classified into these categories:

   (1) Under 18

   (2) 19–45

   (3) 45–65

   (4) Over 65

   a.

   b.

   c.

2. Identify the problems with the plan for coding data in each of the following questions:

   a. From the following list, identify those members of your family who had the flu last year: mother, father, sister, brother, husband, wife, child (coding plan: 1-mother, 2-father, 3-sister, 4-brother, 5-husband, 6-wife, 7-child).

      Problems:

   b. List the name and dosage of drugs administered for nausea and vomiting following surgery (coding plan: ondansetron-1, promethazine-2, droperidol-3).

      Problems:

   c. List length of hospital stay for each family member (plan to code by number of days).

      Problems:

   d. Did you vote last year? _____ Yes _____ No _____ Uncertain

      Problems:

Chapter **17**   **Collecting and Managing Data**

Word Scramble

Directions: Unscramble the sentence by rearranging the letters to form actual words. Note: You will use all the letters in every word.

Plembors nac eb creipeved rethie sa a trustifanor ro sa a leachleng.

Secret Message

Directions: Translate the secret message by substituting one letter for another. For example, if you decide that "m" should really be "t," then "m" will be "t" every time it appears in this puzzle. Hint: Try to translate short words first to establish vowel patterns.

RI bycmpryn fby nw gqwyn, rm grxx, byh bm mpj gwqom uwqqrdxj mrzj.

Crossword Puzzle

Directions: Complete the crossword puzzle. Note: If the answer is more than one word, there are no blank spaces left between the words.

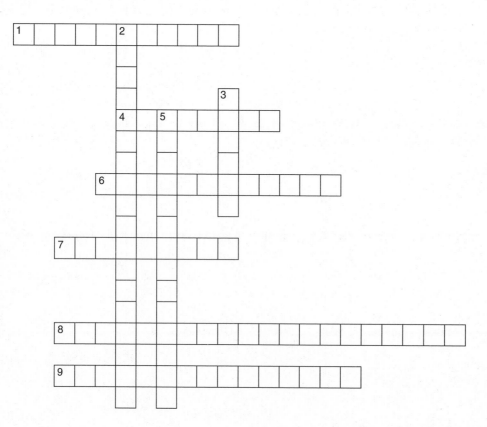

Across

1. The accidental discovery of something valuable or useful during the conduct of a study.
4. Identifies and defines each variable in a study and its range for possible numerical values.
6. Checking raw data to determine errors in data recording, coding, or entry and correcting them.
7. Subjects dropping out of a study before completion.
8. An electronic structured compilation of information that can be scanned, retrieved, or analyzed by computer.
9. A paper form designed to record or code data for rapid entry into a computer.

Down

2. Detailed plan for gathering data in a study.
3. Process of transforming qualitative data into numerical symbols.
5. Precise, systematic gathering of information relevant to research.

EXERCISES IN CRITICAL APPRAISAL

Directions: Review the Bindler, Massey, Shultz, Mills, and Short (2007) and Sethares and Elliott (2004) studies in Appendix B, and answer the following questions.

1. Describe the data collection process for the Bindler et al. (2007) study.

2. What inconsistencies, if any, do you see in the measurement methods? Can you identify any threats to the validity or accuracy of the measures?

3. Describe the data collection process for the Sethares and Elliott (2004) study.

4. What inconsistencies, if any, do you see in the measurement methods? Can you identify any threats to the validity of the measures?

Develop a coding sheet for the data from one of the quantitative studies in Appendix B.

18 Introduction to Statistical Analysis

INTRODUCTION

Read Chapter 18, and then complete the following exercises. These exercises will help you to learn relevant terms and to identify and critically appraise the results sections of published studies. The answers to these exercises are in Appendix A.

RELEVANT TERMS

Theories, Concepts, Statistics, Parameters, and Practical Aspects of Data Analysis
Directions: Match each term with its correct definition.

Terms

a. Calculated variable
b. Decision theory
c. Estimator
d. Exploratory analysis
e. Generalize

f. Infer
g. Inference
h. Parameter
i. Point estimate
j. Post hoc analysis

k. Probability theory
l. Relationship
m. Sampling error
n. Statistic
o. Transform

Definitions

_____ 1. The process whereby specific study results are used to provide an understanding about a general population.

_____ 2. A single figure that is used to estimate a related figure in the population of interest.

_____ 3. A theory that is inductive in nature and based on assumptions associated with the theoretical normal curve; applied when testing for differences between groups.

_____ 4. A statistical test developed specifically to determine the location of differences in studies with more than two groups.

_____ 5. Use of inductive reasoning to move from a specific case to a general truth.

_____ 6. Extend the implications of the findings from the sample that was studied to the larger population or from the situation studied to a larger situation.

_____ 7. A theory that addresses relative rather than absolute causality; a cause will not produce a specific effect each time that particular cause occurs.

_____ 8. Examining all the data descriptively, with the intent of becoming as familiar as possible with the nature of the data.

_____ 9. Two variables have this quality when they occur together in a sample under defined circumstances; the researcher understands that the variables relate to each other in some way.

_____ 10. A variable that is not collected but rather obtained from other variables.

_____ 11. A numerical value obtained from a sample that is used to estimate the parameters of a population.

_____ 12. A statistic that produces a value as a function of the scores in a sample.

_____ 13. The difference between a sample statistic used to estimate a population parameter and the actual but unknown value of the parameter.

_____ 14. A measure or numerical value of a population.

_____ 15. To alter data so that statistical procedures can be used on it or so that it more truly reflects the choices of the subjects.

Distribution of Scores and Shape of Curve

Directions: Match each term with its correct definition.

Terms

a. Alpha	g. Mesokurtic	m. Skewness
b. Bimodal	h. Modality	n. Symmetry
c. Central limit theorem	i. Nonparametric statistics	o. Tails
d. Distribution	j. Normal curve	p. Type I error
e. Kurtosis	k. Parametric statistic	q. Type II error
f. Leptokurtic	l. Platykurtic	r. Unimodal

Definitions

_____ 1. States that even when statistics, such as means, come from a population with a skewed (asymmetrical) distribution, the sampling distribution developed from multiple means obtained from the skewed population will tend to fit the pattern of the normal curve.

_____ 2. Term that indicates a relatively flat curve with the scores having large variance among them.

_____ 3. Occurs when the researcher concludes that the samples tested are from different populations (the difference between groups is significant) when, in fact, the samples are from the same population. The null hypothesis is rejected when it is true.

_____ 4. Symmetrical, unimodal bell-shaped curve that is a theoretical distribution of all possible scores, but no real distribution exactly fits this curve.

_____ 5. Term used to describe an extremely peaked-shape distribution of a curve, which means that the scores in the distribution are similar and have limited variance.

_____ 6. Spread of scores in a study or database.

_____ 7. Property describing a curve that is asymmetrical (positively or negatively) because of an asymmetrical distribution of scores from a study.

_____ 8. Level of significance or cutoff point used to determine whether the samples being tested are members of the same population (nonsignificant) or different populations (significant); commonly set at 0.05 or 0.01, 0.001.

_____ 9. The characteristic of a curve describing whether it has one, two, or multiple peaks.

_____ 10. Term that describes a normal curve with an intermediate degree of kurtosis and intermediate variance of scores.

_____ 11. The most common statistic used when findings are inferred to the parameters of a normally distributed population.

_____ 12. Occurs when the researcher concludes that there is no significant difference between the samples examined when, in fact, a difference exists. The null hypothesis is regarded as true when it is false.

_____ 13. Statistical techniques used when the assumptions of parametric statistics are not met and most commonly used to analyze nominal- and ordinal-level data.

_____ 14. Extremes of the normal curve where significant statistical values can be found.

_____ 15. The degree of peakedness of the curve shape that is related to the spread or variance of scores.

_____ 16. A distribution curve that has two modes or high points; usually indicates an inadequately defined population.

_____ 17. The quality of a curve in which the left side of the curve is a mirror image of the right side; the mean, median, and mode are equal and are the dividing point between the left and right sides of the curve.

_____ 18. A distribution curve that has one peak or mode.

Significance and Confirmations

Directions: Match each term with its correct definition.

Terms

a. Clinical significance
b. Confidence interval
c. Confirmatory analyses
d. Interval estimate

e. Level of statistical significance
f. One-tailed test
g. Power
h. Power analysis

i. Standardized score
j. Two-tailed test
k. Z score

Definitions

_____ 1. Cut-off point used to determine whether the samples being tested are members of the same population (non-significant) or different populations (significant).

_____ 2. Type of analysis used for a nondirectional hypothesis in which the researcher assumes that an extreme score can occur in either tail.

_____ 3. Used to express deviations from the mean (difference scores) in terms of standard deviation units, such as Z scores, where the mean is 0 and the standard deviation is 1.

_____ 4. Established in relation to the difference made in a patient situation and not always the same as statistical significance.

_____ 5. Analyses performed to confirm expectations expressed in hypotheses or to address research questions, or objectives stated in a study.

_____ 6. Analysis that identifies a range of values on a number line where the population parameter is thought to be.

_____ 7. Analysis used with directional hypotheses in which extreme statistical values of interest are thought to occur in a single tail of the curve.

_____ 8. Range in which the value of the population parameter is estimated to be.

_____ 9. Standardized scores developed from the normal curve.

_____ 10. Probability that a statistical test will detect a significant difference or relationship that exists, which is the capacity to correctly reject a null hypotheses.

_____ 11. Analysis that is conducted to determine the likelihood that previously conducted statistical analyses are accurately predicting an event, effectiveness of an intervention, or the extent of a relationship.

KEY IDEAS

Directions: Provide the appropriate responses.

1. List five purposes for the use of statistics.

    a.

    b.

    c.

    d.

    e.

2. List the six steps of the process of data analysis.

    a.

    b.

    c.

    d.

    e.

    f.

3. List four activities of data cleaning.

    a.

    b.

    c.

    d.

Categories

Directions: Match the categories listed here with the statements that follow. Note: You will use some categories more than once.

Categories

a. Decision theory statement
b. Probability theory statement

c. Inference

Statements

_____ 1. "Another interesting observation is that participants who were assigned to the treatment group experienced significantly higher levels of thermal comfort and Thermal Comfort Inventory scores even before the warming unit was activated. This finding suggests that the patient-controlled warming gown itself produces significantly greater levels of thermal comfort and greater preoperative satisfaction" (Wagner, Byrne, & Kolcaba, 2006, p. 444).

_____ 2. "The findings indicated that, among these sheltered battered women, spirituality may be associated with greater internal resources that buffer distressing feelings and calm the mind. This study shows support of spirituality as a means of reducing distress through greater connection to oneself and higher powers" (Humphreys, 2000, p. 273).

_____ 3. "This finding suggests that there is a benefit to using new technology and devices that provide a patient with more control over [his/her] thermal comfort to both decrease anxiety and potentially increase overall patient satisfaction" (Wagner, Byrne, & Kolcaba, 2006, p. 446).

_____ 4. "The difference in mean scores between the treatment groups for perception of the birth experience did not reach the required 0.05 level of significance, $F(1,104) = 3.76$, $p = .055$" (Fawcett, Pollio, Tully, Baron, Henlkein, & Jones, 1993, p. 52).

_____ 5. "The hypotheses were based on the Roy Adaptation Model proposition that management of contextual stimuli promotes adaptation. The study findings provide no support for this proposition, and, therefore, raise a question regarding the credibility of the model" (Fawcett, Pollio, Tully, Baron, Henlkein, & Jones, 1993, p. 52).

_____ 6. "Gastric and intestinal placement of feeding tubes can be differentiated by testing the pH of aspirates from the tubes with a pH-meter (p. 326). ... Discriminant function analysis provided further support for this hypothesis. ... There were 85.2% correct classifications overall, with 80.2% of the 405 gastric aspirates correctly classified and 90.5% of the 389 intestinal aspirates correctly classified (p. 327)" (Metheny, Reed, Wiersema, McSweeney, Wehrle, & Clark, 1993, p. 324).

_____ 7. "Using the protocol described in this study, the pH testing method can predict feeding tube position in the gastrointestinal tract with a relatively high degree of accuracy" (Metheny, Reed, Wiersema, McSweeney, Wehrle, & Clark, 1993, p. 329).

Significance

Directions: For each of the following statistical reports, indicate whether the results were significant or not significant, assuming a level of significance set at 0.05.

Significance

a. Significant
b. Not significant

Chapter **18** **Introduction to Statistical Analysis**

Statistical Reports

_____ 1. "The study investigated whether central nervous system functioning (NACS) has an effect on the normal, term infant's ability to breastfeed in the first day following birth. ... When regression analysis was performed on the individual breastfeeding behaviors and the NACS, $p = .05$ was achieved with breastfeeding behaviors areolar grasp, letdown, and sucking at the initial data collection session" (Radzyminiski, 2005, pp. 335 and 338).

_____ 2. "The study examined the relationship of less restrictive interventions (LRI) with seclusion/restraint usage (S/R) in psychiatric patients, average years of psychiatric experience of nursing staff, and staff mix. The mean years of psychiatric experience was 4.89 ($SD = 1.68$) and the mean number of LRI used was 11.28 ($SD = 5.47$). ... Using Pearson r, the relationship between average year of psychiatric experience and LRI was $r = 0.146$, $p = 0.96$, one-tailed" (Williams & Myers, 2001, pp. 139 and 142).

_____ 3. "The study examined the efficacy of an osteoporosis prevention education program for young adults by measuring osteoporosis knowledge (OKT) in the areas of risk factors, exercise, and calcium. ... Independent t-tests were used to determine statistically significant differences between the experimental and the control group in OKT risk factor (mean = 4.6, SD = 2.6, $p < 0.001$), OKT exercise (mean = 3.3, SD = 1.2, $p < 0.001$), and OKT calcium (mean = 3.0, SD = 1.6, $p < 0.001$)" (Chan, Kwong, Zang, & Wan, 2007, pp. 270, 276–277)

PUZZLES

Word Scramble

Directions: Unscramble the sentence by rearranging the letters to form actual words. Note: You will use all the letters in every word.

Ot eb fuelus, het decineve morf taad yalinass stum eb lulefarcy maxidene, groznadie, dan

venig grnneam.

Secret Message

Directions: Translate the secret message by substituting one letter for another. For example, if you decide that "s" should really be "v," then "s" will be "v" every time it appears in this puzzle. Hint: Try to translate short words first to establish vowel patterns.

Viwievglivw ger riziv tvszi xlmrkw.

Crossword Puzzle

Directions: Complete the crossword puzzle on the next page. Note: If the answer is more than one word, there are no blank spaces left between the words.

Across

2. A finding sufficiently important to change practice.
4. Cut-off point used to determine whether or not samples are part of the same population.
6. A relatively flat curve with values having large variance among them.
8. Used to determine the risk of a type II error.
10. A symmetrical, unimodal bell-shaped figure that is a theoretical distribution of all possible scores.
13. Extremes of the normal curve.
15. A curve that is asymmetric.
16. Extend the implications of the findings from the sample to a larger population.
18. Change from one way of expressing to another.
19. An extremely peaked-shaped distribution of a curve.
20. Spread of values in a data set.
22. The difference between a sample statistic and a population parameter.
23. Statistical tests designed to determine the location of differences in studies with more than two groups.
24. Evenness or balance in a relationship.

Down

1. An association of some kind that exists between or among two or more concepts or variables.
3. Use inductive reasoning to move from a specific case to a general statement.
5. Theory that addresses relative rather than absolute causality.
7. The degree of peakedness of a curve reflecting the spread of scores.
9. The independence of a score's value to vary, given other existing score values and their sum.
11. A normal curve.
12. A calculated numerical value of a sample used to estimate a parameter.
14. A measure or numerical value of a population.
17. Descriptive analyses performed to become familiar with the data.
21. A distribution with two modes.

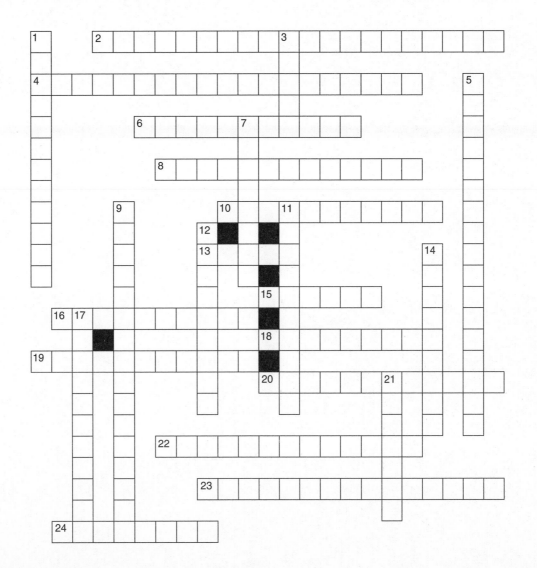

19 Using Statistics to Describe Variables

INTRODUCTION

Read Chapter 19, and then complete the following exercises. These exercises will help you to learn relevant terms, critically appraise the descriptive statistics in the results sections of published studies, and use these analysis techniques to analyze data. The answers to these exercises are in Appendix A.

RELEVANT TERMS

Statistics That Summarize Data

Directions: Match each term with its correct definition.

Terms

a. Average
b. Bimodal
c. Descriptive statistics
d. Frequency distribution
e. Grouped frequency distribution

f. Mean
g. Measures of central tendency
h. Median
i. Mode
j. Outliers

k. Percentage distribution
l. Ungrouped frequency distribution
m. Unimodal

Definitions

_____ 1. The value obtained by summing all the scores and dividing that total by the number of scores being summed.

_____ 2. Summary statistics that allow the researcher to organize the data in ways that give meaning and facilitate insight, such as frequency distributions and measures of central tendency and dispersion.

_____ 3. The extreme scores or values in a set of data that are exceptions to the overall findings.

_____ 4. The score at the exact center of the ungrouped frequency distribution.

_____ 5. A lay term used for a measure of central tendency and not commonly used in statistics because of its vagueness.

_____ 6. A data set that has one mode.

_____ 7. Statistical procedures (mode, median, and mean) for determining the center of a distribution of scores.

_____ 8. A frequency distribution in which all categories of a variable on which you have data are listed and each datum is tallied on the listing.

_____ 9. A statistical procedure that involves tallying each datum and presenting it in a listing.

_____ 10. The percentage of the sample with scores falling in a specific group, as well as the number of scores in that group.

_____ 11. A frequency distribution of continuous variables that are placed in groups based on a classification scheme devised by the researcher.

_____ 12. The numerical value or score that occurs with the greatest frequency in a distribution; however, it does not necessarily indicate the center of the data set.

_____ 13. A data set that has two modes.

Statistics That Explore Deviations and Patterns in Data

Directions: Match each term with its correct definition.

Terms

a. Deviation score
b. Difference score
c. Heterogeneity
d. Homogeneity
e. Least-squares principle

f. Measures of dispersion
g. Modal percentage
h. Pattern
i. Range
j. Standard deviation

k. Sum of squares
l. Summary statistics
m. Survival analysis
n. Time series analysis
o. Variance

Definitions

_____ 1. The quality sought by researchers in attempting to obtain subjects with a wide variety of characteristics to reduce the risk of bias in studies not using random sampling.

_____ 2. A measure of dispersion that is calculated by taking the square root of the variance.

_____ 3. Statistical procedures (range, difference scores, sum of squares, variance, and standard deviation) for examining how scores vary around the mean.

_____ 4. Commonalities or repetition in events as they unfold across time.

_____ 5. The degree to which objects are similar or a form of equivalence.

_____ 6. A technique designed to analyze changes in a variable across time and thus to uncover a pattern in the data.

_____ 7. Appropriate for nominal data and indicates the relationship of the number of data scores represented by the mode to the total number of data scores.

_____ 8. A set of techniques designed to analyze repeated measures from a given time (e.g., the beginning of the study, the onset of a disease) until a certain event (e.g., death, treatment failure) occurs.

_____ 9. Another name for difference score; indicates that extent to which a score deviates from the mean.

_____ 10. Mathematical manipulation involving summing the squares of the difference scores that is used as part of the analysis process for calculating the standard deviation.

_____ 11. A measure of dispersion that is the mean or average of the sum of squares.

_____ 12. The fact that when deviations from the mean are squared, the sum is smaller than the sum of squared deviations from any other value in a sampling distribution.

_____ 13. Descriptive statistics that allow the researcher to organize the data in ways that give meaning and facilitate insight.

_____ 14. The simplest measure of dispersion, obtained by subtracting the lowest score from the highest score.

_____ 15. Deviation score obtained by subtracting the mean from each raw score.

KEY IDEAS

Directions: Fill in the blanks, or provide the appropriate responses.

1. Descriptive statistics may be the only approach to analysis of data in _____ studies.

2. The first strategy used to organize the data for examination is usually creating _____

   _____.

3. Most studies have some categorical data that are presented in the form of _____

   _____ _____.

4. Any method of grouping results in:

5. _____ _____ are particularly useful in comparing the present data with findings from other studies that have varying sample sizes.

6. _____ _____ _____ give some indication of how scores in a sample are dispersed around the mean.

7. A common strategy used to allow meaningful mathematical manipulation of difference in scores is called

   _____.

8. The square root of the variance is called the _____ _____.

9. _____ _____ are a way of comparing a score in one distribution with a score in another distribution.

10. _____ _____ are usually expressed as (38.6,41.4), with 38.6 being the lower end of the interval and 41.4 being the upper end of the interval.

11. _____ _____ _____ is designed to detect the unexpected in the data and to avoid overlooking crucial patterns that may exist.

12. A _____ _____ offers a common way to illustrate graphically the relationship of two variables.

13. List three statistical strategies used to describe the sample.

a.

b.

c.

MAKING CONNECTIONS

Significant Differences

Directions: Perform the following exercises.

In testing for significant differences between groups, the researcher is determining whether the experimental group belongs to the same population as the control group. An initial step in this process is to compare the mean and standard deviation of the control group with those of the experimental group. The normal curve can be used to visually depict differences in these measures between the two groups. For example, Chan, Kwong, Zang, and Wan (2007) examined the effects of an osteoporosis education program on a sample of young adults by comparing knowledge gained, change in health belief, and self-efficacy between the experimental and the control group. For the variable of knowledge of risk factors, the control group mean (*M*) was 3.7 with a standard deviation (SD) of 2.4. Using this information, the distribution of knowledge of risk factors in the control group can be illustrated.

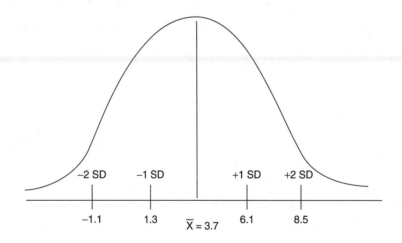

1. The mean of knowledge of risk factors for the treatment group was 10.3, with a standard deviation of 1.0. Using the following curve, illustrate the distribution of values as shown.

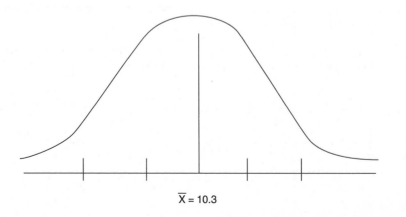

These means look very different with the control group $M = 3.7$ and the experimental group $M = 10.3$. However, statistical analysis is required to determine whether the difference in knowledge of risk factors between the two groups represents two different populations. In this study, an analysis of variance (ANOVA) was conducted to determine differences between the experimental and control groups, and the results were significant at the $p = <0.001$, indicating that the groups were significantly different or from two different populations.

PUZZLES

Word Scramble
Directions: Unscramble the sentence by rearranging the letters to form actual words. Note: You will use all the letters in every word.

Gusni emasreus fo laertnc tencedny ot cebirsed het uatern fo eht aatd soebrsuc eht

ticmpa fo emxetre vsluae ro fo veditanois ni het taad.

Secret Message
Directions: Translate the secret message by substituting one letter for another. For example, if you decide that "t" should really be "g," then "t" will be "g" every time it appears in this puzzle. Hint: Try to translate short words first to establish vowel patterns.

Wzgz zmzobhrh yvtrrnh drgs wvhxirkgrev hgzgrhgrxh rm zmb hgfwb rm dsrxs gsv wzgz ziv

mfnvirx, rmxofwrmt hlnv jfzorgzgrev hgfwrvh.

Crossword Puzzle

Directions: Complete the crossword puzzle. Note: If the answer is more than one word, there are no blank spaces left between the words.

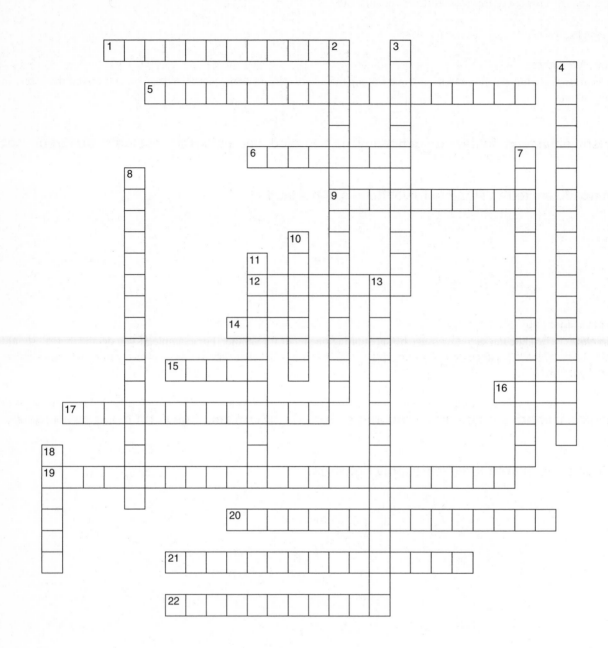

Across

1. Result obtained by adding the squares of different scores.
5. Naturally expected random observations in the extreme ends of the tail.
6. A measure of dispersion that is the mean or average of the sum of the square.
9. Distribution of values.
12. Extreme values in a set of data that are exceptions to the overall findings.
14. Value that occurs with greatest frequency.
15. The simplest measure of dispersion, obtained by subtracting the lowest score from the highest score.
16. Value obtained by summing all the scores and dividing that total by the number of scores being summed.
17. The researcher's attempt to obtain subjects with a wide variety of characteristics to reduce the risk of bias in studies not using random sampling.
19. Designed to detect the unexpected in the data.
20. Designed to analyze repeated measures from a given time until a certain event occurs.
21. Obtained by subtracting the mean from the raw score.
22. List of all values of a variable.

Down

2. The square root of the variance.
3. Graphic illustrations of the point at which each value of x and y intersect.
4. Distribution of categorical data.
7. Mean, median, and mode are measure of this.
8. The difference between what exists in reality and what is measured.
10. A repetitive, regular, or continuous occurrence in time-series analysis.
11. Sample of subjects who are very similar in their scores.
13. An analysis of deviation values in a data set.
18. The score at the exact center of an ungrouped frequency distribution.

EXERCISES IN CRITICAL APPRAISAL

Directions: Review the two quantitative studies in Appendix B—Bindler et al. (2007) and Sethares and Elliott (2004)—and answer the following questions.

1. Identify the descriptive analyses performed in the Bindler, Massey, Shultz, Mills, and Short's (2007) study. What analyses were not reported that you believe should have been included? Why would this information be important to report? Identify exploratory data analyses performed in the study.

2. Identify the descriptive analyses performed in the Sethares and Elliott (2004) study. What analyses were not reported that you believe should have been included? Why would this information be important to report? Identify exploratory data analyses performed in the study.

20 Using Statistics to Examine Relationships

INTRODUCTION

Read Chapter 20, and then complete the following exercises. These exercises will help you to understand and critically appraise bivariate correlational analyses in the results sections of published studies and to conduct these analysis techniques using study data. The answers to these exercises are in Appendix A.

RELEVANT TERMS

Bivariate Correlational Analysis

Directions: Match each term with its correct definition.

Terms

a. Bivariate correlation
b. Coefficient
c. Correlational analyses
d. Correlational matrix
e. Curvilinear relationship
f. Homoscedastic
g. Inverse linear relationship

h. Kendall's tau
i. Linear relationship
j. Negative linear relationship
k. Nonlinear relationship
l. Pearson's product-moment correlation
m. Percentage of variance
n. Perfect correlation

o. Positive linear
p. Regression analysis
q. Scatter plot
r. Spearman rho
s. Spurious correlation
t. Strength of relationship
u. Weak correlation

Definitions

_____ 1. Data are evenly dispersed both above and below the regression line, which indicates a linear relationship on a scatter diagram (plot).

_____ 2. Category of statistical procedures conducted to determine the direction (positive or negative) and magnitude (or strength) of the relationships between two variables.

_____ 3. A relationship easily identifiable in a scatter diagram by the dispersion of plots on the diagram.

_____ 4. The line that best represents the values of the raw scores plotted on a scatter diagram is the line of best fit that is calculated by what type of analysis?

_____ 5. A nonparametric analysis technique for ordinal data that is an adaptation of the Pearson product-moment correlation used to examine relationships among variables in a study.

_____ 6. The relationship between two variables varies depending on the relative values of the variables. The graph of the relationship is a curved line rather than a straight line.

_____ 7. A relationship in which the correlation coefficient is +1.

_____ 8. The relationship between two variables or concepts will remain consistent regardless of the values of each of the variables or concepts.

_____ 9. The amount of variation explained by the relationship.

_____ 10. The analysis technique that determines the extent of the linear relationship between two variables.

_____ 11. The percentage of variability explained by a linear relationship; the value is obtained by squaring Pearson's correlation coefficient (r^2).

_____ 12. Nonparametric test to determine the correlation among variables used when both variables have been measured at least at the ordinal level.

_____ 13. Provides useful preliminary information about the nature of the relationship between two variables. A figure is developed to demonstrate the relationship.

_____ 14. Relationships represented by an r value of < 0.30.

_____ 15. Obtained by performing bivariate correlational analysis on every pair of variables in the data set and putting these values into a table.

_____ 16. Correlations between variables that are not logical; these significant relationships may be a consequence of chance and have no meaning.

_____ 17. The parametric test used to determine the relationship between two variables.

_____ 18. Indicates that as one variable changes (value of the variable increase or decreases), the second variable will also change in the same direction.

_____ 19. Another term for inverse linear relationship

_____ 20. A calculated numerical factor.

_____ 21. Indicates that as one variable or concept changes, the other variable or concept changes in the opposite direction; also referred to as a negative linear relationship.

Multivariate Correlational Analysis
Directions: Match each term with its correct definition.

Terms
a. Beta weight
b. Causal relationship
c. Communality
d. Eigenvalues
e. Exploratory factor analysis
f. Factors

g. Factor analysis
h. Factor loading
i. Factor rotation
j. Factor score
k. Loadings
l. Multivariate correlations

m. Oblique rotation
n. Principal component analysis
o. Scree test
p. Secondary loading
q. Varimax rotation

Definitions

_____ 1. Similar to stepwise regression, in which the variance of the first factor is partialed out before analysis begins on the second factor. It is performed when the researcher has few prior expectations about the factor structure.

_____ 2. This type of relationship may be indicated by a strong correlation and should be tested with inferential statistics.

_____ 3. The regression coefficient of the variable on the factor; indicates the extent to which a single variable is related to the cluster of variables.

_____ 4. Techniques that examine linear relationships among three or more variables.

_____ 5. Used during data analysis in additional studies conducted to examine changes in the phenomenon in various situations and to determine the relationships of the factors with other concepts.

_____ 6. In factor analysis, the lowest loading for a variable when it has high loadings on two factors. When many of these occur, the factoring is not considered clean.

_____ 7. A value in factor analysis used with standardized scores.

_____ 8. The numerical value generated with factor analysis that is the sum of the squared weights for each factor.

_____ 9. An aspect of factor analysis in which the factors are mathematically adjusted or rotated to reduce the factor structure and clarify the meaning.

_____ 10. The second step in exploratory factor analysis that provides the preliminary information that the researcher needs to make decisions before the final factoring.

_____ 11. Symbolized by (h^2), the squared multiple regression coefficient for each variable is closely related to the R^2 coefficient in regression.

_____ 12. A type of rotation in factor analysis used to accomplish the best fit (best-factor solution) when the factors are uncorrelated.

_____ 13. An analysis that examines interrelationships among large numbers of variables and disentangles those relationships to identify clusters of variables that are most closely linked together.

_____ 14. Weights that express the extent to which the variable is correlated with the factor.

_____ 15. One test done to determine the number of factors to be included in a construct.

_____ 16. Variables that are linked together in clusters.

_____ 17. A type of rotation in factor analysis used to accomplish the best fit when the factors are correlated.

KEY IDEAS

Directions: Fill in the blanks in the following sentences.

1. The purpose of correlational analyses is to identify _____ between or among variables.

2. In correlational analyses, all of the data are obtained from _____ group(s).

3. When correlational analyses are planned, sampling and data collection should be designed to maximize obtaining the

_____ _____ of possible values on each variable in the study.

4. A(n) _____ _____ is the line that best represents the values of the raw scores plotted on a scatter diagram.

5. In a negative linear relationship, a(n) _____ score on one variable is related to a

_____ score on the other variable.

6. _____ data will provide the best information when using correlational analyses.

7. _____ can be used when performing correlational analyses on nominal data.

8. Correlational analysis provides information about whether the relationships are _____ or

_____ and also the _____ of the relationship.

9. The data are _____ before conducting the analysis when performing correlational analysis using ordinal data.

10. Performing bivariate correlational analyses on every pair of variables in a data set will provide a(n)

_____ _____ .

11. _____ _____ examines interrelationships among large numbers of variables.

12. Percentage of variance = _____ .

M_____ CONNECTIONS

Ma_____ and McCabe Study

Dire____ In the following statistical report, indicate the strength of the correlation and whether the results were significant, assuming a level of significance set at $\alpha = 0.05$. Use a highlighter to mark significant relationships. A space has been left after each value for you to indicate the strength of the relationship. Indicate H for high, M for moderate, and L for low.

Macnee, C. L. & McCabe, S. (2004). The transtheoretical model of behavior change and smokers in southern Appalachia. *Nursing Research*, *54*(4), 243-250. (The study was supported by a grant from the National Institute of Nursing Research.)

Objective: "To identify, by examining the applicability of the transtheoretical model for southern Appalachian smokers, the percentage of individuals in each of the five stages of change, the use of the processes of change from the transtheoretical model, and the scores on recognized predictors of smoking cessation including the temptation to smoke, the perceived barriers to cessation, the pros and cons of smoking, and nicotine dependence" (Macnee & McCabe, 2004, p. 243).

Nicotine dependence was significantly correlated with the pros of smoking scores ($r = 0.37$; $p < 0.001$) _____, barriers to smoking ($r = 0.32$; $p < 0.001$) _____, and temptation scores ($r = 0.46$; $p. < 0.001$) _____, supporting the theoretical relations proposed in the TTM. However, the levels of nicotine dependence did not vary significantly across the stages of change.

Gary and Yarandi Study
Directions: Review the statistical report, and answer the questions that follow.

Gary, F. A., & Yarandi, H. N. (2004). Depression among southern rural African American women. *Nursing Research*, *54*(4), 251-259.

An iterated principal-factor analysis was performed, in which squared multiple correlations were used for the initial communality estimates, and a Promax (oblique) rotation was used to identify the self-reported dimensions of depression. The minimum 80% variance criterion and the scree plot were used to determine the optimal number of factors. ... Two factors were extracted. ... The coefficient alphas for the factors suggested that the first two common factors were potentially reliable for this sample. The coefficient alphas for the two factors were 0.98 and 0.83, respectively. The two extracted factors explained 89% of the common variance. Two comparably sized eigenvalues of 5.35 and 5.53 were found for the reduced correlation matrix, and the correlation between the two oblique factors was 0.57 ($p < 0.001$). ... Symptoms such as pessimism, worthlessness, punishment feelings, sadness, self-dislike, loss of interest, indecisiveness, and past failure tended to load high on the first factor. All these symptoms were psychological and cognitive in nature. Therefore, Factor I was a cognitive dimension of self-reported depression. Factor II explained somatic symptoms such as tiredness or fatigue, loss of energy, concentration difficulty, irritability, changes in appetite, changes in sleeping pattern, loss of interest in sex, and loss of pleasure. Such factors were thought to represent a "somatic-affective" dimension of self-reported depression.

1. Highlight the terms related to factor analysis that you recognize. Examine the results. Interpret the results based on your understanding of factor analysis.

PUZZLES

Word Scramble
Directions: Unscramble the sentence by rearranging the letters to form actual words. Note: You will use all the letters in every word.

Kawe larrastoonic yam eb rompitnat hewn mobdince thiw roeth blaivarse.

Secret Message
Directions: Translate the secret message by substituting one letter for another. For example, if you decide that "e" should really be "p," then "e" will be "p" every time it appears in this puzzle. Hint: Try to translate short words first to establish vowel patterns.

Ra eijebibmrca lci fciijxbmrcabx babxkrk, hbmb fcxxjfrca kmibmjnrjk kpcoxh dj exbaajh

mc zburzryj mpj eckkrdrxrmw cl cdmbraran mpj lox ibanj cl eckkrdxj qbxojk ca jbfp qbirbdxj

mc dj okjh ra mpj babxwkrk.

Chapter **20**   **Using Statistics to Examine Relationships**

Crossword Puzzle

Directions: Complete the crossword puzzle. Note: If the answer is more than one word, there are no blank spaces left between the words.

Across

1. A type of factor rotation in which factors are allowed to be correlated.
4. A nonlinear relationship.
7. _____ variables—elements external to a theory that are related to variables within the theory.
13. A procedure designed to obtain the best fit of variables to factors.
14. _____ variable—not measurable by direct observation; may be composed of several variables combined.
15. The line that best represents the values plotted on a scatter plot.
16. _____ correlation—a relationship between two variables that makes no sense.
17. Sum of the squared weights for each factor.
18. Created when bivariate correlational analysis is performed on every pair of variables in the data set.
20. Used to determine the number of factors to set in a factor analysis.
21. Multiplying the variable score by the factor loading.

Down

2. _____ correlation—test of relationship between two variables.
3. _____ relationship—a constant relationship between variables with a value greater than zero.
5. The extent to which the variable is correlated with the factor.
6. Nonparametric test to determine the correlation among variables used when both variables have been measured at the ordinal level.
8. A two-dimensional plot designed to illustrate the relationship between two variables.
9. Indicates the extent a variable is related to the cluster of variables.
10. One test done to determine the number of factors to be included in a construct.
11. In path analysis, how well the resulting model fits the data.
12. Equal variance on each side of the line of best fit.
13. A cluster of variables linked closely together.
16. _____ (of a relationship)—increases as the correlation value moves away from zero.
19. _____ correlation—a relationship below 0.3.

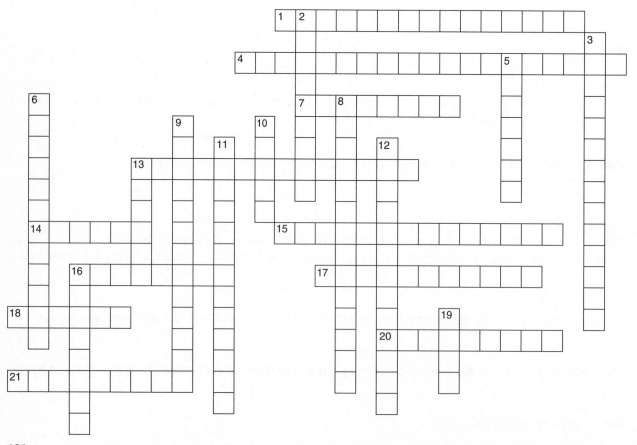

EXERCISES IN CRITICAL APPRAISAL

Directions: Bindler, Massey, Shultz, Mills, and Short (2007) conducted a predictive correlational study (see Appendix B). Please answer the following questions about the correlational results in this study.

1. Review Table 6, and identify the strongest correlation in this table. What two variables were correlated to achieve this relationship? Was this correlation significant, and if so at what level?

2. Review Table 6, and identify the weakest correlation in this table. What two variables were correlated to achieve this relationship? Was this a positive or negative correlation? Was this correlation significant, and if so at what level?

3. What is the *r* value for the correlation between insulin and triglycerides? What percentage of variance was explained by this relationship? Is this relationship statistically significant? Is this relationship clinically important?

4. What is the *r* value for the correlation between insulin and vitamin A (% RDA) (see Table 7)? What percentage of variance was explained by this relationship? Is this relationship statistically significant? Is this relationship clinically important?

5. Bindler et al. (2007, p. 298) formulated the following: "Research Questions 2: What are the relationships between insulin levels and the criteria for metabolic syndrome in a multiethnic sample of children in Central Washington State?" What analysis was conducted to address this question? What were the results?

Identify a recently published study using bivariate correlations, multivariate correlations, factor analysis, or structural equation modeling. Read the study and highlight terms in the study that you are familiar with from this chapter. In the results section, identify and circle significant results. Identify the results with the greatest strength. What was the meaning of these results? Match your findings with those of the author in the findings section.

21 Using Statistics to Predict

INTRODUCTION

Read Chapter 21, and then complete the following exercises. These exercises will help you to understand and critically appraise predictive analysis techniques in the results sections of published studies and to conduct these statistical techniques using study data. The answers to these exercises are in Appendix A.

RELEVANT TERMS

Simple Linear Regression

Directions: Match each term with its correct definition.

Terms

a. Bivariate analysis
b. Estimate
c. Holdout sample
d. Homoscedasticity
e. Horizontal axis
f. Intercept
g. Line of best fit

h. Linear relationship
i. Method of least squares
j. Predicted score
k. Probability
l. Regression analysis
m. Regression coefficient R
n. Regression equation

o. Regression line
p. Scatter plot
q. Simple linear regression
r. Slope
s. Variation
t. Vertical axis
u. Y intercept

Definitions

_____ 1. The relationship between two variables or concepts will remain consistent regardless of the values of each of the variables or concepts.

_____ 2. A mathematical expression of a causal proposition emerging from a theoretical framework.

_____ 3. A sample obtained at the initial data collection period but not included in the initial regression analysis.

_____ 4. The estimate referred to as $\hat{y}$ (expressed y-hat) or occasionally as y' (expressed y-prime).

_____ 5. Represents the y (the dependent or predicted) variable.

_____ 6. Represents the x (independent or predictor) variable.

_____ 7. Provides a means to estimate the value of a dependent variable based on the value of an independent variable.

_____ 8. The point where the regression line crosses the y axis.

_____ 9. An effort to explain the dynamics within the scatter plot by drawing a straight line through the plotted scores.

_____ 10. The independent (predictor) variable or variables cause this in the value of the dependent (outcome) variable.

_____ 11. Analyzes the relationship between two variables.

_____ 12. Addresses relative rather than absolute causality.

_____ 13. Procedure in regression analysis for developing the line of best fit.

_____ 14. Determines the direction and angle of the regression line within the graph; represented by the letter b.

_____ 15. True values are evenly dispersed above and below the linear regression line.

_____ 16. The outcome of simple linear regression.

_____ 17. A common way to illustrate the relationship of variables graphically.

_____ 18. The point where the regression line crosses the axis.

_____ 19. The line that best represents the values of the raw scores plotted on a scatter diagram.

_____ 20. The predicted score or y.

_____ 21. The statistical procedure most commonly used for prediction.

Multiple Regression
Directions: Match each term with its correct definition.

Terms
a. Beta score
b. Coefficient of determination
c. Curvilinear
d. Discriminant analysis
e. Discriminant function

f. Dummy variables
g. Multicollinearity
h. Multiple regression
i. Nonlinearity analysis
j. Prediction equation

k. Predictive validity
l. Shrinkage of R^2
m. Transformed term

Definitions

_____ 1. The relationship between two variables fluctuates depending on the relative values of the variables. The graph of the relationship is a curved line rather than a straight.

_____ 2. Occurs when the independent variables bear relationships to one another aside from their relationship to the dependent variable.

_____ 3. The prediction equation is not sample specific and can be used to predict or perhaps explain values of the dependent variable in the population.

_____ 4. The dependent variable in discriminant analysis that is equivalent in many ways to a factor.

_____ 5. Designed to allow the researcher to identify characteristics associated with group membership and to predict group membership.

_____ 6. The analysis of a relationship that cannot be graphed as a straight line.

_____ 7. A numerical value that indicates the amount of change that occurs in Y for each change in the associated X

_____ 8. Another independent variable that can be added to the regression equation in the case of a curvilinear relationship, a transformation of the original independent variable obtained by squaring the original variable, which may accurately express the curvilinear relationship.

_____ 9. Categorical or dichotomous variables used in regression analysis.

_____ 10. In most cases, R^2 will be lower in the new sample because the original equation was developed to most precisely predict scores in the original sample.

_____ 11. Computed from a matrix of correlation coefficients and provides important information on multicollinearity. The value indicates the degree of linear dependencies among the variables.

_____ 12. The outcome of regression analysis.

_____ 13. The extension of simple linear regression with more than one independent variable entered in to the analysis.

KEY IDEAS

Directions: Fill in the blanks, or provide the appropriate responses.

1. The purpose of regression analysis is to predict as much of the _____ in the value of a dependent variable as possible.

2. Predictive analyses are based on _____ theory.

3. Prediction is one approach to examining _____ relationships.

4. The _____ variable(s) cause(s) variation in the value of the _____ variable.

5. In plotting a regression line, the horizontal axis represents _____ and the vertical axis

   represents _____.

6. What is the procedure for developing the line of best fit?

7. The outcome of a regression analysis is the regression coefficient _____.

8. R^2 indicates the amount of _____ in the data that is explained by the regression equation.

9. Simple linear regression provides a means to _____ the value of a dependent variable based on the value of an independent variable.

10. Multiple regression analyses are closely related mathematically to _____

   _____ (ANOVA).

11. In multiple regression, more than one _____ variable is entered into the analysis.

12. Multicollinearity can be minimized by careful selection of _____ variables.

13. Multicollinearity causes problems with _____.

14. With multicollinearity, the amount of variance explained by each variable in the equation will be

   _____.

15. A _____ of types of variables may be used in a single regression equation.

16. The outcome of a regression analysis is referred to as a(n) _____ _____.

17. Discriminant analysis is designed to predict _____ _____.

18. What are the outcomes of a discriminant function analysis called? _____

_____ _____.

MAKING CONNECTIONS

Regression Analysis

1. List the three assumptions of regression analysis.

   a.

   b.

   c.

2. What is the algebraic equation for a straight line?

3. List four types of variables that can be used in a regression equation.

   a.

   b.

   c.

   d.

Matching

Directions: Match each term with its description.

Terms

a. Coefficient R
b. *t*
c. *t* will increase as
d. *t* will decrease as

e. Least squares method
f. ANOVA
g. R^2
h. multicollinearity

Descriptions

_____ 1. Amount of variance explained in regression equation.

_____ 2. *b* moves farther from zero.

170

_____ 3. Based on decision theory.

_____ 4. Statistic to test significance of regression equation.

_____ 5. Outcome of regression analysis.

_____ 6. Sum of squared deviations increases.

_____ 7. Procedure to develop line of best fit.

_____ 8. Reduces capacity to generalize regression findings.

PUZZLES

Word Scramble

Directions: Unscramble the following sentence by rearranging the letters to form actual words. Note: You will use all the letters in every word.

Eht gloa fo onerigress sainisly si ot mintedeer who trulycarae noe nac dripcet het evual fo a

tendneped raibleva dabes no eth aluve ro sualve fo neo ro rome pendnindeet raveblias.

Secret Message

Directions: Translate the following secret message by substituting one letter for another. For example, if you decide that "b" should really be "d," then "b" will be "d" every time it appears in this puzzle. Hint: Try to translate short words first to establish vowel patterns.

Hrofqrzrybym bybxcoro ro hjornyjh mw hjmjqzryj pwg bffkqbmjxc wyj fby uqjhrfm mpj ibxkj

wq ibxkjo wl wyj wq zwqj ryhjujyhjym ibqrbdxjo.

Crossword Puzzle

Directions: Complete the crossword puzzle. Note: If the answer is more than one word, there are no blank spaces left between the words.

Across

1. The *x* axis.
3. The product of two terms that expresses the joint effect of both.
11. The point on the *y* axis where the line of best fit interfaces.
12. The *y* axis.
13. Two variables.
14. The outcome of a regression analysis.
15. *b*, the coefficient of *x*.
16. Best subset of discriminating variables.

Down

1. Sample data not included in first analysis.
2. Independent variable.
4. The accuracy of a predictive equation.
5. Predicts group membership.
6. Analyzes more than one independent variable.
7. Equal scatter of values of *y* above and below the regression line.
8. Categorical variables.
9. A straight line drawn through plotted scores that provides the best explanation of the linear relationship between two variables.
10. Test of the ability of the regression equation to predict in a new sample.

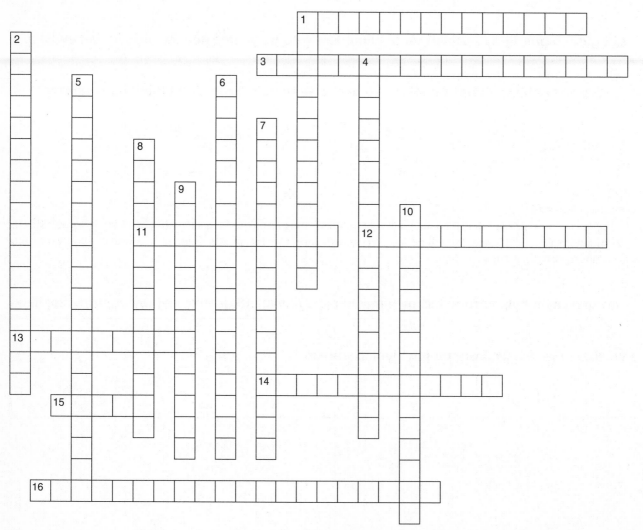

Directions: Review Bindler et al.'s (2007) study in Appendix B, and answer the following questions.

1. Which of the five research questions is answered using regression analysis?

2. List the variables that will be used in statistical analyses to answer the previous research question, and state the level of measurement of each variable.

Variable	Level of Measurement

3. What forms of regression analyses were used in the study and why?

4. Multiple linear regression was performed first and analyzed how much of the variance in the insulin levels (dependent variable) is predicted by the independent variables listed in question 2. What was the outcome of this regression analysis?

5. Of the nine variables tested in the regression model, which did not significantly contribute to the variance in insulin levels?

6. Bindler et al. (2007) went on to use a more sophisticated regression analysis (backward stepwise regression) in which the variables that did not contribute significantly to the variance of insulin were removed. The model that resulted explained how much of the variance in insulin levels?

7. Circle the appropriate categorization of the initial results of the simple linear regression.

   a. Significant and predicted

   b. Nonsignificant

   c. Significant and not predicted

   d. Mixed results

   e. Unexpected

GOING BEYOND

Search the current issues of nursing research journals for studies using regression analyses. Evaluate the adequacy of descriptions of the procedures performed.

INTRODUCTION

Read Chapter 22, and then complete the following exercises. These exercises will help you to understand and critically appraise statistics used to examine causality included in the results sections of published studies and to conduct these inferential analysis techniques using study data. The answers to these exercises are in Appendix A.

RELEVANT TERMS

Contingency Tables

Directions: Match each term with its correct definition.

Terms

a. Causality
b. Cell
c. Chi-square
d. Chi-square test of independence
e. Contingency coefficient (C)
f. Contingency table
g. Cramer's *V*

h. Critical value
i. Dichotomous
j. Distribution-free
k. Interval data
l. Lambda
m. Nominal data
n. Observed cell frequency

o. Ordinal data
p. Parametric procedure
q. Partitioning
r. Phi coefficient
s. Statistical assumptions
t. Statistical power

Definitions

_____ 1. A statistical test that is used with two nominal variables and is the most commonly used of the chi-square-based measures of association.

_____ 2. Nonparametric analysis technique that measures the degree of association (or relationship) between two nominal-level variables.

_____ 3. The value of the statistic that must be obtained to indicate that a difference exists in the two populations represented by the groups under study.

_____ 4. Data that can be ranked but the intervals between the ranked data are not necessarily equal.

_____ 5. Data at the lowest level of measurement that can be organized into categories that are exclusive and exhaustive but the categories cannot be compared or rank ordered.

_____ 6. Includes three conditions: (a) there must be a strong relationship between the proposed cause and effect, (b) the proposed cause must precede the effect in time, and (c) the cause has to be present whenever the effect occurs.

_____ 7. Analysis technique used to determine relationships in dichotomous, nominal data. It is also used with the chi-square test to determine the location of a difference or differences among cells.

_____ 8. Analysis technique for nominal data that is a modification of phi for contingency tables larger than 2×2.

_____ 9. Characteristics of the data that must be met in order for certain statistical procedures to be appropriately used.

_____ 10. A statistical analysis technique that tests whether the two variables being examined are independent or related.

175

_____ 11. Data that are measured on scales having intervals that are numerically equal but without a meaningful zero point.

_____ 12. A statistical procedure used when three assumptions are met: (a) the sample was drawn from a population for which the variance can be calculated and the distribution is normal or near normal, (b) the level of measurement should be interval or ratio with an approximately normal distribution, and (c) the data can be treated as though they were obtained from random samples.

_____ 13. The intersection between the row and column in a table where a specific numerical value is inserted.

_____ 14. The probability that a statistical test will detect a significant difference or relationship that exists, which is the capacity to correctly reject a null hypothesis.

_____ 15. Variables that have only two categories (e.g., Male or Female).

_____ 16. Used to examine the data statistically to determine in exactly which categories the differences exist.

_____ 17. Cross-tabulation table that allows visual comparison of summary data output related to two variables within a sample.

_____ 18. No assumption has been made of a normal distribution of values in the population from which the sample was taken.

_____ 19. The actual number of frequencies in a cell when data are being examined.

_____ 20. Used to analyze nominal data to determine significant differences between observed frequencies within the data and frequencies that were expected.

and ANOVA

_s:_ Match each term with its correct definition.

	h. Difference scores	o. Post hoc analysis
	i. Escalation of significance	p. Robust
procedure	j. _F_ statistic	q. Sampling distribution
ups variance	k. Grand mean	r. Standard error
e.	l. Independent samples or variable groups	s. _t_-test
f.	m. Independent variable	t. Total variance
g. Do ble	n. Location of significant difference	

Definiti

_____ 1.   rocedure designed to reduce the error term (or variance within groups) by partialing out the variance n a confounding variable by performing regression analysis before performing analysis of variance.

_____ 2. The   behavior, or outcome that is predicted and measured in research.

_____ 3. Sample.   ns in which the selection of one subject is totally unrelated to the selection of other subjects.

_____ 4. Inflation of   e that happens with the use of multiple _t_-tests and results in increased risk of type I error.

_____ 5. Statistical tests   specifically to determine the location of differences in studies with more than two groups, such as w   VA results are significant in a study that has three or more groups.

_____ 6. A parametric analysis technique that controls for escalation of significance and can be used if various *t*-tests must be performed on different aspects of the same data.

_____ 7. Description of an analysis procedure that will yield accurate results even if some of the assumptions are violated by the data being analyzed.

_____ 8. A statistic used in ANOVA to determine if the groups are statistically different.

_____ 9. A parametric analysis technique used to determine significant differences between measures of two samples. This test can be used to examine differences between dependent and independent groups.

_____ 10. The value of the statistic that must be obtained to indicate that a difference exists in the two populations represented by the groups under study.

_____ 11. The combination of the variance from within and between the groups.

_____ 12. Deviation scores obtained by subtracting the mean from each raw score.

_____ 13. Because of sampling error, each sample mean is likely to deviate somewhat from the true population mean.

_____ 14. The variance of the group means around the grand mean (the mean of the total sample) that is examined in ANOVA.

_____ 15. Post hoc tests have been developed specifically to determine this after ANOVA is performed to analyze data from more than two groups.

_____ 16. Determined by using statistical values (such as means) of many samples obtained from the same population.

_____ 17. The freedom of a score's value to vary given the other existing scores' values and the established sum of the scores ($df = N - 1$).

_____ 18. The treatment, intervention, or experimental activity that the researcher manipulates or varies to create an effect on the dependent variable.

_____ 19. The mean of the total sample.

_____ 20. The statistical technique used to examine differences among two or more groups by comparing the variability between the groups with the variability within the groups.

KEY IDEAS

Directions: Fill in the blanks in the following sentences.

1. If subjects are randomly assigned to treatment and control groups, the groups are _____.

2. If subjects serve as their own control by using the pretest as a control, the observations (and therefore the groups) are

   _____.

3. Use of _____ _____ allows visual comparison of summary data output related to two categorical variables within the sample.

4. One assumption of the chi-square test of independence is that there is only _____

   _____ of data for each subject in the sample.

5. The *t*-test is _____ to moderate violation of its assumptions.

6. ANOVA compares the variance _____ each group with the variance

_____ groups.

7. ANOVA is relatively sensitive to variations in the size of the _____.

8. ANCOVA partials out the variance resulting from a confounding variable by performing _____

_____ before performing ANOVA.

PUZZLES

Word Scramble

Directions: Unscramble the following sentence by rearranging the letters to form actual words. Note:
You will use all the letters in every word.

Het t-sett nac eb sued yonl noe emit rundig lanisysa ot mixenea tada mofr wot mapless ni a

yustd.

Secret Message

Directions: Translate the following secret message by substituting one letter for another. For example, if you decide
that "c" should really be "y," then "c" will be "y" every time it appears in this puzzle. Hint: Try to translate short
words first to establish vowel patterns.

Ry zbyc fbojo, dribqrbmj bybxcoro hwjo ywm uqwirhj b fxjbq urfmkqj wl mpj hcybzrfo wl mpj

ormkbmrwy.

Crossword Puzzle

Directions: Complete the crossword puzzle. Note: If the answer is more than one word, there are no blank spaces left
between the words.

Across

1. A numerical value obtained from a sample.
5. Uses cut-off point to judge the significance of differences.
8. Results that are unlikely due to chance.
11. Probability that an analysis will detect a difference that exists.
12. Exclude incomplete data from analysis.
14. Analysis used to predict the value of one variable if values of other variables are known.
15. Test that uses variance to compare differences between groups.

Down

2. Analysis technique used to determine differences between two samples.
3. Statistical procedures used to examine the data descriptively.
4. Measure of central tendency for nominal data.
5. The spread of the scores around the mean is referred to as the _____ of scores.
6. Sample that is like the population.
7. Meanings of conclusions for the body of nursing knowledge.

178

Across

16. Groups in which selection of one subject is related to selection of another subject.
17. Determines an outcome.
18. Measure of central tendency for interval data.
19. Extreme of the normal curve.
20. Dispersion of values in sample.
21. Difference between lowest value and highest value.
22. Subjects with extreme values unlike the rest of the sample.
23. Measure of central tendency for ordinal data.
24. Outcome of data analysis.
25. Judgment based on evidence.

Down

9. Theoretical symmetrical distribution of all possible values.
10. Statistical test used to analyze nominal data.
13. Tests performed after initial analyses to identify specific groups that are different.

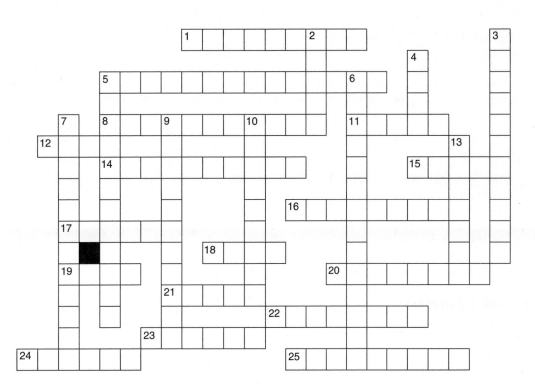

EXERCISES IN CRITICAL APPRAISAL

Directions: Review Sethares and Elliott's (2004) study in Appendix B, and answer the following questions. Consider the hypotheses for Sethares and Elliott's study: (1) Persons who receive the intervention will have lower HF readmission rates. (2) Persons who receive the intervention will report better quality of life. (3) Intervention subjects will report fewer barriers and more benefits to performing self-care of HF after receiving the tailored message intervention.

1. List the variable that will be analyzed to test hypothesis 1, and identify the level of measurement of this variable as nominal, ordinal, or interval/ratio.

Variable   Level of Measurement

2. Identify the two groups included in the first analysis.

   a.

   b.

3. Are these groups dependent or independent? Provide a rationale for your answer.

4. What statistical procedure was used to test this hypothesis?

5. Why was this procedure chosen?

6. State the results of the first analysis, providing numerical value.

7. Circle the appropriate response for the results listed in question 6.

   a. Significant and predicted

   b. Nonsignificant

   c. Significant and not predicted

   d. Mixed results

   e. Unexpected

8. Provide a rationale for the HF readmission results.

9. List the variable that was analyzed to test hypothesis 2, and identify the level of measurement of this variable.

   Variable   Level of Measurement

10. Identify the groups included in the second analysis.

    a.

    b.

11. Are these groups dependent or independent?

12. What statistical procedure was used to test hypothesis 2?

13. Why was this procedure chosen?

14. State the results of the second analysis, providing numerical values.

15. Circle the response that indicates the results identified in question 14.

    a. Significant and predicted

    b. Nonsignificant

    c. Significant and not predicted

    d. Mixed results

    e. Unexpected

16. List the variables that were analyzed to test hypothesis 3 and the level of measurement of each variable.

    Variables   Level of Measurement

17. Identify the groups included in the analyses to address hypothesis 3.

   a.

   b.

   c.

18. Are these groups dependent or independent?

19. What statistical procedure was used to test hypothesis 3?

20. State the results of the third analysis, providing numerical values.

21. Circle the response that indicates the results identified in question 20.

   a. Significant and predicted

   b. Nonsignificant

   c. Significant and not predicted

   d. Mixed results

   e. Unexpected

GOING BEYOND

Search current issues of nursing research journals for studies using inferential statistical procedures to examine the effectiveness of nursing interventions. Critically appraise the adequacy of the descriptions of the procedures performed.

INTRODUCTION

Read Chapter 23, and then complete the following exercises. These exercises will help you to learn relevant terms and to read and comprehend published qualitative studies. The answers for these exercises are in Appendix A.

RELEVANT TERMS

Data Collection in Qualitative Studies

Directions: Match the terms with the following definitions.

Terms

a. Case study
b. Data triangulation
c. Focus group
d. Life story

e. Moderator
f. Segmentation
g. Story
h. Storytakers

i. Storytelling
j. Unstructured interview
k. Unstructured observations

Definitions

_____ 1. A skilled facilitator of focus groups.

_____ 2. An event or series of events, encompassed by temporal or spatial boundaries, that are shared with others using an oral medium or sign language.

_____ 3. A group that is designed to obtain participants' perceptions in a specific (or focused) area in a setting that is permissive and nonthreatening.

_____ 4. Those listening to a story.

_____ 5. A collection of data from multiple sources in the same study.

_____ 6. Involved in spontaneously observing and recording what is seen with a minimum of prior planning.

_____ 7. A narrative analysis designed to reconstruct and interpret the life of an ordinary person. This methodology emerged from history, anthropology, and more recently from phenomenology.

_____ 8. The process or interaction used to share stories.

_____ 9. Sorting participants into focus groups with common characteristics to facilitate more open discussion.

_____ 10. Intensive exploration of a single unit of study, such as a person, family, group, community, or institution.

_____ 11. Initiated with a broad question, and subjects are usually encouraged to further elaborate on particular dimensions of a topic.

Data Management and Reduction (A)

Directions: Match the terms with the following definitions.

Terms

a. Causal network
b. Codes
c. Chronolog
d. Coding
e. Cognitive mapping
f. Conceptual/ theoretical coherence

g. Connecting findings to theory
h. Content analysis
i. Critical incident chart
j. Data-reducing devices
k. Decentering devices
l. Descriptive codes

m. Displaying data
n. Dwelling with the data
o. Eliminative induction
p. Enumerative induction

Definitions

_____ 1. A visual representation of the information provided by a participant. It represents the researcher's conceptualizations and interpretations of the participant.

_____ 2. A tentative theory that is vague and poorly pieced together that develops as the researcher begins to understand the processes being studied.

_____ 3. Ways of forcing the viewer to step back from the mass of particular observations to see the larger picture.

_____ 4. Qualitative analysis technique to classify words in a text into a few categories chosen because of their theoretical importance.

_____ 5. A theory developed from a qualitative study is connected with other existing theories in the body of knowledge, adding strength to the newly developed theory.

_____ 6. A means of summarizing qualitative data through highly condensed versions of the outcomes of qualitative research.

_____ 7. The type of unstructured observation that provides a detailed description of an individual's behavior in a natural environment.

_____ 8. Data management methods that help decrease the volume of data by generalizing from the particulars.

_____ 9. A qualitative data analysis technique that is part of a process referred to as *analytic induction* in which a number and variety of instances must be collected to verify a model that was developed from the research process.

_____ 10. The process of transforming qualitative data into numerical symbols that can be computerized.

_____ 11. A qualitative data analysis technique that is part of a process referred to as *analytic induction* and requires that the hypothesis generated from the analysis be tested against alternatives.

_____ 12. The researcher thinks in more general terms and moves from particular observations (findings) to the larger picture.

_____ 13. Immersion in the data as part of the process of data management and reduction in phenomenology.

_____ 14. The term used for "concepts" in cognitive mapping.

_____ 15. Terms used to organize and classify qualitative data.

_____ 16. A data display method that indicates particularly important events that occurred during data collection, the subgroup in which they occurred, and the time they occurred.

Data Management and Reduction (B)

Directions: Match the terms with the following definitions.

Terms

a. Event-time matrix
b. Explanatory code
c. Factoring
d. Immersion in the data
e. Interpretative code
f. Logical chain of evidence

g. Marginal remarks
h. Memoing
i. Metaphors
j. Narrative analysis
k. Pattern-making devices
l. Pattern

m. Premature parsimony
n. Propositions
o. Reflective remarks
p. Splitting variables
q. Themes

Definitions

_____ 1. Figurative language to suggest a likeness or analogy of one kind of idea used in the place of another; provides a strong image with a feeling tone that is powerful in communicating meaning.

_____ 2. Another term for dwelling in the data.

_____ 3. Abstract statements that further clarify relationships among categories, participants, actions, and events.

_____ 4. Devising this activity assumes the prior development of a tentative theory and requires the researcher to go back and carefully trace evidence from the data through development of the tentative theory.

_____ 5. A composite of traits or features characteristic of the data.

_____ 6. Particularly important during the initial stages of data analysis to allow more detailed examination of the processes that are occurring.

_____ 7. Developed late in the data collection process after theoretical ideas from the qualitative study have begun to emerge.

_____ 8. A qualitative means of formally analyzing text including stories. When stories are analyzed, the researcher "unpacks" the structure of the story.

_____ 9. An organizational system developed late in the qualitative data collection and analysis process as the researcher gains insight into the processes occurring.

_____ 10. Repeated ideas emerging from the data that allow the researcher to more clearly explain what is going on in the data.

_____ 11. General themes within the list of characteristics that allow one to explain more clearly what is going on. When clusters have been identified, they must be named.

_____ 12. One function of a metaphor places patterns in the data in a larger context.

_____ 13. The act on the part of the researcher of writing down conceptual ideas immediately as data are being reviewed.

_____ 14. As the researcher works with the data and makes notes, thoughts or insights often emerge; these are recorded in the notes in double parentheses.

_____ 15. A qualitative analysis technique that can facilitate comparisons of events occurring in different sites during particular time periods.

_____ 16. Occurs when concepts are integrated too quickly without thorough investigation of the need for differentiation.

_____ 17. As the researcher's notes about the data are being reviewed, observations about them need to be written immediately. These remarks are usually placed in the right-hand margin of the notes.

Qualitative Research Methods

Directions: Match the terms with the following definitions.

Terms

a. Critical social theory
b. Ethical analysis
c. Ethnographic methodology
d. External criticism
e. Feminist research method
f. Field research

g. Foundational inquiry
h. Going native
i. Grounded theory methodology
j. Historical research
k. Immersion in the culture
l. Internal criticism

m. Intuiting
n. Phenomenological research
o. Philosophical analysis
p. Philosophical inquiry

Definitions

_____ 1. The purpose of this methodology is transformational and directed at social structures and social relationships that marginalize women.

_____ 2. A qualitative research method that includes a narrative description or analysis of events that occurred in the remote or recent past.

_____ 3. In ethnographic research, when the researcher becomes part of the culture and loses all objectivity and, with it, the ability to observe clearly.

_____ 4. A qualitative research methodology in which the researcher seeks to understand how people communicate and develop symbolic meanings in a society.

_____ 5. The process of actually looking at the phenomenon in qualitative research; the individual focuses all awareness and energy on the subject of interest.

_____ 6. A qualitative research method used to examine the foundations for a science, such as studies that provide analysis of the structure of a science and the process of thinking about and valuing certain phenomena held in common by the science.

_____ 7. A qualitative research method that uses concept or linguistic analysis to examine meaning and develop theories of meaning in philosophical inquiry.

_____ 8. A qualitative research methodology developed within the discipline of anthropology for investigating cultures that involves collection, description, and analysis of data to develop a theory of cultural behavior.

_____ 9. An inductive, descriptive qualitative methodology for the purpose of describing experiences as the study participants live them.

_____ 10. Involves gaining increasing familiarity with such elements as language, sociocultural norms, traditions, communication patterns, religion, work patterns, and expression of emotion in a selected culture.

_____ 11. A method of determining the validity of source materials in historical research that involves knowing where, when, why, and by whom a document was written.

_____ 12. A qualitative research method using intellectual analysis to clarify meanings, manifest values, identify ethics, and study the nature of knowledge.

Chapter **23** **Qualitative Research Methodology**

_____ 13. An analysis related to obligation, rights, duty, right and wrong, conscience, justice, choice, intention, and responsibility.

_____ 14. Involves examination of the reliability of historical documents.

_____ 15. The activity of collecting the data that requires taking extensive notes in ethnographic research.

_____ 16. A qualitative, inductive research technique based on symbolic interaction theory that is conducted to discover what problems exist in a social scene and the processes persons use to handle them.

Qualitative Research Issues

Directions: Match the terms with the following definitions.

Terms

a. Auditability
b. Bracketing
c. Complete observer
d. Complete participation
e. Interpretation
f. Observer as participant
g. Participant as observer
h. Participatory research
i. Reflexivity
j. Researcher-participant relationship

Definitions

_____ 1. The researcher becomes a member of the group and conceals the researcher role.

_____ 2. A strategy that includes representatives from all groups that will be affected by the change (stakeholders) as collaborators.

_____ 3. A qualitative research technique of suspending or laying aside what is known about an experience being studied.

_____ 4. The contact or interchange that has an impact on the data collected and the interpretation.

_____ 5. The researcher's time is spent mainly observing and interviewing subjects and less in the participation role.

_____ 6. The researcher is passive and has no direct social interaction in the setting.

_____ 7. Critically thinking through the dynamic interaction between the self and the data during the analysis of qualitative data.

_____ 8. The rigorous development of a decision trail that is reported in sufficient detail to allow a second qualitative researcher, using the original data and the decision trail, to arrive at conclusions similar to those of the original qualitative researcher.

_____ 9. A special form of observation in which researchers immerse themselves in the setting so they can hear, see, and experience the reality as the participants do; participants are aware of the researcher's dual role.

_____ 10. An analysis that involves more than just stringing events together; events should be linked in a way that the researcher can create theoretical sense.

Directions: Fill in the blanks, or provide the appropriate responses.

1. Qualitative data analysis occurs _____ _____ data collection.

2. Qualitative data analysis uses _____ rather than _____ as the basis for analysis.

3. In qualitative analysis, the flow of reasoning moves from _____ to increasing _____.

4. Auditability requires that the researcher establish _____ _____ for categorizing data, arriving at ratings, or making judgments.

5. The researcher's _____ is a key factor in qualitative research.

6. Memos move the researcher toward _____.

7. Findings are often described from the orientation of the _____.

8. List four types of researcher-participant relationships. You can review the section on "Terms Related to Qualitative Research Issues" for definitions of these relationships.

   a.

   b.

   c.

   d.

9. List three characteristics of researcher-participant relationships in qualitative research.

   a.

   b.

   c.

10. List four methods of reducing data in qualitative research.

   a.

   b.

   c.

   d.

11. List six methods of drawing conclusions in analyzing qualitative data.

a.

b.

c.

d.

e.

f.

MAKING CONNECTIONS

Directions: Match the qualitative methodology types listed here with the examples that follow.

Qualitative Methodology Types
a. Phenomenology
b. Grounded theory
c. Ethnography
d. Historical
e. Philosophical
f. Critical social theory

Examples

_____ 1. Ask questions that reveal flaws in logic

_____ 2. Reveal power relations

_____ 3. Check the fit between the emerging theory and the original data

_____ 4. Dwell with the data

_____ 5. Clarify the validity and reliability of data

_____ 6. Emergence of the core variable

_____ 7. Acquire informants

_____ 8. Develop an inventory of sources

_____ 9. Intuiting

_____ 10. Search for negative instances of categories

_____ 11. Gain entrance

_____ 12. Examine principles to guide conduct

_____ 13. Analyze constraints on human action

_____ 14. Use archival data

_____ 15. I-Thou being with the participant

_____ 16. Avoid "going native"

_____ 17. Questions more important than answers

PUZZLES

Word Scramble
Directions: Unscramble the following sentence by rearranging the letters to form actual words. Note: You will use all the letters in every word.

Salyasin squirere scros-hicknecg heac tib fo taad thiw lal het throe stib fo adat.

Secret Message
Directions: Translate the following secret message by substituting one letter for another. For example, if you decide that "t" should really be "q," then "t" will be "q" every time it appears in this puzzle. Hint: Try to translate short words first to establish vowel patterns.

Rqh ipsruwdqw gliihuhqfh ehhwzhhk txdqwlwdwlyh dqg txdolwdwlyh uhvhdufklv wkh

qdwxuh ri uhodwlrqvklsv ehwzhhq wkh uhvhdufkhu dqg wkh iqglylgxdov ehlqj vwxglhg.

Crossword Puzzle
Directions: Complete the crossword puzzle. Note: If the answer is more than one word, there are no blank spaces left between the words.

Across
2. Explanation.
5. Developing graphic map of concepts and relationships.
9. Divide into parts.
11. Intensive exploration of a single unit of study.
12. Tale.
14. Have a feeling.
15. Decreasing volume of information.
16. Suspending or laying aside what is known.
17. Person who hears a story.
18. Making written note of.
19. Instructive.
20. Rigorous development of a decision trail.
21. Developing categories.

Down
1. Interaction between self and data.
3. Reducing categories too soon.
4. Relating a story.
6. Premises.
7. Method of retracing choices.
8. _____ (with) _____ abiding.
10. Involve oneself.
13. Using a combination of methods.

190

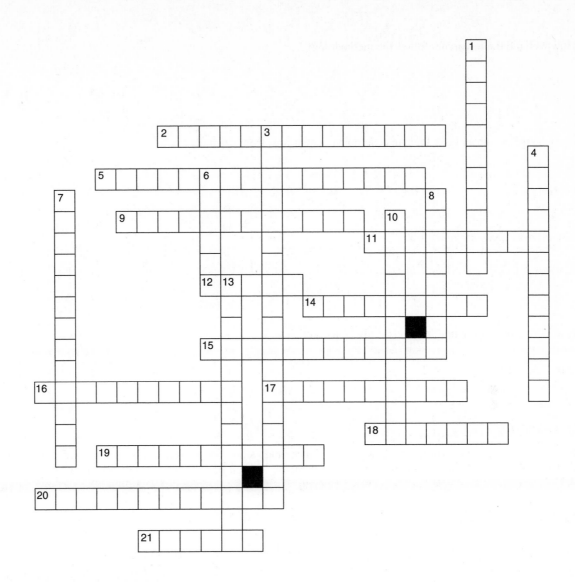

EXERCISES IN CRITICAL APPRAISAL

Directions: Read the Wright (2003) article in Appendix B, and answer the following questions.

1. Identify the philosophical base of the study.

2. Identify the methodology using to collect and analyze the data.

3. Did the philosophical base influence the selection of methods?

4. How well did the researcher follow the methodology?

5. Can you follow the author's logic in developing conclusions from the study?

6. What flaws do you see in the study?

7. How could the information from this study be used clinically?

GOING BEYOND

Identify full-text qualitative studies in CINAHL. Read them and identify the methodology used in each study. How well do you think the researcher(s) did in following the methodology? What flaws do you see in each study?

24 Interpreting Research Outcomes

INTRODUCTION

Read Chapter 24, and then complete the following exercises. These exercises will help you to learn relevant terms and identify and critically appraise the content of the discussion section of published studies. The answers to these exercises are in Appendix A.

RELEVANT TERMS

Types of Study Results

Directions: Match each type of study result with its correct definition.

Result Types

a. Mixed results
b. Nonsignificant results
c. Significant and not predicted results
d. Significant and predicted results
e. Unexpected results

Definitions

_____ 1. Results that are in keeping with those that the researcher has identified. Thus, these results support the logical links developed among the purpose, framework, questions or hypotheses, variables, and measurement tools of the study.

_____ 2. Results that are significant but were not identified by the researcher in the study framework and research questions or hypotheses.

_____ 3. Results that are negative or inconclusive, which are often the most difficult to explain.

_____ 4. Results about the relationships between the variables that were not hypothesized and not predicted from the framework being used. These results are serendipitous.

_____ 5. Results that include both significant and nonsignificant findings, which are the most common outcomes of studies.

Content Areas of the Discussion Section of a Study

Directions: Match each content area listed here with its correct definition.

Content Areas

a. Conclusions
b. Findings
c. Generalization
d. Implications of study finding for nursing
e. Limitations
f. Recommendations for further research

Definitions

_____ 1. The methodological and theoretical problems identified before or during a study that can impact the quality of the study findings.

_____ 2. The researcher provides suggestions for further study that might include replicating the current study with a larger sample or with a different population.

_____ 3. The synthesis and clarification of the meaning of the study findings.

_____ 4. The meaning of research conclusions for the body of nursing knowledge, theory, and practice.

_____ 5. Extends the implications of the findings from the sample that was studied to the larger population or from the situation studied to a larger situation.

_____ 6. The translated and interpreted results from a study.

KEY IDEAS

Directions: Fill in the blanks, or provide the appropriate responses.

1. To be useful, the evidence from data analysis needs to be:

2. When the results of the study are being interpreted, the researcher must use the following intellectual skills:
   a.

   b.

   c.

   d.

   e.

3. The initial evidence for the validity of the study results is derived from:

4. An assumption often made in interpreting study results is that the study variables were:

5. Only the researcher knows how _____ the measures were taken.

6. List four questions that need to be asked regarding data analysis.

   a.

   b.

   c.

   d.

7. The value of evidence in any study is dependent on the:

8. Any report of nonsignificant results needs to indicate:

9. _____ results are usually relationships found between variables that were not hypothesized and not predicted from the framework being used.

10. It is important to remember that research never _____ _____.

11. What is one of the risks in developing conclusions in research?

12. Identify three characteristics of significant studies.

   a.

   b.

   c.

13. From the conservative perspective, one cannot generalize beyond the _____

    _____.

14. Currently, nursing has few _____ generalizations.

15. To formulate empirical generalizations, one must have evidence from:

16. Conclusions need to address the relationships in the study _____.

MAKING CONNECTIONS

Directions: Match each term with its definition.

Terms

a. Translate
b. Fidelity of data collection
c. Validation of qualitative analysis

d. Synthesis of findings
e. Interpret
f. Measures with poor validity and reliability

Definitions

_____ 1. Decision trail

_____ 2. Explain the meaning of information

_____ 3. Undetectable by computers

_____ 4. Use terms that can be more easily understood

_____ 5. Conclusions

_____ 6. Dependent on integrity of the researcher

PUZZLES

Word Scramble

Directions: Unscramble the following sentence by rearranging the letters to form actual words. Note: You will use all the letters in every word.

Laveguatin het cherreas sproces duse ni eth dusty, cuprigdon gimeann morf teh strusle, nad

torceginfas eth lusessfune fo teh dingfins, lal fo chiwh rae dinvlove ni treationinpert, errique

gihh-veell tillteencula sporesecs.

Secret Message

Directions: Translate the following secret message by substituting one letter for another. For example, if you decide that "x" should really be "a," then "x" will be "a" every time it appears in this puzzle. Hint: Try to translate short words first to establish vowel patterns.

Oe vp qmpnqb, ojp pshrpctp nkea rxox xcxbmhm cpprm oe vp txkpnbbz pwxahcpr, xchypr,

xcr lhspc apxchcl, xcr veoj moxohmohtxb xcr tbhchtxb mhlchnhtxctp cpprm oe vp pwxahcpr.

Crossword Puzzle

Directions: Complete the crossword puzzle. Note: If the answer is more than one word, there are no blank spaces left between the words.

Across

3. Generate knowledge that influences a discipline.
7. Substantiation.
9. Synthesis and clarification of the meaning of study findings.
10. Change from one language to another.
11. Meaning of findings for clinical practice.

Down

1. Important information that is immediately useful.
2. Noteworthy.
4. Extending the conclusions beyond the sample.
5. Elucidation of study findings.
6. Interpreted results.
8. Products of research.

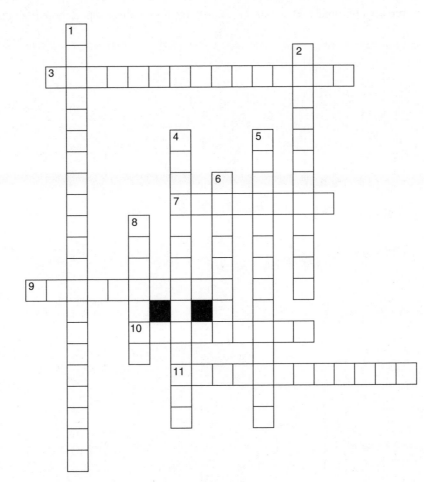

Directions: Review the Bindler, Massey, Shultz, Mills, and Short (2007) study in Appendix B, and answer the following questions. Consider the research questions formulated by Bindler et al. (2007, p. 296) for their study:

a. "What are the fasting serum insulin levels in a multiethnic sample of schoolchildren in central Washington State?

b. What are the relationships between insulin levels and the criteria for metabolic syndrome in a multiethnic sample of children in central Washington State? See the operational definition of metabolic syndrome criteria.

c. What are the relationships between reported dietary intake and metabolic syndrome criteria?

d. Which data predict insulin levels in this multiethnic sample of children?

e. How can the information learned in this study be used by pediatric nurses in clinical settings?"

1. Identify the findings reported by Bindler et al. (2007). Identify the results that support these findings.

2. Identify conclusions made by the author based on the findings.

3. Were the conclusions warranted in this study? Provide a rationale for your answer.

4. Did the researchers identify the methodological or theoretical limitations of their study? If so, what were those limitations?

5. Identify the implications for nursing made by the Bindler et al. (2007).

6. Are these study findings clinically significant? Provide a rationale for your response.

7. Were the findings generalized? If so, to what populations?

8. What recommendations did the researchers make for further studies?

25 Disseminating Research Findings

INTRODUCTION

Read Chapter 25, and then complete the following exercises. These exercises will help you to understand the process for developing the final research report and to disseminate this report through presentations and publications to audiences of nurses, other health care professionals, policy makers, and health care consumers. The answers to these exercises are in Appendix A.

RELEVANT TERMS

Directions: Match each term with its correct definition.

Terms

a. Abstract
b. Disseminating research findings
c. Duplicate publication
d. Intervention fidelity

e. Poster session
f. Presentation
g. Publication

h. Query letter
i. Referred journal
j. Research report

Definitions

_____ 1. A visual presentation of a study using pictures, tables, and illustrations on a display board.

_____ 2. Developing a research report and communicating it through presentations and publications to a variety of audiences.

_____ 3. A journal that uses expert reviewers to determine whether a manuscript is of acceptable quality for publication.

_____ 4. A letter sent to determine an editor's interest in reviewing a manuscript; it usually includes the research problem, a brief discussion of the major findings, the significance of the findings, and the researchers' qualifications for writing the article.

_____ 5. A clear, concise summary of a study that is usually limited to 100 to 250 words and briefly identifies the problem, purpose, framework, methodology, and results.

_____ 6. The practice of publishing the same article or major portions of the article in two or more print or electronic media without notifying the editors or referencing the other publications in the reference list.

_____ 7. Through this mechanism, research findings are permanently recorded in a journal or book.

_____ 8. Through this mechanism, research findings are verbally communicated at conferences and meetings.

_____ 9. A document that describes the research project and includes four major sections: introduction, methods, results, and discussion of the findings; this document is developed to communicate the research findings through presentation and publication.

_____ 10. The reliable and competent implementation of an experimental treatment.

KEY IDEAS

Directions: Fill in the blanks, or provide the appropriate responses.

1. Identify three elements of the introduction section of a quantitative research report.

   a.

   b.

   c.

2. Identify four content areas covered in the methods section of a quantitative research report.

   a.

   b.

   c.

   d.

3. A discussion of the level of significance (0.05, 0.01, or 0.001) selected for a study is usually discussed in the

   _____ section of a research report.

4. The results section of a quantitative research report includes the following:

   a.

   b.

5. Nursing research reports sometimes include figures to provide a picture of the results. Commonly used

   figures in nursing research reports include _____ _____ and

   _____ _____.

6. The American Psychological Manual (APA, 2001) provides direction for the development of figures and tables used

   to display the _____ of a study.

7. The figures and tables in a research report _____ (*do* or *do not*) need to be referred to in the written text of the report.

8. The means and standard deviations for study variables should be included in the published study for use in future

   _____ and in conducting a(n) _____ _____ to determine sample size of future studies.

9. Nonsignificant findings are usually not presented in _____ and _____ but are discussed in the narrative of the research report.

10. Identify four major content areas covered in the discussion section of a research report.

a.

b.

c.

d.

11. The theoretical importance of the study is determined by linking the study findings and conclusions to the study

_____.

12. The discussion section has a link to practice by providing what?

13. The methods section of a qualitative research report includes a description of the researcher's role. What are the key parts of this role?

a.

b.

c.

d.

14. Identify the six elements that are usually covered in the introduction section of a qualitative research report.

a.

b.

c.

d.

e.

f.

15. The results of qualitative research might include the development of a(n) _____

or _____, or the description of a(n) _____, an historical

_____, or a particular phenomenon.

16. _____ and _____ are research reports that students develop in depth as part of their requirements for a degree.

17. Nurses need to report their research findings to a variety of audiences, including the following:

    a.

    b.

    c.

    d.

18. More nurses need to be aware of research findings and their potential to provide evidence-based practice; therefore, research reports need to be communicated to all nurses, including _____,

    _____, and _____.

19. The _____ has greatly increased electronic access to research findings as well as other health-related information.

20. Presenting research findings at a conference includes the following steps:

    a.

    b.

    c.

    d.

21. Acceptance as a presenter at most research conferences requires the submission of a(n) _____.

22. An effective poster is a complete presentation of the study's contents, yet it is easily comprehended in

    _____ minutes or less.

23. An advantage of a poster session is the opportunity for _____ interaction between the researcher and those viewing the poster.

24. Selecting a journal for publication of a study requires knowledge of the following:

    a.

    b.

    c.

25. The *Nursing Research* journal editor prefers to receive a _____ regarding the possible publication of a manuscript.

26. Review of a manuscript by a potential publisher results in one of four possible decisions:

    a.

    b.

c.

d.

27. The most common reason manuscripts are rejected is that they are _____.

28. Complex qualitative studies might be published in _____ or in _____.

29. In a survey, 41 of 77 authors had published at least one form of duplicate article. Thus, _____

_____ is a serious concern in nursing literature.

30. Authors need to avoid unethical duplication by submitting original manuscripts or by providing full disclosure of any portion of a manuscript that has been previously published. Previous publications must be cited in the text of the

manuscript and also in the _____ _____.

MAKING CONNECTIONS

Directions: Match the sections of the quantitative research report listed here with the specific statements or elements from a research report.

Quantitative Research Report Sections
a. Introduction
b. Methods
c. Results
d. Discussion

Statements or Elements of a Research Report

_____ 1. This is a significant problem for nursing because the number of elderly is increasing, they are living longer, and they are experiencing more chronic illnesses and self-care deficits.

_____ 2. The sample was randomly selected from the seniors' Sunday school classes in four churches in a large metropolitan area.

_____ 3. The findings supported the study framework.

_____ 4. The framework for the study was Orem's theory of self-care.

_____ 5. The data were analyzed using means, standard deviations, ranges, and analysis of variance to determine the differences among the three groups.

_____ 6. The purpose of the study was to examine the effects of a low-intensity weight-lifting program on the muscle strength, balance, and performance of self-care behaviors in the elderly.

_____ 7. Tables and figures were used to present the results.

_____ 8. The limitations of the study were the small sample and the limited reliability and validity of the scale to measure self-care behaviors.

_____ 9. The quasi-experimental design of this study was an untreated control group design with pretest and posttest.

_____ 10. Future studies need to examine the impact of other interventions on the self-care and functional capacity of the elderly.

205

Bindler, Massey, Shultz, Mills, and Short Study

Directions: Review the Bindler et al. (2007) research article in Appendix B, and answer the following questions.

1. Did the study include the major sections of a research report? Identify the sections of the research report.

2. Identify the audiences most likely to have read this journal article.

Sethares and Elliott Study

Directions: Review the Sethares and Elliott (2004) research article in Appendix B, and answer the following questions.

1. Did the study include the major sections of a research report? Identify the sections of the research report.

2. Identify the audiences most likely to have read this journal article.

Wright Study

Directions: Review the Wright (2003) research article in Appendix B, and answer the following questions.

1. Did the study include the major sections of a research report? Identify the sections of the research report.

2. Identify the audiences most likely to have read this journal article.

26 Critical Appraisal of Nursing Studies

INTRODUCTION

Read Chapter 26, and then complete the following exercises. These exercises will help you to understand the quantitative and qualitative research critical appraisal processes. The answers to these exercises are in Appendix A.

RELEVANT TERMS

Directions: Match each term with its correct definition.

Terms

a. Analysis step of critical appraisal
b. Analytic preciseness
c. Auditability
d. Comparison step of critical appraisal
e. Comprehension step of critical appraisal

f. Conceptual clustering
g. Context flexibility
h. Critical appraisal of research
i. Descriptive vividness
j. Evaluation step of critical appraisal
k. Heuristic relevance

l. Reasoning skills of research
m. Methodological congruence
n. Theoretical connectedness
o. Transforming ideas across levels of abstraction

Definitions

_____ 1. Standard for evaluating qualitative research, in which documentation rigor, procedural rigor, ethical rigor, and auditability of the study are examined.

_____ 2. Rigorous development of a decision trail that is reported in sufficient detail to allow a second researcher to use the original data and the decision trail to arrive at conclusions similar to those of the original researcher.

_____ 3. Critical appraisal step that involves determining the strengths and limitations of the logical links connecting one study element with another.

_____ 4. Theoretical schema developed from a qualitative study; is clearly expressed, logically consistent, reflective of the data, and compatible with the knowledge base in nursing.

_____ 5. Critical appraisal step in which the ideal for each step of the quantitative research process is compared with the real steps in a published study.

_____ 6. Performing a series of transformations during which concrete data are transformed across several levels of abstractions to develop a theoretical schema that imparts meaning to the phenomenon under study.

_____ 7. Critical appraisal step during which the reader gains understanding of the terms in the research report; identifies the study elements; and grasps the nature, significance, and meaning of these elements.

_____ 8. Standard for evaluating a qualitative study in which the study's intuitive recognition, relationship to the existing body of knowledge, and applicability are examined.

_____ 9. Description of the site, subjects, experience of collecting data, and the researcher's thoughts during the qualitative research process presented clearly enough that the reader has the sense of personally experiencing the event.

_____ 10. A skill needed to critically appraise qualitative studies that involves the capacity to switch from one context or worldview to another, to shift perception in order to see things from a different perspective.

_____ 11. Involves a careful examination of all aspects of a study to judge the merits, limitations, meaning, and significance.

_____ 12. Last step of the critical appraisal process for quantitative research that involves the synthesis of study findings to determine the current body of knowledge in an area.

_____ 13. A skill needed to critically appraise qualitative research that includes both deductive and inductive reasoning in order to follow the researcher's logic.

_____ 14. Critical appraisal step in which the reader examines the meaning and significance of a study according to set criteria and compares it with previous studies conducted in the area.

_____ 15. A skill needed to critically appraise qualitative research that involves moving from specific pieces of information and ideas to a synthesis of these ideas and a broader understanding of the phenomenon examined. An example of this skill is reviewing the literature, organizing the ideas from the review, and summarizing these ideas to determine the existing body of knowledge in a selected area.

KEY IDEAS

Directions: Fill in the blanks, or provide the appropriate responses.

1. Critical appraisal of research involves careful examination of all aspects of a study to judge the

   _____, _____, _____ and _____,

   of the study.

2. Identify three important questions that are part of a critical appraisal of a study.

   a.

   b.

   c.

3. Describe your role in conducting critical appraisals of research.

4. Identify four criteria that are usually addressed in critical appraisal of an abstract.

    a.

    b.

    c.

    d.

5. Conducting a critical appraisal of a quantitative study involves applying some basic guidelines that are outlined in your text. Identify three of these basic guidelines.

    a.

    b.

    c.

6. List the five steps of the quantitative research critical appraisal process.

    a.

    b.

    c.

    d.

    e.

7. Identify the five standards used to critically appraise qualitative studies.

    a.

    b.

    c.

    d.

    e.

Directions: Read the research articles in Appendix B. Conduct critical appraisals of these three studies using the guidelines in Chapter 26 of your text.

1. Conduct a critical appraisal of the Bindler, Massey, Shultz, Mills, and Short (2007) study using the guidelines outlined in your text. Many parts of this study were critically appraised in Chapters 5 through 11 and Chapters 14 through 24 of this study guide.

   a. Conduct the comprehension step of the critical appraisal process. Questions are outlined in your text to direct you in this process.

   b. Do a critical appraisal that includes the comparison, analysis, and evaluation steps of the quantitative research critical appraisal process.

2. Conduct a critical appraisal of the Sethares and Elliott (2004) study using the guidelines outlined in your text. Many parts of this study were critically appraised in Chapters 5 through 11 and Chapters 14 through 24 of this study guide.

   a. Conduct the comprehension step of the critical appraisal process. Questions are outlined in your text to direct you in this process.

   b. Do a critical appraisal that includes the comparison, analysis, and evaluation steps of the quantitative research critical appraisal process.

3. Conduct a critical appraisal of the Wright (2003) study using the guidelines outlined in your text. Many parts of this study were critically appraised in Chapters 4 through 9, 14 through 17, and 23 of this study guide.

   a. Conduct a critical appraisal of this study using the five standards of qualitative research: descriptive vividness, methodological congruence, analytical preciseness, theoretical connectedness, and heuristic relevance. Questions are outlined in your text to direct your critical appraisal of this study.

INTRODUCTION

Read Chapter 27, and then complete the following exercises. These exercises will help you to understand and implement the process of synthesizing and using research knowledge to promote evidence-based practice for nursing. The answers to these exercises are in Appendix A.

RELEVANT TERMS

Directions: Match each term with its correct definition.

Terms

a. Best research evidence
b. Communication of research findings
c. Evidence-based practice
d. Evidence-based practice centers
e. Evidence-based practice guidelines
f. Grove Model for Implementing Evidence-Based Guidelines in Practice
g. Integrative review of research
h. Iowa Model of Evidence-Based Practice
i. Meta-analysis
j. Qualitative research synthesis
k. Stetler Model of Research Utilization to Facilitate Evidence-Based Practice
l. Systematic review

Definitions

_____ 1. A structured, comprehensive synthesis of quantitative studies in a particular health care area to determine the best research evidence available for expert clinicians to use to promote evidence-based practice.

_____ 2. Developing a research report and disseminating it through presentations and publications to practicing nurses, other health care professionals, policy makers, and consumers.

_____ 3. A process of statistically pooling the results from previous studies into a single quantitative analysis that provides the highest level of evidence for an intervention's efficacy.

_____ 4. Quality research knowledge produced by the conduct and synthesis of numerous high-quality studies in a health-related area.

_____ 5. Patient care guidelines that are based on synthesized research findings from meta-analyses, integrative reviews of research, systematic reviews, and extensive clinical trials; supported by consensus from recognized national experts; and affirmed by outcomes obtained by clinicians.

_____ 6. A process that includes the identification, analysis, and synthesis of research findings from independent quantitative and sometimes qualitative studies to determine the current knowledge (what is known and not known) in a particular area.

_____ 7. This is a comprehensive framework to enhance the use of research findings by nurses that includes the phases of preparation, validation, comparative evaluation/decision making, translation/application, and evaluation.

_____ 8. Model developed by one of the textbook authors to promote the use of evidence-based guidelines in practice.

_____ 9. Centers designated by the Agency for Healthcare Research and Quality for the development or research in designated areas and the translation of the evidence-based research findings into clinical practice.

_____ 10. A process and product of systematically reviewing and formally integrating the findings from qualitative studies.

_____ 11. A model developed by Titler and colleagues in 1994 and revised in 2001 that directs the development of evidence-based practice in a clinical agency.

_____ 12. A practice that involves the conscientious integration of best research evidence with clinical expertise and patient values and needs in the delivery of quality, cost-effective health care.

KEY IDEAS

Directions: Fill in the blanks, or provide the appropriate responses.

1. List three reasons nursing needs to develop an evidence-based practice.

   a.

   b.

   c.

2. Identify three sources you might access to keep current with the research literature.

   a.

   b.

   c.

3. Identify the three criticisms of evidence-based practice in nursing.

   a.

   b.

   c.

4. Identify three reasons why nursing lacks the research evidence needed for implementing an evidence-based practice.

   a.

   b.

   c.

5. Identify and describe three ways that research findings might be implemented in nursing practice that were discussed in Stetler's Model of Research Utilization to Facilitate Evidence-Based Practice.

   a. Identify:

   Description:

   b. Identify:

   Description:

   c. Identify:

   Description:

6. Identify two sources of summaries of nursing research knowledge.

   a.

   b.

7. Identify the five phases of the Stetler Model of Research Utilization to Facilitate Evidence-Based Practice.

   a.

   b.

   c.

   d.

   e.

8. The comparative evaluation phase of Stetler's Model includes four parts: substantiating evidence, fit of the setting,

   _____, and _____ _____.

9. Identify the three options of the decision-making phase of the Stetler's Model.

   a.

   b.

   c.

10. The _____ Model was developed in 1994 and revised in 2001 to promote evidence-based practice in nursing.

11. The Joint National Committee on Prevention, Detection, Evaluation, and Treatment of High Blood Pressure (JNC VII)

    guideline that was published in 2003 is an example of _____ _____.

Chapter **27**   **Strategies for Promoting Evidence-Based Nursing Practice**

12. The National Guideline Clearinghouse (NGC) website was developed by the Agency for _____

_____ and _____.

13. The NGC is maintained by a partnership with two organizations:

a.

b.

14. In 1997, the Agency for Healthcare Research and Quality established 12 _____

_____ centers to promote the conduct of research and the development of evidence-based guidelines for practice.

15. The goal of the Grove Model for Implementing Evidence-Based Guidelines in Practice is _____.

MAKING CONNECTIONS

Directions: Match the phase in Stetler's Model with the appropriate description or example.

Phase
a. Comparative evaluation/decision making
b. Evaluation
c. Preparation
d. Translation/application
e. Validation

Descriptions

_____ 1. The phase where nurses evaluate the feasibility of using the Braden scale to prevent pressure ulcers in their clinical agency.

_____ 2. The phase where nurses develop a formal protocol for treatment of stage IV pressure ulcers in the elderly.

_____ 3. The first awareness of the existence of an exercise program for severely disabled children obtained from attending a research conference and reading the study and similar studies in research journals.

_____ 4. Research knowledge about prevention of hospitalized infections is synthesized and evaluated using specific criteria.

_____ 5. The incidence of hospital-acquired infections is examined following the implementation of a new protocol to prevent infections.

GOING BEYOND

1. Answer the following questions about the clinical agency where you are currently doing your clinical hours or where you are working:

a. Are the agency's policies, protocols, or algorithms based on the best research evidence?

b. What is the basis of the policies, protocols, or algorithms if not research?

c. Who are the innovators in this agency who want to base practice on the best research evidence? (Identify them by their positions.)

d. Who might be resistant to change based on current research evidence?

e. Does the agency provide research publications and access to evidence-based websites for nurses? Provide some examples of the publications and websites that you use.

f. Does the agency have the goal of evidence-based practice?

g. Is the agency seeking magnet status?

2. Conduct a project to promote evidence-based practice in a selected area of your practice. Use the following steps as a guide:

a. Identify a clinical problem that might be improved by using the most current research knowledge.

b. Locate and review the studies and evidence-based websites in this problem area. (A list of integrated reviews of research and meta-analyses is provided on the textbook website.) If possible, locate a synthesis of the research literature in this problem area.

c. Select a model or theory to direct your use of research evidence in practice, such as Stetler's Model of Research Utilization to Facilitate Evidence-Based Practice or the Iowa Model of Evidence-Based Practice.

d. Assess your agency's readiness to make the change.

e. Communicate the evidence-based change proposed to the nursing personnel, other health professionals, and administration.

f. Support those persons involved in making the evidence-based change in practice.

g. Implement the evidence-based change by developing a protocol, algorithm, or policy to be used in practice.

h. Develop evaluation strategies to determine the effect of the evidence-based change on patient, provider, and agency outcomes.

i. Evaluate overtime to determine whether the evidence-based change should be continued. You might also extend the change to additional units or clinical agencies.

3. Use the Grove Model for Implementing Evidence-Based Guidelines in Practice to implement an evidence-based guideline from the Agency for Healthcare Research and Quality website in your practice.

Chapter **27**   **Strategies for Promoting Evidence-Based Nursing Practice**

28 Writing Research Proposals

INTRODUCTION

Read Chapter 28, and then complete the following exercises. These exercises will help you to understand the process of writing a research proposal and receiving approval to conduct the study. The answers to these exercises are in Appendix A.

RELEVANT TERMS

Directions: Match each term with its correct definition.

Terms

a. Approval process
b. Condensed proposal
c. Preproposal

d. Research proposal
e. Verbal defense of a proposal

Definitions

_____ 1. A written, detailed plan for conducting a study that includes the elements of a study, such as problem, purpose, literature review, framework, and methodology.

_____ 2. Presentation and clarification of the proposed research project to the members of the agency's institutional review board.

_____ 3. A short document (four to five pages plus appendixes) written to explore the funding possibilities for a research project.

_____ 4. A process implemented by a researcher to obtain permission to conduct a study.

_____ 5. A proposal of limited length that is developed for review by clinical agencies and funding institutions.

KEY IDEAS

Directions: Fill in the blanks, or provide the appropriate responses.

1. A quality proposal is clear, _____, and _____.

2. Writing a quality proposal involves the following:

   a.

   b.

c.

d.

3. A commonly used format in developing a nursing research proposal is the _____ (APA) format.

4. A quantitative research proposal usually includes the following sections:

a.

b.

c.

d.

5. Identify at least four areas included in presenting a design for quasi-experimental and experimental studies:

a.

b.

c.

d.

6. Conducting research in a clinical agency requires approval by the _____ (IRB).

7. Identify at least three content areas covered in the introduction section of a qualitative research proposal.

a.

b.

c.

8. List at least three areas that are included in a preproposal:

a.

b.

c.

9. Clinical agencies and health care corporations review studies for the following reasons:

    a.

    b.

    c.

10. As part of the approval process, the researcher must determine the agency's policy regarding presentation and publication of the study that include the following:

    a.

    b.

    c.

11. If a study is funded, changes in a study must be discussed with the _____

    _____.

12. List the questions that a researcher needs to address before revising a research project.

    a.

    b.

    c.

MAKING CONNECTIONS

Directions: Match the processes listed here with the steps that follow. Select the process that is most likely to be linked to each step.

Processes
a. Proposal development process
b. Approval process for research

Steps

_____ 1. Requires developing an esthetically appealing copy.

_____ 2. Involves examining the impact of conducting the study on the reviewing institution.

_____ 3. Includes an introduction, review of relevant literature, framework, and methods and procedures sections.

_____ 4. Involves examining the social and political factors in an agency where the study is to be conducted.

_____ 5. Includes a verbal defense of the proposed study to the agency's institutional review board (IRB).

1. Identify a significant nursing problem, and develop a research proposal to direct the investigation of this problem. Use the guidelines in Chapter 28 of your text as a basis for developing the proposal, and seek the assistance or your instructor in revising and formulating the final proposal. Also review the example proposals on the Evolve Learning Resources website: http://evolve.elsevier.com/Burns/practice.

2. Identify an agency where your proposed study might be conducted. Seek approval from that agency to conduct your study.

29 Seeking Funding for Research

INTRODUCTION

Read Chapter 29, and then complete the following exercises. These exercises will help you to learn relevant terms and understand the process of seeking funding for research. The answers to these exercises are in Appendix A.

RELEVANT TERMS

Directions: Match each term with its correct definition.

Terms

a. Developmental grant
b. Funded research
c. Grantsmanship
d. Foundation grant
e. Mentor
f. Networking
g. Pink sheet
h. Query letter
i. Reference group
j. Request for application (RFA)
k. Request for proposals (RFP)
l. Research grant
m. Researcher-initiated proposal

Definitions

_____ 1. Research that is supported financially and possibly in other ways (e.g., technically) by a government or private agency.

_____ 2. A letter indicating rejection of a research grant proposal and a critique by the scientific committee that reviewed the proposal.

_____ 3. A process of developing channels of communication between people with common research interests throughout the country.

_____ 4. Published in the Federal Register, this announcement calls for researchers to develop a proposal for a study around a topic of interest to a federal government agency. Researchers have the freedom to design the study as they see fit, and the proposals are judged competitively.

_____ 5. Skills needed to obtain external funding for research.

_____ 6. In these proposals, the idea for the study comes from the researcher who contacts the appropriate government agency or foundation to investigate the organization's interest in and likelihood of funding the researcher's proposal.

_____ 7. Individuals who share common values, ways of thinking, or activities, or any combination of these traits.

_____ 8. A grant from a private organization that funds research based on its own set priorities.

_____ 9. Funding awarded specifically for conducting a study.

_____ 10. Proposals written to obtain funding for the development of a new program in a discipline.

_____ 11. A contract for which researcher's bid consisting of identification of a researchable problem by a government agency and identification by that agency of the design to be followed in the study of the problem.

_____ 12. Someone who provides information, advice, and emotional support to a novice or protégé.

_____ 13. A letter sent to an editor of a journal to determine interest in publishing an article or a letter sent to a funding agency to determine interest in funding a study.

KEY IDEAS

Directions: Fill in the blanks, or provide the appropriate responses.

1. As the control of variance and the complexity of the design increase, the cost of the study tends to

   _____.

2. _____ _____ and funding for research are interrelated.

3. _____ _____ may be stepping stones to larger grants.

4. Funding agencies are usually more supportive of researchers who do what?

5. An aspiring researcher needs to initiate a(n) _____ of _____ in a specific area of study.

6. What can help researchers become better able to critique their own proposals and revise them?

7. Obtaining _____ _____ often provide the first step in becoming recognized as a credible researcher.

8. The book most useful in determining funding available from foundations is the _____

   _____.

9. In preparing a proposal to submit to a foundation, the _____ _____ need to be followed carefully.

10. The largest source of grant monies is the _____ _____.

11. The most complete source of information on federal funding sources is the _____

    _____ _____ _____.

12. If a researcher is preparing a researcher-initiated proposal for federal funding, it is useful to:

13. RFPs are published in the _____ _____.

14. Because a number of researchers will be responding to the same RFP and only one or a few proposals will be

    approved, these proposals are considered _____ _____.

15. An RFA is similar to an RFP except that with the RFA, the government agency:

    a.

    b.

16. After submission, a federal proposal is assigned to a(n) _____ _____ for scientific evaluation.

17. Receipt of money to initiate a federal grant may not occur for up to _____ after submission of the proposal.

18. When must a researcher begin to seek funding for a second grant?

MAKING CONNECTIONS

1. List four strategies that can be used to gain skills in grantsmanship.

   a.

   b.

   c.

   d.

2. List four sources of small grant funding.

   a.

   b.

   c.

   d.

PUZZLES

Word Scramble
Directions: Unscramble the following sentence by rearranging the letters to form actual words. Note: You will use all the letters in every word.

Lewl-geseddin dusties nac eb sexpivene.

Chapter **29** **Seeking Funding for Research**

Secret Message

Directions: Translate the following secret message by substituting one letter for another. For example, if you decide that "x" should really be "t," then "x" will be "t" every time it appears in this puzzle. Hint: Try to translate short words first to establish vowel patterns.

Xfi ukeizxehek kvijelebexo yh xfi xvyhiuueyz eu vibmtij xy xfi wsmblxo yh uxsjeiu kyzjskxij

lo exu viuimvkfivu.

Crossword Puzzle

Directions: Complete the crossword puzzle. Note: If the answer is more than one word, there are no blank spaces left between the words.

Across

1. Grant-supported study.
6. Form sent from government agency rejecting and critiquing a proposal.
8. Advisor.
9. Calls for research on a government-identified topic.
10. Skill in writing proposals.
11. Funds intended to pay for a study.
12. Proposal to fulfill government contract.

Down

2. A number of people with common interests and aspirations.
3. Connection with researchers who have common interests.
4. Funding by a private agency.
5. Proposal to implement a new program.
7. Inquiry about the interest of a journal in publishing an article.

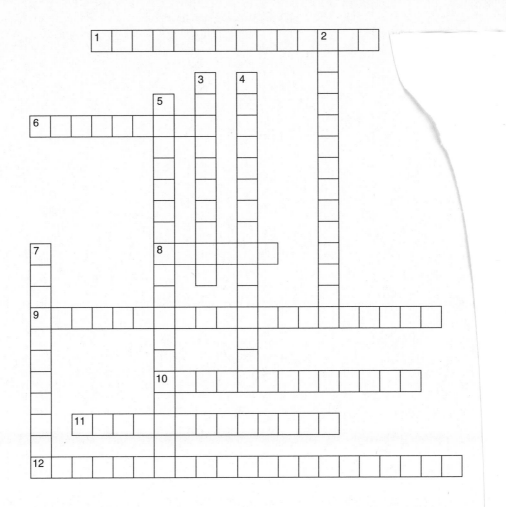

GOING BEYOND

1. Ask a faculty member for permission to read a research proposal for which he or she has received fundi

2. Ask a faculty member for permission to read a research proposal that was not funded and the associated   sheet.

Appendix A: Answers to Study Guide Exercises

CHAPTER 1

Relevant Terms
Framework for Nursing Research
1. i   6. l   11. f
2. j   7. n   12. g
3. b   8. d   13. k
4. m   9. e   14. c
5. h   10. a

Types of Reasoning
1. c   4. f
2. e   5. d
3. a   6. b

Key Ideas
1. Description involves identifying the nature and attributes of nursing phenomena. Descriptive knowledge generated through research can be used to identify and describe what exists in nursing practice, discover new information, promote understanding of situations, and classify information for use in the discipline. Some examples of research evidence developed from studies focused on description include identification of the responses of individuals to a variety of health conditions; description of the health promotion and illness-prevention strategies used by a variety of populations; determination of the incidence of a disease locally, nationally, and internationally; identification of the cluster of symptoms for a particular disease; and description of the effects and side effects of selected pharmacological agents in a variety of populations.
2. Explanation focuses on clarifying relationships among phenomena and identifies the reasons why certain events occur. Research focused on explanation provides the following types of evidence essential for practice: the determination of the assessment data (both subjective data from the health history and objective data from physical exam) that need to be gathered to address a patient's health need; the link of assessment data to determine a diagnosis (both nursing and medical); the link of causative risk factors or etiologies to illness, morbidity, and mortality; and the determination of the relationships among health risks, health status, and health care costs.
3. Prediction involves estimating the probability of a specific outcome in a given situation. With predictive knowledge, nurses can anticipate the effects certain nursing interventions might have on patients and families. Knowledge generated from research focused on prediction is critical for evidence-based practice and includes examples such as prediction of the risk for a disease in different populations; prediction of the accuracy and precision of a screening instrument, such as mammogram, to detect a disease; prediction of the prognosis once an illness is identified in a variety of populations; prediction of behaviors that promote health and prevent illness; and prediction of the health care required based on a patient's need and values.
4. Control is the ability to manipulate a situation to produce the desired outcome(s). With research evidence at the control level, nurses could provide evidence-based care to produce the desired quality health outcomes. Examples of research focused on control include testing interventions to improve the health status of individuals, families, and communities; testing interventions to improve health care delivery; determining the quality and cost-effectiveness of interventions; and implementing an evidence-based intervention to determine if it is effective in managing a patient's health need (health promotion, illness prevention, acute and chronic illness management, and rehabilitation) to produce quality outcomes.

Making Connections
1. You could have identified any of the following ways of acquiring knowledge in nursing. Some possible examples of each way of acquiring nursing knowledge are provided.
   a. Tradition: giving patients a bath everyday in the morning.
   b. Authority: expert clinical nurses, educators, and authors of articles or books.
   c. Borrowing: using knowledge from medicine or psychology to provide nursing care.
   d. Trial and error: trying a particular position to reduce a patient's discomfort during labor.
   e. Personal experience: obtaining knowledge by being in a clinical agency and providing care to patients and families.
   f. Role modeling: a new graduate in an internship is mentored by an expert nurse who role-models quality nursing care behaviors for the new graduate.
   g. Intuition: knowing that a patient's condition is deteriorating but having no concrete data to support this feeling or hunch.
   h. Reasoning: reasoning from the general to the specific (deductive reasoning); reasoning from the specific to the general (inductive reasoning).
   i. Research: quantitative and qualitative research methods.
2. personal experience
3. Novice, advanced beginner, competent, proficient, and expert
4. borrow
5. Research or empirical
6. intuition
7. Traditions
8. mentors or role models
9. role-model
10. inductive and deductive
11. Deductive reasoning

12. Use the content in your textbook on Acquiring Knowledge in Nursing to determine the knowledge base for each of the interventions you identified. Nursing knowledge is acquired through tradition, authority, borrowing, trial and error, personal experience, role-modeling, intuition, reasoning, and research. Some of the interventions you identified include more than one type of knowledge to implement.

13. You need to examine the interventions you use in clinical practice and decide which way of acquiring knowledge you use most frequently: tradition, authority, borrowing, trial and error, personal experience, role-modeling, intuition, reasoning, or research. It is important that you increase your use of research-based interventions to promote evidence-based practice.

14. Examine the care you provide your patients, and indicate if this care is based on the best research evidence or on other types of knowledge. Provide a rationale for the care delivered. There is an increasing emphasis in medicine and nursing on evidence-based practice.

15. Evidence-based practice is essential for the delivery of the highest quality of care to and to ensure quality outcomes for patients, families, providers, and health care agencies.

16. The American Nurses Association (2003) identified the following areas of focus for nursing knowledge: promotion of health and safety; care and self-care processes; physical, emotional, and spiritual comfort, discomfort, and pain; adaptation to physiological and pathophysiological processes; emotions related to experiences of birth, growth, and development, health, illness, disease, and death; meanings ascribed to health and illness; decision making and ability to make choices; relationships, role performance, and change processes within relationships; social policies and their effects on the health of individuals, families, and communities; health care systems and their relationships with access to and quality of health care; and the environment and the prevention of disease (Burns & Grove, 2009).

17. The types of research conducted in nursing include quantitative, qualitative, outcomes, and intervention research.

18. A variety of philosophical beliefs could be identified, including the holistic perspective in providing health care, the importance of the family in caring for a patient, providing access to care for patients regardless of their financial status, and providing physical, emotional, and social care to the patient and family.

19. evidence-based practice

20. Evidence-based practice includes best research evidence, clinical expertise of the health care professional, and values and needs of the patient and family.

Puzzles

Theory, empirical world (nursing practice), science, and abstract thought processes. (There are *indirect* links of nursing research to philosophy, knowledge, and ways of knowing.)

Word Scramble

"Nursing research is directly linked to the world of nursing."

CHAPTER 2

Relevant Terms
Methodologies Used to Develop Research Evidence in Nursing

1. c	6. a	11. k
2. e	7. f	12. d
3. j	8. l	13. b
4. m	9. n	14. i
5. o	10. g	15. h

Processes for Synthesizing Research Evidence for Practice

1. e	3. b	5. d
2. c	4. a	

Key Ideas

1. Nightingale
2. 1952
3. ANA Council of Nurse Researchers
4. research
5. Archie Cochrane
6. *Research in Nursing & Health*
7. *Scholarly Inquiry for Nursing Practice, Applied Nursing Research*, or *Nursing Science Quarterly*
8. Conduct and Utilization of Research in Nursing (CURN)
9. Summaries of current research knowledge in the areas of nursing practice, nursing care delivery, nursing education, and the profession of nursing
10. 1985
11. National Institute for Nursing Research (NINR)
12. Quantitative research
13. You may have identified any of the following areas of emphasis in the NINR mission:
    a. Conduct of biological research
    b. Conduct of clinical research
    c. Communication of research findings
    d. Promotion of evidence-based practice for nursing
14. outcomes
15. research evidence
16. Agency for Health Care Policy and Research (AHCPR)
17. evidence-based
18. Agency for Healthcare Research and Quality (AHRQ)
19. The goals of AHRQ are as follows:
    a. Support improvements in health outcomes
    b. Strengthen quality measurements and improvements
    c. Identify strategies to improve access, foster appropriate use of health care resources, and reduce unnecessary expenditures
20. Foci of *Healthy People* 2010 are health promotion and illness prevention.
21. Systematic review of experimental studies (well-controlled randomized clinical trials)
22. Opinions of respected authorities based on clinical evidence, reports of experts, and committees
23. Meta-analyses of experimental (randomized clinical trials) and quasi-experimental studies

Making Connections
Synthesis Processes

1. b	5. e	8. b
2. c	6. a	9. e
3. a	7. c	10. d
4. d		

Research Methods

1. b	5. a	8. a
2. b	6. a	9. b
3. a	7. a	10. a
4. b		

Nurses' Educational Preparation

1. a	5. b
2. e	6. c
3. b	7. d or e
4. d	

Puzzles
Word Scramble

"Both quantitative and qualitative research methods are essential to nursing knowledge. Research knowledge is needed to promote evidence-based nursing practice."

Exercises in Critical Appraisal
Research Types

1. b
2. b
3. a

CHAPTER 3

Relevant Terms
Steps of the Research Process

1. q	8. m	14. b
2. c	9. o	15. r
3. l	10. s	16. d
4. g	11. p	17. k
5. n	12. j	18. i
6. a	13. h	19. e
7. f		

Types of Study Settings

1. b	3. a	5. c
2. c	4. a	6. b or c

Key Ideas
Control in Quantitative Research

1. highly controlled
2. quasi-experimental, experimental
3. Descriptive, correlational
4. Experimental
5. nonrandom, random
6. Basic research
7. highly controlled
8. experimental
9. partially controlled
10. Quasi-experimental

Steps of the Research Process

1. Quantitative research process
2. Step 1: Formulate a research problem and purpose
   Step 2: Review relevant literature
   Step 3: Develop a framework
   Step 4: Formulate research objectives, questions, or hypotheses
   Step 5: Define research variables
   Step 6: Make assumptions explicit
   Step 7: Identify limitations
   Step 8: Select a research design
   Step 9: Define the population and sample
   Step 10: Select methods of measurement
   Step 11: Develop a plan for data collection and analysis
   Step 12: Implement the research plan
   Step 13: Communicate research findings
3. You could identify any of the following assumptions (Williams, 1980, p. 48):
   a. People want to assume control of their own health problems.
   b. Stress should be avoided.
   c. People are aware of the experiences that most affect their life choices.
   d. Health is a priority for most people.
   e. People in underserved areas feel underserved.
   f. Most measurable attitudes are held strongly enough to direct behavior.
   g. Health professionals view health care in a different manner than do laypersons.
   h. People operate on the basis of cognitive information.
   i. Increased knowledge about an event lowers anxiety about the event.
   j. People would rather receive health care at home than in an institution.
4. a. Methodological limitations
   b. Theoretical limitations
5. Methodological limitations include such factors as a nonrepresentative sample, small sample size, weak design with threats to design validity, single setting, instruments with limited reliability and validity, limited control over data collection, weak implementation of the treatment, and improper use of statistical analyses.
6. theoretical limitation
7. You could identify any of the following reasons for conducting a pilot study:
   a. To determine whether the proposed study is feasible (e.g., Are the subjects available? Does the researcher have the time and money to do the study?)
   b. To develop or refine a research treatment
   c. To develop a protocol for the implementation of a treatment
   d. To identify problems with the design
   e. To determine whether the sample represents the population or whether the sampling technique is effective
   f. To examine the reliability and validity of the research instruments
   g. To develop or refine data collection instruments

h. To refine the data collection and analysis plan
i. To give the researcher experience with the subjects, setting, methodology, and methods of measurement
j. To try out data analysis

Making Connections

1. c	8. b	15. c
2. a	9. c	16. a
3. b	10. d	17. c
4. a	11. b	18. c
5. c	12. a	19. a
6. d	13. c	20. c
7. a	14. a	

Puzzles

Word Scramble

"Quantitative research methods include descriptive, correlational, quasi-experimental, and experimental studies."

Crossword Puzzle

Across	Down
2. Design	1. Outcome
4. Quantitative	2. Data
8. Problem	3. Study
9. Hypothesis	5. Assumptions
10. Basic	6. Variable
12. Measurement	7. Literature
14. Framework	11. Control
16. Setting	13. Process
17. Rigor	15. Applied
18. Sample	
19. Question	

Exercises in Critical Appraisal

1. b. Bindler et al. conducted a correlational study to examine the relationships of serum insulin levels to metabolic syndrome criteria in schoolchildren.
2. c. Sethares and Elliott conducted a quasi-experimental study with a treatment for patients with heart failure.
3. e. Wright conducted a phenomenological qualitative study of recovery from substance abuse.
4. a
5. a
6. a

Going Beyond

The section on making connections includes several ideas for quantitative studies.

CHAPTER 4

Relevant Terms

1. a	4. g	7. d
2. b	5. c	8. j
3. i	6. h	

Key Ideas

1. discovering
2. wholes or holistic
3. outside, phenomenon
4. stance or philosophy
5. lived
6. reality
7. created, situations or events
8. "portrait of a people"
9. culture
10. have we come from, are we, are we going
11. structure, valuing
12. principles, ethical
13. critical social theory
14. a. Phenomenological research
    b. Grounded theory research
    c. Ethnographic research
    d. Historical research
    e. Philosophical inquiry
    f. Critical social theory
15. a. Foundational inquiry
    b. Philosophical analysis
    c. Ethical analysis

Making Connections

Any three of the following characteristics would be correct.
a. Openness
b. Scrupulous adherence to a philosophical perspective
c. Thoroughness in collecting data
d. Consideration of all the data

Understanding Qualitative Research Methods

1. c	6. c	11. b
2. a	7. d	12. d
3. b	8. d	13. a
4. c	9. d	14. b
5. a	10. c	15. d

Linking Qualitative Philosophies and Methods with Types of Qualitative Research

a. Critical social theory
b. Grounded theory research
c. Phenomenological research
d. Historical research
e. Philosophical inquiry
f. Ethnographic research

Puzzles

Crossword Puzzle

Across	Down
1. Emergent fit	2. Foundations
3. Ethnonursing	4. Culture
5. Deconstruct	9. Reconstructing
6. Material	11. Philosophical
7. Participatory	12. Intervention
8. Grounded	13. Ethnographic
10. Rigor	15. Cognitive
14. Ethics	17. Context
16. Phenomenological	19. Discovery
18. Being	
20. Ethnoscientific	
21. Descriptive	
22. Sedimented	
23. Embodied	
24. Situated	

Word Scramble

"Once you have ascended to the open context, you cannot go back to the idea that the phenomenon you have observed can be seen only one way."

Secret Message

"It is critical to understand the philosophy on which each qualitative method is based." (Do you know your Greek letters?)

Exercises in Critical Appraisal

1. The philosophical perspectives of Frankl provide the conceptual orientation for this study—the meaning of life differs from person to person, day to day, and hour to hour

2. Journaling and discussing preconceived ideas, past experiences, and thoughts after interviewing may be indicative of the internal process of ascending to an open construct.

3. Giorgi's method.

4. Credibility was established via prolonged engagement with the subject matter: Bracketing (journaling) throughout data collection and analysis.

   Notes regarding beliefs, presuppositions, and past experiences with spirituality and recovery from substance abuse as well as thoughts after interviews were recorded and discussed with senior researchers.

   Journaling served to establish confirmability as an audit trail was established by presenting data from the beginning where naive meaning units were identified, to clustering, to themes, and finally to essential descriptions.

Going Beyond

Select two to three qualitative studies from nursing research journals. Identify the philosophical base, research questions, sampling process, data collection and analysis strategies, and outcomes for these studies. Ask your instructor to review your work, or collaborate with another student to increase your understanding of the types of qualitative research.

CHAPTER 5

Relevant Terms

1. b	5. f	8. j
2. h	6. i	9. d
3. g	7. c	10. e
4. a		

Key Ideas

1. a. Goal of the study
   b. Variables
   c. Population
   d. Setting

2. Any of the following responses might be given:
   a. Has an impact on nursing practice
   b. Builds on previous research
   c. Is used to develop evidence-based practice
   d. Promotes theory development
   e. Promotes theory testing
   f. Addresses current concerns or priorities in nursing and health care

3. landmark, Agency for Healthcare Research and Quality (AHRQ)

4. replicated

5. approximate or operational

6. a. Researchers' expertise
   b. Money commitment
   c. Availability of subjects, facility, and equipment
   d. Study's ethical considerations

7. educational preparation, research, clinical.

8. The common sources of research problems include, but are not limited to, the following:
   a. Nursing practice
   b. Researcher and peer interactions
   c. Literature review: replicating previous studies, using study ideas generated by previous researchers and identifying gaps in the knowledge base of a selected research topic
   d. Theoretical propositions or relationships expressed in theories
   e. Research priorities identified by funding agencies and specialty groups and organizations

9. The priority goals of outcomes research include the following, but other goals might be listed that would improve the outcomes for patients, families, providers, and health care agencies:
   a. Avoid adverse effects of care
   b. Improve the patient's physiological, mental, and social status
   c. Reduce the patient's signs and symptoms of illness
   d. Improve the patient's functional status and well-being
   e. Achieve patient satisfaction
   f. Minimize the cost of care
   g. Maximize revenues of care
   h. Improve access to care
   i. Improve the quality of care delivered by providers
   j. Improve the quality of care provided by health care agencies

231

10. research topics
11. research purposes

Making Connections

1. g	6. j	11. h
2. c	7. e	12. a
3. h	8. i	13. j
4. f	9. d	14. g
5. a	10. c	15. d

Exercises in Critical Appraisal

Bindler, Massey, Shultz, Mills, and Short Study

1. a. Significance of the problem: "One in four Americans is at risk for developing metabolic syndrome (Ford, Giles, & Diets, 2002; Roberts, Dunn, Jean, & Lardinois, 2000). Life-style, environment, and genetic component are influential in the syndrome.... Due to an epidemic in youth obesity and sedentary behaviors, there is an increasing need to describe the factors associated with the development of insulin resistance in youths" (Bindler et al., 2007, p. 293).

   b. Background of the problem: "Metabolic syndrome, also known as dysmetabolic syndrome, syndrome X, or insulin resistance syndrome, is characterized by a group of risk factors and is often a precursor to both diabetes and cardiovascular disease. These risk factors cluster in individuals and populations, both in adults and in youths.... These criteria reflect the major metabolic components of the syndrome, which are abdominal obesity, atherogenic dyslipidemia, increased blood pressure (BP), insulin resistance, proinflammatory state, and prothrombotic state (Grundy, Brewer, Cleeman, Smith, & Lenfant, 2004). Other groups have recommended somewhat different criteria, leading to confusion among clinicians (see Table 1 for a summary of adult criteria recommendations for metabolic syndrome) (Zimmet, Magliano, Matsuzawa, Alberti, & Shaw, 2005)" (Bindler et al., 2007, p. 293).

   c. Problem statement: "Children in general, and those from Native American and Hispanic groups, in particular, are underrepresented in diabetes and cardiovascular disease origins research. There is scant application of identification methods for metabolic syndrome in the nursing literature. More information is needed to establish the contribution of various characteristics to insulin resistance in children, and translational research is needed so that findings can be applied by nurses and other health professionals in pediatric settings. Descriptive data about children, particularly from disparate ethnic groups, will help to identify children at highest risk so that appropriate interventions can be identified. Clear guidelines for nurses will assist in applying findings about metabolic syndrome to pediatric settings with youths" (Bindler et al., 2007, p. 296). This study includes several problem statements that clearly indicate what is not known and provide a basis for this study.

2. Study purpose: "The purpose of this study was to describe serum insulin levels and to investigate their relationships to metabolic syndrome criteria in a multiethnic sample of school children" (Bindler et al., 2007, p. 296).

3. The problem and purpose are significant because of the increasing number of obese, sedentary school-age children who are at risk for developing metabolic syndrome. Research has documented that those developing this insulin-resistance syndrome are at increased risk for diabetes and cardiovascular disease. Because metabolic syndrome is caused by lifestyle choices of diet and exercise that can be altered, it is important to identify the children at risk and to provide appropriate interventions. Care of children requires a unique knowledge base for nurses to provide interventions that promote health and prevent illness, such as metabolic syndrome. In addition, identifying and treating children with metabolic syndrome can greatly improve their future health and decrease health care costs.

4. Yes, the variables, population, and settings are identified.
   a. This is a predictive correlational study. The dependent variable of insulin level was predicted using the independent variables of metabolic syndrome criteria of gender, age, race, BMI percentile, glucose, triglycerides, HDL-C, systolic blood pressure, and diastolic blood pressure.
   b. Population: School-age children attending fourth to eighth grades.
   c. Settings: Public elementary and middle schools in a predominately agricultural area of central Washington State.

5. The problem and purpose are feasible because (1) the study was funded by a Sigma Theta Chapter and Washington State University College of Nursing; (2) Bindler had previous research in this area and clinical expertise and the other researchers had educational and clinical expertise to conduct this study, as discussed in Chapter 2 of this study guide; (3) adequate subjects were available to participate in the study because the population was school-age children and the settings were public elementary and middle schools; (4) school personnel were supportive of the study; (5) arrangements were made to obtain the blood samples needed for the study and to conduct the laboratory analysis of the serum; and (6) the study was ethical and protected the rights of the subjects.

Sethares and Elliott Study

1. a. Significance of the problem: "Cardiovascular disease, the leading cause of death in the United States today, is one of the most prevalent chronic illnesses of adulthood. A common clinical endpoint of many cardiovascular disorders if heart failure (HF).... The American College of Cardiology/American Heart Association Task Force reports that 4.8 million Americans experience HF, with 550,000 new cases and 50,000 deaths reported annually. In 1999, 962,000 Americans were discharged from acute care facilities with a primary diagnosis of HF, the most prevalent diagnosis in those aged more than 65 year" (Sethares & Elliott, 2004, p. 270).

   b. Background of the problem: "HF is characterized by an unstable course of illness with unpredictable exacerbations and progression of symptoms, often without further damage to the myocardium....Because HF is a chronic condition, most lifestyle change is made on an outpatient basis, necessitating follow-up in the home setting to evaluate

232

medication effectiveness, monitor symptoms, and promote self-care behaviors. However, current capitation rates fiscally limit the quality of nursing care provided in the home" (Sethares & Elliott, 2004, p. 270).

c. Problem statement: "It is imperative that nurses develop innovative methods to improve the self-care behaviors of this population while attempting to decrease costly rehospitalizations. A tailored message intervention is one proposed alternative" (Sethares & Elliott, 2004, p. 270).

2. Study purpose: The purpose of this study is to "determine the efficacy of a tailored message intervention administered during hospital admission and at 1 week and 1 month after discharge on HF readmission rates, reported quality of life, and perceived benefit and barrier beliefs in elderly patients with HF" (Sethares & Elliott, 2004, p. 270).

3. The problem and purpose are significant because a large number of adults are affected by HF and this is such a costly chronic illness. Nurses are uniquely positioned to educate patients and assist them in coping with chronic illnesses such as HF. Research is needed to find more effective interventions to assist patients with HF.

4. Yes, the variables, population, and settings are identified in the study purpose.

   a. The independent variable is tailored message intervention, and the dependent variables are HF readmission rates, reported quality of life, and perceived benefit and barrier beliefs. Thus, the study had one intervention and four outcome variables.

   b. Population: Elderly patients with HF.

   c. Settings: Both hospital and homes of patients.

5. The problem and purpose are feasible because (1) the study was funded by a grant from the University of Massachusetts Dartmouth Foundation; (2) researchers had research and clinical expertise, as discussed in Chapter 2 of this study guide; (3) adequate subjects were available to participate in the study; (4) hospital personnel were supportive of the study; (5) no special equipment was needed for the study; and (6) the study was ethical and protected the rights of the subjects.

Wright Study

1. a. Significance of the problem: "Recovery from substance abuse is a recovery phenomenon that is of importance to nursing. Reports in the literature indicate that recovery from substance abuse is a complex multidimensional process that occurs both with and without expert assistance.... The recidivism rate for substance abusers has been reported to be at 90% 12 months after treatment, with most relapses occurring after 3 months" (Wright, 2003, p. 281).

   b. Background of the problem: "For many African American women recovering from substance abuse, current treatment modalities, and self-help groups do not meet their needs (Hooks, 1993; Nelson-Zlupko, Dore, Kauffman, & Kaltenbach, 1996), because mainstream treatment of substance abuse has traditionally been developed and implemented by male providers for male clients (Abbott, 1994; Reed, 1985). ... Research suggests that women may benefit from substance abuse programs that include a residential component, as well as gender-specific services (Dempsey

& Wenner, 1996; Nelson-Zlupko et al., 1996). Spirituality has often been noted in the health care literature to affect recovery (Ellison & Levin, 1998; McNichol, 1996; Sloan, Bagiella, & Powell, 1999)" (Wright, 2003, p. 281).

   c. Problem statement: "Whereas a combination of human, social, and economic costs of substance abuse have led to a plethora of research on topics such as the epidemiology of substance abuse, treatment outcomes such as client functioning, relapse phenomena, and most recently matching individual and treatment characteristics (Murphy, 1993), very little is known about recovery from substance abuse in African American women" (Wright, 2003, p. 281).

2. Study purpose: "A qualitative phenomenological research study was designed to explore the essential elements of the lived experience of spirituality among African American women recovering from substance abuse and to describe the meanings made of this phenomenon by the person experiencing it" (Wright, 2003, p. 282).

3. The problem and purpose are significant because they focus on a common problem of substance abuse, which is complex and requires extensive understanding and a variety of strategies to treat. In addition, limited research has been done to facilitate understanding of women and substance abuse treatment and the impact of spirituality on the recovery process. Wright (2003) clearly indicated that the problem is significant to nursing and encouraged nurses to increase their involvement in recognizing and treating African-American women with substance abuse problems.

4. The research concept and population are identified, but not the setting in the study purpose.

   a. Research concept is the lived experience of spirituality in recovery from substance abuse.

   b. Population: African-American women recovering from substance abuse.

   c. Setting: Not identified in the study purpose.

5. The problem and purpose are feasible because (1) the study was conducted on a National Institute of Health (NIH) Unit; (2) researcher had research and clinical expertise, as discussed in Chapter 2 of this study guide; (3) adequate subjects were available to participate in the study; (4) NIH personnel were supportive of this study; (5) no special equipment was needed for the study; and (6) the study was ethical and protected the rights of the subjects.

Going Beyond

Do the exercises as identified, and seek feedback from peers and your instructor. Be sure to select a research problem and purpose that are significant to nursing and of interest to you.

CHAPTER 6

Relevant Terms

1. g		6. h		11. i	
2. k		7. e		12. j	
3. f		8. o		13. a	
4. n		9. c		14. m	
5. l		10. d		15. b	

Key Ideas

1. Choose any five of the following:
   a. Clarify the research topic
   b. Clarify the research problem
   c. Verify the significance of the research problem
   d. Specify the purpose of the study
   e. Describe relevant studies
   f. Describe relevant theories
   g. Summarize current knowledge
   h. Facilitate development of the framework
   i. Specify research objectives, questions, or hypotheses
   j. Define major variables
   k. Identify limitations and assumptions for the study
   l. Select a research design
   m. Identify methods of measurement
   n. Direct data collection and analysis
   o. Facilitate interpretation of findings
2. Advantages of electronic databases:
   a. internationally
   b. quickly, easily, or reliably
   c. full-text
3. a. along paths you have already searched.
   b. retrace.
   c. new
4. theoretical, empirical
5. primary
6. computer, manual
7. 3, 1, 4, 6, 2, 5
8. a. Catalog listings
   b. Indexes
   c. Abstracts
   d. Bibliographies
9. Nursing Studies Index
10. a. Cumulative Index to Nursing and Allied Health (CINAHL)
    b. MEDLINE (MEDical literature analysis and retrieval system onLINE)
11. *Annual Review of Nursing Research*
12. synthesis
13. To store information related to literature sources and to provide in-text citations and reference lists in the correct format.
14. a. Introduction
    b. Theoretical literature
    c. Empirical literature
    d. Summary
15. Key terms to direct the literature review include acute myocardial infarction symptoms, delay treatment for women, and rate of mortality and morbidity for women.
16. Key terms to direct the literature review include smoking prevalence, Appalachian states, heart disease rates, cancer rates, smoking cessation, and transtheoretical model.
17. Key terms to direct the literature review include cancer-related pain, untreated pain, and cancer pain management.
18. a. Limit to English language
    b. Limit the years of your search
    c. Limit the search to only papers that are research, are reviews, are published in consumer health journals, include abstracts, or are available in full text.

19. Identify any four of the following research journals:
    a. *Advances in Nursing Science*
    b. *Applied Nursing Research*
    c. *Biological Research for Nursing*
    d. *Clinical Nursing Research*
    e. *Journal of Nursing Scholarship*
    f. *Nurse Researcher*
    g. *Nursing Inquiry*
    h. *Nursing Research*
    i. *Nursing Science Quarterly*
    j. *Qualitative Health Research*
    k. *Research and Theory for Nursing Practice*
    l. *Research in Nursing & Health*
    m. *Scholarly Inquiry for Nursing Practice*
    n. *Western Journal of Nursing Research*
20. a. Introduction
    b. Methods
    c. Results
    d. Discussion
21. skimming, comprehending, analyzing, synthesizing
22. paraphrase

Making Connections

Purpose of the Literature Review

1. d
2. c
3. a
4. b

Theoretical and Empirical Literature

1. T	5. T	9. T
2. E	6. E	10. T
3. E	7. E	11. E
4. T	8. E	

Primary and Secondary Sources

1. S	3. P	5. S
2. P	4. S	6. P

Exercises in Critical Appraisal

1. a. Title of the journal.
   b. Year the study was published.
   c. Volume number of the journal.
   d. Pages of the article.
   e. Issue number of the journal.
   f. Sethares and Elliott.
2. Bindler, R. C. M., Massey, L. K., Schultz, J. A., Mills, P. E., & Short, R. (2007). Metabolic syndrome in a multiethnic sample of school children: Implications for the pediatric nurse. *Journal of Pediatric Nursing, 22*(1), 43–58.
3. a. Title and page numbers of the article are missing.
   b. Volume number of the journal and page numbers of the article are missing.
   c. Year the article was published and volume and issue numbers of the journal are missing.
4. a. Literature Review.
   b. Part of introduction; no title given.
   c. Review of Literature.

5. Yes. You may have identified any of the following: Ford, Giles, & Dietz, (2002); Roberts, Dunn, Jean, & Lardinois, (2000); Kelley (2000); Ludwig et al. (1999); Mayer-Davis et al., (1997); Cruz et al., (2004); Valdez (2000); Falkner, Hassink, Ross, & Gidding (2002); Golley, Magarey, Steinback, Baur, & Daniels (2006); Steinberger & Daniels (2003).

6. No theories are clearly identified in the article; however, the researchers provided concepts from physiological and pathological theories and link these concepts to the variables.

7. Secondary source.

8. Yes the sources are current. The article was published in 2007. The reference dates range from 1985 to 2006, with the majority of the sources published in the past 5 years.

9. Sethares and Elliott clearly summarized the current knowledge base in intervention studies and transitional care models. These are consistent with the problem and purpose of the study.

10. Yes. You may have listed any of the following: Rich, Beckham, Wittenberg, Leen, Freedland, & Carney (1995); Naylor & McCauley (1999); Bennett, Hays, Embree, & Arnould (2000); Naylor, Brooten, Campbell, Jacobsen, Mezey, Pauly, et al. (1999).

11. a. Becker (1974).
    b. No theory is clearly identified as the framework for the study, but the researchers present concepts from physiological and pathological theories as a basis for their study. These concepts are linked to the study variables.

12. Secondary source.

13. This study was published in 2004, and the reference dates range from 1974 to 2003. The 1974 publications are theoretical papers. Most of the studies cited are in the past 10 years. Thus, the current literature is well covered in the literature review.

14. Yes, the knowledge base of factors that contribute to metabolic syndrome are carefully reviewed and synthesized, particularly as they relate to children of different ethnic origin.

15. Yes. You may have mentioned Prochaska, DiClemente, & Norcross (1992); Murphy (1993); Davis (1997); and Jackson (1995).

16. Yes. You may have mentioned: Watson (1988); Roy (1984); Neuman (1989); and Reed (1992).

17. a. Primary.
    b. Secondary.

18. Yes the sources are current. The study was published in 2003 and the literature cited ranges from 1962 to 2001. Most of the studies were published in the past 5 years with the older sources being predominately theoretical or textbooks describing qualitative research methodology.

19. Yes. However, the knowledge base for African American women recovering from drug addiction was limited. Knowledge of spirituality has been examined for a variety of situations, but none had examined spirituality in relation to recovery from drug addiction in women, particularly not African American women.

Going Beyond

Conduct a literature review using the steps outlined in your study guide. Ask your instructor or a fellow student to review your work and give you feedback. This literature review might become the basis for a thesis, dissertation, or study in your clinical agency.

CHAPTER 7

Relevant Terms

Terms Related to Theory

1. e	6. f
2. b	7. g
3. i	8. j
4. h	9. d
5. a	10. c

Terms Related to Relational Statements

1. g	9. p	17. q
2. c	10. j	18. d
3. w	11. o	19. s
4. m	12. l	20. f
5. e	13. r	21. u
6. t	14. n	22. b
7. a	15. k	23. v
8. h	16. i	

More Terms Related to Statements and Theory

1. d	6. e	11. c
2. n	7. g	12. m
3. b	8. j	13. l
4. a	9. i	14. k
5. f	10. h	

Key Ideas

1. theories	8. constructs
2. validity	9. variable
3. Conceptual models	10. proposition(s) or relationships
4. theory	11. hypotheses
5. effect size	12. contribute, cause
6. framework	13. concepts, arrows, relationships
7. concepts	14. research tradition

Making Connections

1. c	4. f	7. h
2. b	5. a	8. d
3. e	6. i	9. g

Levels of Abstraction

Construct (highest level of abstraction)
Concept
Variable
Operational definition (lowest level of abstraction)

Puzzles

Word Scramble

"Many studies are required to validate all of the statements in a theory."

Secret Message

"You need to determine links among the conceptual definitions, the variables in the study, and the related measurement methods."

Crossword Puzzle

Across	Down
1. Conceptual model	1. Concrete
4. Implicit	2. Theory testing
6. Framework	3. Map
7. Hypothesis	5. Theory
11. Self-care	8. Proposition
12. Abstract	9. Statement
13. Variable	10. Adaptation
14. Tradition	

Exercises in Critical Appraisal

1. Concepts:
   a. Metabolic syndrome
   b. Lifestyle factors
   c. Environment
   d. Genetic component
2. Conceptual definitions:
   a. Metabolic syndrome: a syndrome typified by a decrease in the number of insulin receptors and in their functional abil- ity at the cellular level (insulin resistance) with resultant hyperinsulinemia and development of type 2 diabetes.
   b. Lifestyle factors: high-saturated-fat and low-fiber diets, stress, and physical activity.
   c. Environment: limited opportunity for physical activity and access to fresh and nutritious food choices.
   d. Genetics: certain population groups, such as Native Americans and Hispanic Americans, are at higher risk for metabolic syndrome.
3. Variables:
   a. Glucose   e. Triglycerides   i. Physical   m. Ethnicity
   b. TC   f. Insulin level   fitness
   c. HDL-C   g. Blood   j. Body fat
   d. LDL-C   pressure   k. Diet
                h. Smoking   l. Family
                   history   history
4. Relationship between concepts and variables:
   a. Metabolic syndrome:
      Glucose   Insulin
      TC, HDL-C, LDL-C   Blood pressure
      Triglycerides
   b. Lifestyle and environmental factors:
      Smoking history
      Physical fitness
      Body fat
      Diet
   c. Genetic component:
      Family history
      Ethnicity

5.

Concepts	Variables	Measurement Methods
Metabolic syndrome	Glucose	Blood draw
	TC, HDL-C, LDL-C	Blood draw
	Triglycerides	Blood draw
	Insulin level	Blood draw
	BP	BP cuff
Lifestyle	Smoking hx	Questionnaire
	Physical fitness	Canadian Aerobic Fitness Test $\rightarrow$ VO$_{2max}$ Godon Leisure Time Questionnaire $\rightarrow$ MET
	Body fat	Height & weight $\rightarrow$ BMI Calipers $\rightarrow$ Triceps skinfold thickness
	Diet	Youth/Adolescent Questionnaire (YAQ) Interview for 24 hour recall $\rightarrow$ Healthy Eating Index (HEI)
Genetics	Family history	Medical history form
	Group/ethnicity	Parental interview/questionnaire

6. The study does not have a clearly identified framework but draws on physiological and pathological theories as a theoretical basis for the study. The concepts are clearly identified and defined. Many of the variables are not conceptually defined, but all the variables are operationally defined. Not all of the variables are clearly associated with the concept they were to represent in the study (i.e., smoking history, VO_{2max}, MET, and BMI, although BMI is broadly recognized as a measure of body fat). Environmental influences on the development of metabolic syndrome are difficult to separate from lifestyle factors as they appear to play interactive parts in the emergence of metabolic syndrome. The study indirectly examined environmental factors by asking questions about lifestyle and habits.

7. Statements:

   a. *Lifestyle, environment,* and *genetic components* are influential in *metabolic syndrome:*

   $$\text{lifestyle} + \text{environment} + \text{genetics} \rightarrow \text{metabolic syndrome}$$

   b. If there is limited opportunity for daily physical activity or limited access to fresh and nutritious food choices, then the *environment* promotes *metabolic syndrome:*

   $$\text{If A1 or A2 then B} \rightarrow \text{C}$$

   c. *Environment* and *lifestyle* are closely related, but both may play independent and interactive parts in the emergence of *metabolic syndrome.*

   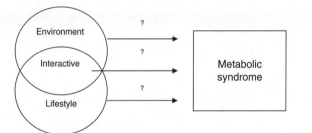

   d. Lifestyle factors of high-saturated-fat and low-fiber diets, stress, and lack of physical activity contribute to *metabolic syndrome.*

   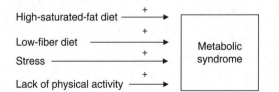

   e. Membership in Native American and Hispanic American ethnic groups increases risk for diabetes and insulin resistance.

   Native Americans and Hispanic Americans → ↑ diabetes and insulin resistance

   When these relational statements are combined, they can be shown as a map expressing the existing knowledge base and providing some validity for the researcher's framework map shown here.

8. Links between propositions and statements.

   a. *Proposition*: Ethnicity/genetics is influential in metabolic syndrome.

   Research question: What are the fasting serum insulin levels in schoolchildren in central Washington state?

   b. *Proposition*: Metabolic syndrome is characterized by ↓ in insulin receptors + ↑ insulin levels + compensation by the pancreas = Type 2 DM.

   Research question: What are the relationships between insulin levels and the criteria for metabolic syndrome in a multiethnic sample of children in central Washington state?

   c. *Proposition*: High saturated fat diet + low fiber diet = metabolic syndrome.

   Research question: What are the relationships between reported dietary intake and metabolic syndrome criteria?

   d. *Proposition*: Metabolic syndrome is associated with: ↑ triglycerides + ↓ HDL + ↑ BP + ↑obesity + ↑fasting blood glucose + ↑hyperinsulinemia.

   Research question: Which data predict insulin levels in this multiethnic sample of children?

9. Yes, the study used a descriptive correlational design to address the five research questions formulated for the study (Bindler et al., 2007, p. 296). See above the link of propositions to research questions.

   a. Describe the sample and the biophysiological measures related to metabolic syndrome.

   b. Examine the relationship of insulin levels with criteria for metabolic syndrome.

   c. Examine the relationship between dietary intake and metabolic syndrome.

   d. Determine which data are highly correlated with insulin levels.

10. The researcher does not provide a conceptual map. A proposed map is provided on the next page.

11. The author provides statements for each linkage on the map. References to support each linkage include the following:

    a. Genetic factors place certain population groups, such as Native Americans and Hispanic Americans, at higher risk for diabetes and insulin resistance (Cruz et al., 2004; Valdez, 2000).

    b. Lifestyle factors that contribute to the problem are high-saturated-fat and low-fiber diets, stress, as well as a lack of physical activity (Kelley, 2000; Ludwig et al., 1999; Mayer-Davis et al., 1997).

    c. The environment promotes metabolic syndrome when there is limited opportunity for daily physical activity or limited access to fresh and nutritious food choices (Cruz et al., 2004; Valdez, 2000).

    d. Lifestyle and environmental factors are closely related, but both may play independent and interactive parts in the emergence of metabolic syndrome (Cruz et al., 2004; Valdez, 2000).

237

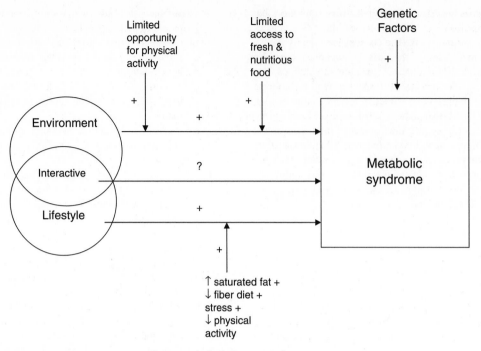

Proposed study framework map

12. Bindler et al. (2007) did not clearly indicate the framework for their study. However, the unidentified framework was a combination of physiological and pathological theories. The introduction and review of literature sections clearly identified the concepts and the propositions that provided the theoretical basis for this study. But the researchers did not provide a conceptual map to guide their study. However, linkages among the components of the framework are clearly delineated. Some of the linkages were not validated in previous studies. Operationalization of some of the theoretical concepts is not strong, because it measures, in a sense, low levels of the concept rather than its fullness.

Going Beyond

Critique of the Sethares and Elliott (2004) study in Appendix B: Model of the conceptual framework described in the article:

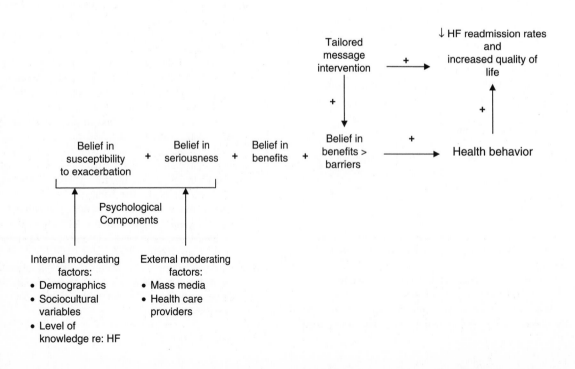

Diagram of the relationship posited in each of the three hypotheses of the study:

a. Tailored message intervention → ↓ HF readmission rates
b. Tailored message intervention → ↑ Quality of life
c. Tailored message intervention → ↓ barriers and ↑ benefits to performing self-care of HF

Concept(s)	Variable(s)	Measurement Method(s)
Belief in benefits > barriers	a. Benefits and barriers of taking HF medication	a. Beliefs about Medication Compliance Scale
	b. Benefits and barriers of following sodium-restricted diet	b. Beliefs about Diet Compliance Scale
	c. Benefits and barriers to self-monitoring for signs of fluid overload	c. Beliefs about Self-Monitoring Compliance Scale
Health behaviors	a. HF readmission rates	a. Count of total number of admission for HF in each group during 3-month study interval
	b. Quality of life	b. Minnesota Living with Heart Failure questionnaire

CHAPTER 8

Relevant Terms

General Concepts

1. b 3. a
2. d 4. c

Types of Hypotheses

1. h 4. e 7. d
2. g 5. c 8. f
3. b 6. a

Types of Variables

1. a 4. c 7. h
2. d 5. e 8. g
3. f 6. b

Key Ideas

1. Objectives, questions, hypotheses
2. independent, dependent
3. directions
4. null hypothesis
5. Contains variables that can be measured or manipulated in a study
6. Treatment, intervention, experimental variable, predictor (in a predictive correlational design), or stimulus
7. Outcome variable, criterion, or response variable
8. concepts
9. confounding
10. Environmental
11. age, gender, ethnicity

Making Connections

Types of Hypotheses

1. b, c, d, g
2. a, c, e, g
3. b, c, e, f
4. a, d, g, h
5. b, d, g, h
6. b, c, d, g

7. a, c, e, g
8. b, c, e, f
9. a, c, e, g
10. b, d, g, h
11. Increased age, decreased family support, and decreased health status are related to decreased self-care abilities of nursing home residents. OR Decreased age, increased family support, and increased health status are related to increased self-care abilities of nursing home residents.
12. Low-back massage is no more effective in decreasing perceptions of low-back pain than no massage in patients with chronic low-back pain.

Types of Variables

1. a 7. c
2. b 8. c
3. c 9. a
4. a 10. b
5. a or b 11. a
6. b 12. a

Exercises in Critical Appraisal

Bindler, Massey, Shultz, Mills, and Short Study

1. Bindler et al. (2007, p. 296) stated research questions to guide their study: "1. What are the fasting serum insulin levels in a multiethnic sample of school children in central Washington State? 2. What are the relationships between insulin levels and the criteria for metabolic syndrome in a multiethnic sample of children in central Washington State? 3. What are the relationships between reported dietary intake and metabolic syndrome criteria? 4. Which data predict insulin levels in this multiethnic sample of children? 5. How can the information learned in this study be used by pediatric nurses in clinical settings?"

239

2. The research questions are clearly stated and direct the development of the design, the data analysis, and interpretation of the findings. This is a correlational study with a descriptive, predictive correlational design. (See Ch. 11 for a discussion of the predictive correlational design and the independent and dependent variables included in this type of design.) The first research question focuses on description of insulin levels in children, questions 2 and 3 focus on examining relationships among study variables, and question 4 focuses on prediction of insulin levels. Question 5 is not linked to the study design and might have been omitted. The link to practice or "Clinical Implications" are best included in the "Discussion" section and do need a research question. The "Results" section clearly identifies the research questions and descriptive analyses are conducted to address question 1, bivariate correlational analyses for questions 2 and 3, and regression analysis is conducted to address question 4. Question 5 is addressed in the "Discussion" section.

3. Independent variables of gender, age, race, BMI percentile, glucose, triglycerides, HDL-C, systolic blood pressure, and diastolic blood pressure were used to predict the dependent variable serum insulin levels. Normally the term *independent variable* is used to describe a treatment that is manipulated in a study. However, in a predictive correlational design, the term *independent variable* is used to identify the variables that are measured and used to predict the dependent or outcome variable in the study. (Review predictive correlational design in Ch. 11 of your text.)

4. Fasting serum insulin levels
   a. Conceptual definition: "Serum insulin levels are a physiological indicator of metabolic functioning and health status and high insulin levels have been linked to metabolic syndrome or insulin resistance" (Bindler et al., 2007, p. 297).
   b. Operational definition: Fasting serum insulin levels were obtained from blood draws "completed in the early morning by the licensed phlebotomist after the children had fasted for at least 10 hours . . . Insulin was measured by solid-phase radioimmunoassay with the Coat-A-Count Insulin System" (Bindler et al., 2007, p. 297). Although the article describes the operational definition as "Elevated fasting insulin ≥ 15 μU/ml" on page 296, this definition does not describe how the variable will be measured. Thus the section of "operational definitions" might be more clearly developed in the article (Bindler et al., 2007, p. 297).

5. Demographic variables included in this study were gender, age, family history (cardiovascular disease, diabetes, overweight, and smoking), and smoking history (see Table 3). Age and gender were also used as independent variables in the regression analysis (see Table 8).

Sethares and Elliott Study

1. Sethares and Elliott (2004) included three research questions and three hypotheses. "The following research questions are the basis for the study: 1. Do individuals who receive the tailored message intervention have lower HF readmission rates than a control group at 3 months? 2. Do individuals who receive a tailored message intervention report better quality of life at baseline and 1 month after discharge than a

control group? 3. What is the effect of the tailored message intervention on the perceived benefit and barrier beliefs of the treatment group at baseline, 1 week, and 1 month?

There were three hypotheses for the study. The first two hypotheses were that persons who received the intervention would have lower HF readmission rates and report better quality of life. The third hypothesis was that intervention subjects would report fewer barriers and more benefits to performing self-care of HF after receiving the tailored message intervention" (Sethares & Elliott, 2004, p. 271).

2. The study really does not need both questions and hypotheses; these are redundant. Because this is a quasi-experimental study, the hypotheses are most appropriate to guide the study. Three separately stated hypotheses would be the clearest. The hypotheses provided reflect the study purpose, clearly indicate the focus of the study, include the study variables, and identify the proposed outcomes for the study.

3. Sethares and Elliott (2004) have one independent variable of tailored message and four dependent variables of readmission rate for HF, reported quality of life, perceived barrier beliefs, and perceived benefit beliefs.

4. Independent variable: Tailored message intervention
   a. Conceptual definition: Tailored message is an intervention "focused on decreasing client-identified barriers to self-care. Individualized teaching by a nurse focused on enhancing the benefits and decreasing the barriers to self-care of a person with HF.... By changing perceived beliefs [benefits and barriers] related to self-care, it is anticipated that persons with HF will improve self-care behaviors, which may lead to improved quality of life and lower readmission rates" (Sethares & Elliott, 2004, p. 271).
   b. Operational definition: The tailored message was "based on the perceived benefits and barriers to self-care of HF that were identified by persons with HF" (Sethares & Elliott, 2004, p. 274). The specifics of the intervention are provided under the heading Intervention (p. 274), and the tailored messages for diet and medications are in Table III (p. 274) in the article.

5. The demographic variables are identified in Tables I and II and include the following: age, NYHA, EF, number of comorbidities, education, marital status, race, gender, medications, and VNA services.

Wright Study

1. Wright (2003) used the purpose to guide her study and had no objectives, questions, or hypotheses, which is appropriate in qualitative research.

2. The purpose of this study is clearly stated and provides direction to the study. Often in qualitative studies, the research purpose is used to direct the study. Qualitative studies sometimes have research questions and occasionally objectives but do not include hypotheses.

3. Wright (2004) has one research concept: lived experience of spirituality in recovery from substance abuse.

4. Lived experience of spirituality in recovery from substance abuse
   a. Conceptual definition: This definition was provided in the results section of the article in Tables 1 and 2 (Wright, 2003, pp. 284–285), which include the major meaning units and themes in the study. Often in qualita-

tive research, the theoretical understanding of the concept is provided in the results and discussion section of the article.

   b. Operational definition: The lived experience of spirituality is measured by in-depth, unstructured interviews with subjects recovering from substance abuse.

5. Demographic variables included in this study were age, marital status, religious affiliation, age of onset of substance abuse, past legal problems, and abstinence time in years or months (Wright, 2003, p. 283).

Going Beyond

Develop objectives, questions, or hypotheses for a proposed study and conceptually and operationally define the variables. Share your results with peers and your instructor for feedback.

CHAPTER 9

Relevant Terms

1. l	8. b	15. t
2. a	9. i	16. s
3. m	10. d	17. k
4. o	11. p	18. r
5. e	12. q	19. h
6. n	13. g	20. j
7. f	14. c	

Human Rights Based on Ethical Principles

1. b
2. a
3. c

Types of Institutional Review of Research

1. c
2. b
3. a

Key Ideas

1. justice
2. You may have identified any of the following:
   a. Children (minors)
   b. Mentally impaired individuals (mentally ill and those with dementia)
   c. Unconscious patients
   d. Terminally ill patients
   e. Those confined to institutions (prisoners)
3. competent
4. assent
5. a. Best interest standard: The decision to participate in the study is based on what is therapeutically in the best interest of the mentally incompetent patient and also to ask the patient for his or her assent to participate in the study.
   b. Substituted judgment standard: The decision to participate in the study is based on what the patient would have probably wanted if he or she were mentally competent to give consent and also to ask the patient to assent to participate in the study.
6. qualitative
7. a. Disclosure of essential study information to the subject

   b. Comprehension of this information by the subject
   c. Competency of the subject to give consent
   d. Voluntary consent by the subject to participate in the study
8. You may have identified any of the following:
   a. Introduction of the research activities
   b. Statement of the research purpose
   c. Explanation of study procedures
   d. Description of study risks and discomforts
   e. Description of study benefits
   f. Disclosure of alternatives
   g. Assurance of anonymity and confidentiality
   h. Offer to answer questions
   i. Option to withdraw
9. Voluntary
10. institutional review board
11. Short written consent form, long written consent form, tape recording of consent process, or a videotape of the consent process
12. research (or scientific) misconduct
13. Promoting the integrity of biomedical and behavior research in approximately 4000 institutions worldwide
14. You may have identified any of the following:
    a. Defining research misconduct
    b. Developing policies aimed at preventing misconduct and promoting the conduct of ethical research
    c. Identifying mechanisms to distribute the policy to scientists
    d. Designating membership of committees investigating research misconduct
    e. Identifying the administrative actions for acts of research misconduct
    f. Developing a process for notifying funding agencies and journals
    g. Providing for public disclosure of the incidents of research or scientific misconduct
    h. Identifying legal ramifications
    i. Prevention and the role of peer review
15. a. Exempt from review
    b. Expedited review
    c. Complete or full review
16. a. Should animals be used as subjects in a research project?
    b. If animals are used in research, what mechanisms ensure that they are treated humanely?
17. American Association for Accreditation of Laboratory Animal Care (AAALAC)
18. To determine the benefit-risk ratio, you need to assess the benefits and risks of the sampling method, consent process, procedures, and outcomes of the study. Informed consent must be obtained from the subjects, and selection and treatment of the subjects during the study must be fair. The type of knowledge generated from the study also needs to be examined to determine how this knowledge will influence nursing practice. If the benefits outweigh the risks, it is often recommended that the studies be conducted.
19. You must obtain voluntary, informed consent from the children's parents or legal guardians and the assent of each child. The consent needs to be documented on a short or long consent form. You also must obtain the approval of the school to conduct the study.
20. protected health information

Making Connections
Levels of Discomfort or Harm

1. b	5. e	8. c or d
2. a	6. b	9. e
3. c	7. a	10. c or d
4. c or d		

Unethical Studies

1. b	5. c	8. b
2. c	6. a	9. a
3. d	7. d	10. c
4. b		

Puzzles
Crossword Puzzle

Across	Down
1. Confidentiality	2. Fair treatment
4. Institutional review	3. Risk
6. Autonomous	5. IRB
7. Nuremberg	8. Deception
10. Self-determination	9. Consent
11. Ethics	12. Children
13. Assent	
14. Privacy	
15. Anonymous	

Exercises in Critical Appraisal

1. Bindler, Massey, Shultz, Mills, and Short (2007) received approval to conduct their study from both the university and the school as indicated by the following quote: "The protocol was approved by the Institutional Review Boards of Spokane, Washington, and Washington State University, and the school board of the district where the study was conducted" (p. 296). The researchers obtained consent from the parents and assent from the children to participate in their study, and the study information was provided in both English and Spanish to ensure communication with the parents: "If they signed a consent, their children were informed about the study and could choose whether to sign an assent and participate" (Bindler et al., 2007, p. 296).

2. Sethares and Elliott (2004) received approval from the institutional review board (IRB) at the community hospital where the study was conducted: "After stabilization of HF [heart failure], hospitalized subjects were invited to participate in the study, and written informed consent was obtained" (p. 274). The study was ethical because the researchers obtained institutional approval from the hospital and written informed consent from the subjects who voluntarily participated in the study. In additional, the potential subjects were not approached until their HF was stabilized, which strengthens the ethics of this study. The results and discussion sections of the study protect the privacy of the subjects and do not reflect the protected health information of any one subject.

3. Wright (2003) indicated that the purpose of the study was explained and informed consent was obtained from the subjects. The subjects were also given a rationale for the researcher's interest in the phenomenon studied. Wright

recognized that "the recall of painful memories can trigger anxiety and other emotional distress. Therefore, the emotional state of each participant was evaluated throughout the interviews by stopping when the participant was upset and offering support" (p. 284). Thus, Wright (2003) documented the informed consent process and the method for protecting subjects from discomfort and harm. However, she did not document the institutional review of this study by the shelter where the data were collected or by the National Institute of Health (NIH) that provided support for the study. The ethics of this study would be strengthened by the inclusion of the IRB process that was implemented before the study was conducted.

Going Beyond

Use the content in Chapter 9 to discuss the benefit-risk ratio for a proposed study, develop a consent form, and complete a preliminary IRB form from the university where you are conducting a thesis or dissertation.

CHAPTER 10

Relevant Terms
Terms Related to Triangulation

1. d	4. c	7. h
2. i	5. a	8. e
3. b	6. g	9. f

Concepts Important to Design

1. i	5. f	9. d
2. a	6. h	10. e
3. g	7. j	
4. c	8. b	

Terms Important to Design Validity

1. m	6. d	11. a
2. l	7. k	12. h
3. b	8. g	13. c
4. i	9. f	
5. e	10. j	

Controlling Extraneous Variables

1. d	5. e	9. c
2. a	6. b	10. h
3. j	7. g	
4. i	8. f	

Key Ideas

1. effects
2. cause, effect, cause
3. biases
4. control
5. treatment or intervention
6. threats, validity
7. cause and effect
8. selection, setting, history
9. comparisons

Making Connections

1. h	5. j	8. m
2. b	6. d and g	9. d and f
3. f	7. a	10. b and l
4. b and l		

Puzzles

Word Scramble

"Just as the blueprint for a house must be individualized to the specific house being built, so must the design be made specific to a study."

Secret Message

"The purpose of a design is to set up a situation that maximizes the possibilities of obtaining accurate answers to objectives, questions, or hypotheses."

Crossword Puzzle

Across

1. Matching
4. Comparisons
7. Effect
8. Counterbalancing
10. Equivalence
12. Treatment
16. Validity
17. Threat
18. Probability
19. Design
20. Stratification
21. Experimental

Down

2. Heterogeneity
3. Map
5. Manipulation
6. Sample
8. Control
9. Blocking
11. Correlational
13. Random
14. Bias
15. Descriptive
17. Trend

Exercises in Critical Appraisal

1. You may have identified any of the following ideas, or you may have identified other biases in these studies.

   a. The researchers used only subject recall for measuring diet intake possibly leading to mono-operation bias or only one measurement method being used to measure the variable (in addition, subject recall has been criticized as not accurately reflecting diet intake).

   The sample was not randomly selected; it was a non-probability sample of convenience. The parents volunteered for the study in response to a flyer sent home with their children, and they may be different from those who did not volunteer (e.g., must have been able to read the flyer). However, the researchers provided the flyer in both English and Spanish to increase the representativeness of the sample.

   Only children with no identified illnesses or medications were included; the sample, therefore, did not represent the population, which would include children with identified illnesses.

   No power analysis was addressed to determine the sample size needed for the study. Was the sample size large enough to prevent a type II error? What was the effect size for the study?

Only 88 of the 100 subjects identified their ethnicity, and the sample included 64 Hispanics, 15 Native Americans, and 9 Caucasians. The group sizes for the Native Americans and Caucasians are really too low for this study.

   b. The sample was not randomly selected; it was a nonprobability sample of convenience. The subjects volunteering may be different from those who did not volunteer.

   Subjects were limited to patients who planned to be discharged home, rather than a nursing home or other facilities. This strategy provided a more homogeneous sample but suggests a possible bias of the patients having a stronger support system than those who were not discharged home. A strong support system might have altered the perception of benefits and barriers.

   The subjects were obtained from a single hospital.

   It was not really a control group but a comparison group because the sample was not random and the subjects received usual care. Half of the subjects in the control group received referrals to local visiting nurse agencies. This could also influence the findings in the study because they have more support.

2. Identify any three of the following methods of control:

   a. Controlling measurement: Blood pressures were measured the same way, and three times and the average value was used.

   Controlling extraneous variables: Blood draws were in early morning by licensed phlebotomist after fasting 10 hours.

   Controlling environment: All measurements were completed in 1 day at the same setting.

   Controlling measurement reliability: Interrater reliability was established among all researchers by training and evaluating them for reliability on measurement and for assistance to children during questionnaire completion.

   Controlling for the effects of maturation: Fed students after fasting blood draws so that increasing hunger did not effect study results.

   Controlling analysis: Completed questionnaires were returned to YAQ developers at the Harvard School of Public Health for the calculation of the dietary intake of nutrients and percentage of recommended dietary allowance (RDA) for each nutrient.

   b. Controlling measurement: Valid and reliable instruments were used.

   Controlling extraneous variables and promoting equivalent groups: Subjects were randomly assigned to treatment and control groups.

   Controlled extraneous variables by waiting for patients' heart failure to be stabilized before approaching them for inclusion in the study.

   Homogeneity: Subjects had documented diagnoses of systolic or diastolic heart failure confirmed by echocardiography and were free from serious cognitive deficits.

   Controlled the implementation of the treatment: All subjects in the treatment group received the consistently implemented tailored message intervention during hospitalization and one week and one month following discharge.

3. Populations generalized to the following:
   a. Ethnically mixed populations of children in fourth to eighth grade from small rural farm communities with limited access to fast food
   b. Adults with a primary diagnosis of chronic heart failure who were discharged home. No information is provided on subject's ethnicity or socioeconomic status.
4. Threats to external validity:
   a. Generalization limited to ethnically mixed populations of children in fourth to eighth grade who live in small rural farm communities with limited access to fast food and who speak and write English or Spanish. The small number of Caucasians (9 subjects) and Native Americans (15 subjects) included in the study limit the generalizability of the findings to these two ethnic groups. Study findings really are best generalized to Hispanics.
   b. Generalization limited to English-speaking adults with heart failure who are free from serious cognitive deficits and anticipate returning to a community setting. There were only six African Americans included in the study and no mention of Hispanic subjects. Therefore generalization to minority groups would be questionable. Lack of information on socioeconomic status makes generalizability to low-income patients questionable.

Going Beyond

Critically appraise the design of a current quantitative study, and address the questions in the study guide in this section. Ask your instructor or another student to evaluate your work.

CHAPTER 11

Relevant Terms
Types of Designs (A)

1. g	5. l	9. k	12. b
2. d	6. a	10. n	13. m
3. e	7. f	11. j	14. h
4. i	8. c		

Types of Variables and Designs

1. m	4. g	7. a	10. l	13. f
2. j	5. d	8. c	11. e	
3. b	6. i	9. h	12. k	

Types of Designs (B)

1. j	5. h	9. f	13. p	17. n
2. a	6. c	10. r	14. g	18. q
3. b	7. d	11. l	15. o	19. k
4. s	8. e	12. i	16. m	

Key Ideas

1. To achieve greater control over the conduct of the study and thus improve the validity of the study in addressing the research problem and examining the research purpose.
2. nursing philosophy
3. time
4. self-report
5. The full range of scores possible on the variables being measured.
6. causality
7. highly, not highly
8. Improved outcomes of the experimental group or improvement or change in the dependent or outcome variable.
9. The experimental treatment or independent variable can cause an effect on the dependent or outcome variable and the extent to which the effect of the treatment can be detected by measuring the dependent variable.
10. random assignment
11. nested variables
12. Valid answers to the research purpose and the objectives, questions, or hypotheses that the researchers have posed.

Making Connections
Designs

1. g	4. a	6. j
2. h	5. i	7. f
3. b, c		

Mapping the Design

1. Treolar (1994):

	Pretest (before heelstick)	During heelstick	Treatment (pacifier inserted)	Posttest (5 minutes after heelstick)
Experimental group NNS infants	O_1	O_2	T	O_3
Control group ONNS infants	O_1	O_2		O_3

Note: O = Observation or measurement of trancutaneous oxygen and behavioral state.

2. Guiffre, Heidenreich, and Pruitt (1994):

	Pretest Temperature Measured	Treatment	Repeated Posttests Temperature Measured
Radiant heat group	O_1	T_1	$O_2 O_3 O_4 O_5 O_6 O_7...$
Forced warm air group	O_1	T_2	$O_2 O_3 O_4 O_5 O_6 O_7...$
Warm blanket group	O_1	T_3	$O_2 O_3 O_4 O_5 O_6 O_7...$

Note: O = Observation or measurement of temperature.

Exercises in Critical Appraisal

1. Design:
   a. Bindler et al.'s (2007) study has a predictive correlational design.
   b. Sethares and Elliott's (2004) study was a randomized controlled trial.
2. Group comparisons:
   a. Bindler et al.'s (2007) study mainly focused on relationships but did make comparisons among three ethnic groups, Native American, Hispanic, and Caucasian groups, on the following characteristics:
      - Demographic variables (i.e., age, sex, family history) (see Table 3)
      - Physical fitness variables (i.e., VO_{2max}, MET score) (see Table 3)
      - Smoking history (see Table 3)
      - BP (see Table 3)
      - Measures of body fat (i.e., height, weight, BMI, skinfold percentile) (see Table 3)
      - Biophysiological measures of serum cholesterol, triglycerides, and glucose (see Table 4)
      - Multiple dietary intake factors (e.g., carbohydrates, proteins, total fat, saturated fat, fiber (see Table 4)
      - Some other comparisons were made on the insulin levels of different genders and age groups.
   b. Sethares and Elliott's (2004) study:
      - Health Belief Scale scores of experimental group during hospitalization and 7 to 10 days later
      - Quality of life Scores 1 month after hospitalization comparing experimental group and control group
      - Readmission rate at 3 months comparing experimental and control groups
      - Readmission rate with quality of life
      - Readmission rate with health beliefs 7 to 10 days after discharge in experimental group
3. Strengths of the design:
   a. Bindler et al.'s (2007) study:
      - Data collected at one time in same setting
      - Subjects obtained from a racially mixed population
      - Sample size of Hispanics is strong, but the numbers of Native Americans and Caucasians were limited
      - Content experts (e.g., dietitian) used to collect data related to their expertise
      - Training of data collectors
      - Objective measurement of many variables with physiological measurement methods, such as insulin levels, cholesterol values, blood pressure
      - Multiple methods used to measure some variables
      - Steps were taken with data collection to ensure accuracy and precision of physiological measures and reliability and validity of the diet data
   b. Sethares and Elliott's study:
      - Carefully designed and implemented intervention (intervention fidelity)
      - Description of care received by control subjects
      - Protocol reviewed with research nurses weekly to maintain consistency in treatment
      - Random assignment to groups
      - Interview and measurements guided by theoretical framework

Going Beyond

Share the article you chose and your paragraph with your instructor, and ask for feedback.

CHAPTER 12

Relevant Terms

Outcomes Research Terms (A)

1. g	5. h	9. j	13. f	17. i
2. b	6. l	10. p	14. o	
3. d	7. n	11. c	15. q	
4. e	8. a	12. k	16. m	

Outcomes Research Terms (B)

1. k	5. a	9. m	13. c
2. e	6. h	10. j	14. i
3. n	7. d	11. b	15. o
4. l	8. p	12. g	16. f

Key Ideas

1. The end results of patient care
2. a. The Hospital and Medical Facilities Study Section
   b. The Nursing Study Section
3. The Medical Outcomes Study (MOS)
4. a. The effect of nursing interventions on medical outcomes
   b. The effect of staffing patterns on medical outcomes

c. The effects of nursing practice delivery models on medical outcomes

5. a. Coordination of care
   b. Counseling
   c. Referrals

6. You may have identified any of the following questions:
   a. Do patients benefit from the care provided?
   b. What treatments work best?
   c. Has the patient's functional status improved? According to whose viewpoint?
   d. Are health care resources well spent?

7. Incorporate available evidence on health outcomes into sets of recommendations concerning appropriate management strategies for patients with the studied conditions.

8. Inclusion of nursing data in the large databases used to analyze outcomes.

9. clearly linked, process; caused

10. subjects of care

11. a. Clinical guidelines
    b. Critical paths
    c. Care maps

12. Large heterogeneous

13. a. Information about the patient such as disease severity, comorbidity, and types of outcomes
    b. Processes of care provided
    c. Patient status over time
    d. Follow-up information

14. a. Decisions can be quantified.
    b. All possible courses of action can be identified and evaluated.
    c. The different values of outcomes—viewed from the perspective of the physician, patient, payer, and administrator—can be examined.
    d. The analysis allows the selection of an optimal course of therapy.

15. a. What proportion of people experiencing a specific cluster of symptoms were diagnosed (correctly or not) as having a particular condition, and of this group, who received what treatment?
    b. Should a treatment or procedure have been performed?
    c. Did persons with a particular diagnosis receive appropriate treatment?
    d. What proportion of people with the cluster of symptoms received no treatment?

16. Most consistent with nursing theory and practice

17. Change across time in subjects

18. The American Nurses Association

19. a. In change, regression toward the mean is an unavoidable law of nature.
    b. The difference score between pre- and postmeasurement is unreliable.
    c. ANCOVA is the way to analyze change.
    d. Two points (pretest and posttest) are adequate for the study of change.
    e. The correlation between change and initial level is always negative.

20. a. Mean improvement score for all patients' treatment
    b. The percentage of patients who improve
    c. Whether all patients improve slightly, or there is a divergence among patients, with some improving greatly while others do not improve at all
    d. Characteristics of patients who experience varying degrees of improvement
    e. Characteristics of outliers

21. a. Variance
    b. Comorbidities
    c. The identity of at-risk patients

Making Connections

1. h	6. l	10. a
2. e	7. m	11. d
3. j	8. i	12. g
4. c	9. f	13. k
5. b		

Puzzles

Word Scramble

"The momentum propelling outcomes research is coming from policy makers, insurers, and the public."

Secret Message

"The strategies used in outcome research are, to some extent, a departure from the accepted scientific method."

Crossword Puzzle

Across
1. Standard of care
4. Cost benefit
6. Patient
8. Person
11. Cohort
16. Numerical method
20. Efficiency
21. Variance
22. Individual
23. Research tradition

Down
2. Out of pocket cost
3. Measurement error
5. Structures of care
7. Geographic
9. Intermediate end point
10. Providers of care
12. Opportunity cost
13. Sampling error
14. Subjects of care
15. Primordial cell
17. Multilevel
18. Aggregate
19. Small area

Going Beyond

Discuss your ideas about the recently published outcomes studies with your instructor and class members.

CHAPTER 13

Relevant Terms

Intervention Studies (A)

1. e	4. f	7. a	10. j
2. c	5. i	8. h	11. d
3. g	6. k	9. l	12. b

Intervention Studies (B)

1. c	4. l	7. k	10. e
2. f	5. g	8. d	11. i
3. a	6. h	9. j	12. b

Interventions Studies (C)

1. c	5. a	9. f	13. o	17. b
2. g	6. l	10. i	14. r	18. n
3. k	7. p	11. q	15. h	19. j
4. m	8. e	12. d	16. s	

Interventions Studies (D)

1. b	5. l	9. e	13. c
2. f	6. g	10. m	14. j
3. i	7. h	11. a	
4. d	8. k	12. n	

Key Ideas

1. Designing and testing nursing interventions
2. true experiment
3. a. Single act
   b. Series of actions at a given point in time
   c. Series of actions over time
   d. Series of acts performed collaboratively with other professionals
4. clinical trial
5. explain why the intervention causes changes in outcomes, how it does so, or both
6. all groups that will be affected by the change
7. a. The components, intensity, and duration of the intervention required
   b. The human and material resources needed
   c. The procedures to be followed to produce the desired outcomes
8. amount, frequency, duration
9. independent
10. confounding variables

Making Connections

1. e	5. c	8. f
2. b	6. i	9. j
3. a	7. h	10. g
4. d		

Puzzles

Word Scramble

"Interventions must be described more broadly as all of the actions required to address a particular problem."

Secret Message

"There is currently little consistency in the performance of an intervention."

Crossword Puzzle

Across
1. Treatment matching
3. Moderator variable
6. Intensity
8. Disadvantaged group
12. Intervener
13. Complexity
15. Effectiveness
16. Dose
17. Strength
18. Integrity
19. Reinvention
20. Duration
21. Observation system
22. Intermediate outcome

Down
2. Adaptation
4. Key informant
5. Prescriptive theory
7. Stakeholders
9. Extraneous factors
10. Logical positivist
11. Taxonomy
12. Intervention
14. True experiment

Exercises in Critical Appraisal

Note: Although this study was not designed using an intervention theory approach, the authors do describe the intervention in their study sufficiently to allow you to critically appraise the intervention.

1. No, the intervention is not sufficiently described to implement the intervention without contacting the researchers.
2. The intervention is theory based but not in the manner of intervention theory methods. The framework for the Sethares and Elliott (2004) quasi-experimental study provides the theoretical basis for the study intervention. The Health Belief Model provides the organizing framework for this study.

Going Beyond

1. Planning a program of intervention research:
   - Determine the makeup and function of the project team.
   - Begin with an extensive search for relevant information that is applied to the development of an intervention theory.
   - Decide whether or not to use participatory research methods.
   - Define the intervention and obtain evidence of its effectiveness.
   - Carry out field testing of the intervention to further refine the intervention and improve clinical application.
   - Design an observation system allowing the researcher to observe events related to the intervention naturalistically.
   - Plan for extensive dissemination of the newly refined intervention.
2. Share your paragraph and the study you've critically appraised with your instructor, and ask for feedback.

CHAPTER 14

Relevant Terms

1. j
2. a
3. n
4. g
5. k
6. f
7. m
8. i
9. l
10. b
11. d
12. e
13. h
14. c
15. o

Key Ideas

1. elements, subjects
2. target population
3. sample, accessible population, target population
4. You might have identified any two of the following ideas:
   a. Identify the sampling method. Probability sampling methods increase the representativeness of the sample.
   b. Determine the acceptance rate for a study; the higher the acceptance rate, the more representative the sample.
   c. Determine sample mortality; the lower the sample mortality, the more representative the sample.
   d. Compare the demographic characteristics of the sample to those of the target population or the samples of similar previous studies.
   e. Compare mean sample values of study variables to the values of the target population determined from previous research.
   f. Evaluate the possibilities of systematic bias in the sample in terms of the setting, characteristics of the sample, and ranges of values on measured variables.
5. The expected difference in values that occurs when different subjects from the same sample are examined
6. sampling frame
7. Strategies used to obtain a sample for a study
8. You could choose any of the following:
   a. Did the researcher successfully implement the sampling plan?
   b. Was the sampling plan effective for representing the target population?
   c. Were the subjects selected from a sampling frame?
   d. What sampling method was used to determine the sample?
   e. Were the subjects randomly selected?
   f. Was power analysis used to determine sample size?
   g. What sample size was achieved?
   h. Were the characteristics of the sample consistent with the characteristics of the accessible and the target populations?
9. homogeneous
10. heterogeneous
11. sample criteria
12. sample characteristics
13. sample mortality or attrition
14. random or probability
15. nonrandom or nonprobability
16. a. Simple random sampling
    b. Stratified random sampling
    c. Cluster sampling
    d. Systematic sampling
17. probability or random
18. You could choose any four of the following:
    a. Convenience sampling
    b. Quota sampling
    c. Purposive sampling
    d. Network sampling
    e. Theoretical sampling
19. nonprobability
20. accidental sampling
21. judgmental sampling
22. power analysis
23. differences, relationships
24. 0.8 or 80%
25. power analysis
26. null hypothesis
27. a. Effect size of a study
    b. Type of study
    c. Number of variables
    d. Measurement sensitivity
    e. Data analysis techniques
28. a. Purposive sampling
    b. Network sampling
    c. Theoretical sampling
29. purposive
30. You could choose from the following:
    a. Scope of the study
    b. Nature of the topic studied
    c. Quality of the data collected
    d. Study design
31. a. Natural settings
    b. Partially controlled settings
    c. Highly controlled settings
32. natural
33. highly controlled
34. partially controlled
35. inclusion, exclusion

Making Connections
Sampling Methods

1. f
2. b
3. c
4. a
5. i
6. g
7. h
8. b
9. e
10. d
11. f
12. c
13. d
14. i
15. f

Types of Settings

1. a
2. b
3. b or c
4. c
5. a

Puzzles
Crossword Puzzle

Across	Down
2. Comparison group	1. Criteria
5. Random	3. Probability
6. Power analysis	4. Sample size
7. Elements	5. Representative
9. Sampling methods	8. Subjects

11. Bias
12. Accessible
13. Target
14. Network
15. Purposive

10. Population

Exercises in Critical Appraisal
Bindler, Massey, Shultz, Mills, and Short Study

1. The population was school-age children.
2. Inclusion sample criteria were children "attending fourth to eight grades at public elementary and middle schools" and "Participants who spoke English or Spanish were eligible" (Bindler et al., 2007, p. 296). Exclusion sample criteria were children with identified illnesses or medications were excluded.
3. The results section of the study included a subsection titled "Description of Sample" that identified the sample characteristics for the study, as well as Table 3 in the study. "The age range of the sample was 9–15 years ($M = 12$ years). The sample included 52 boys and 48 girls. Sixty-four (64%) claimed to be purely Hispanic, 15 (15%) claimed to be purely Native American, and 9 (9%) claimed to be purely Caucasian. Twelve (12%) additional subjects claimed to have mixed-race ethnic heritage. All Hispanic children had Mexico as origin of the family and were employed in farming or food processing industries. There were no significant differences among ethnic groups regarding age or gender; reported family history of cardiovascular disease, diabetes, overweight, or smoking; physical activity; weight percentiles; BMI percentiles; or triceps skin fold percentiles. Table 3 shows the demographic data and physical measurements of the total sample and of the ethnic sub-sample (those children identifying with just one major ethnic group)" (Bindler et al., 2007, pp. 297–298). Table 3 is on page 299 of the study.
4. The sample size was "100 children (representing approximately 15% of eligible students) attending fourth to eight grades at public elementary and middle schools" (Bindler et al., 2007, p. 296). No power analysis was mentioned to determine sample size.
5. The adequacy of the sample size is questionable because the researchers conducted analyses on small groups formed based on ethnic origin with only 15 Native Americans, 9 Caucasians, and 12 participants of mixed tace. Some of the study results were not significant, which might be because of an inadequate sample size and would be considered a type II error. Sample size is also limited for the large number of variables that are examined in this study. The lack of a power analysis to determine the sample size limits the ability of the reader to judge the adequacy of a sample.
6. The sample attrition or mortality was not discussed in this study, but the researchers did mention in the results section that blood samples were not obtained on two children so they were omitted from this aspect of the analyses. This study would have been strengthened by a discussion of sample attrition or mortality.
7. Nonprobability sampling, and the sampling method is sample of convenience.
8. The representativeness of the sample is limited because only 15% of the eligible students attending the public elementary and middle schools participated. The researchers did not address the acceptance rate or the attrition rate, which would have been useful in determining the representativeness of the sample. The sample included 64 Hispanic students, which is more representative for that group than for the Caucasians with 9 subjects and the Native Americans with 15 subjects. Based on the information provided, the representativeness of the sample of the target population is limited.
9. The generalization of the study findings is decreased by the nonprobability sampling method and the limited representativeness of the sample for selected ethnic groups. However, because some of these study findings were consistent with the findings of other studies, this increases the generalizability of the findings. Because this is a relatively new area of research for children, the findings can be generalized to the sample and probably the accessible population but not to the target population. Additional research is needed in this problem area before the findings are ready for generalization.

Sethares and Elliott Study

1. The population was adults with a primary diagnosis of chronic heart failure.
2. Sample inclusion criteria were as follows: "(1) primary diagnosis of either systolic or diastolic HF listed in the medical record, confirmed by the presence of symptoms of HF for 3 months or longer; (2) echocardiography for confirmation of ejection fraction; (3) English speaking; (4) freedom from serious cognitive deficits, as determined by the Mini Mental Status Exam; and (5) anticipated return to a community setting, rather than long-term care" (Sethares & Elliott, 2004, pp. 271–272).
3. Sample or demographic characteristics are presented in Table I (p. 272) and Table II (p. 273) in the article.
4. Sample size was 70: "a power analysis with an effect size of .35, an alpha of .05, and a power of .80" was conducted (Sethares & Elliott, 2004, p. 272).
5. The sample size was adequate to examine most of the variables in this quasi-experimental study, because most of the findings were significant. Power analysis indicated that the sample size was adequate to detect differences if they existed. In the power table in appendix 9 on the Evolve website, an effect size of 0.34, alpha = 0.05, and a sample of 70 yields a power of 0.90, which is more than adequate to detect the significant differences in the sample. Sethares and Elliott (2004, p. 272) stated that "the sample size provided adequate power for all outcome variables."
6. Sample attrition or mortality was 18 subjects (8 subjects withdrew and 10 subjects died), or 25.7%. "A t test was run to compare the 2 groups of patients (those who died within 3 months of the discharge and those who survived). … There were no significant differences on any of the measures between the 2 groups" (Sethares & Elliott, 2004, p. 272). This indicates the researchers did attempt to determine whether the mortality rate had an impact on the two groups (treatment and control), and none was found. This strengthens the sampling plan and indicates less potential for sampling error.

249

7. Nonprobability convenience sampling was used in this study.
8. Because the sample is not random, this has a potential to decrease its representativeness of the target population. However, actively recruiting subjects and including all subjects that met the sample criteria increases the representativeness of this sample. The sample size of 70 is a strength, but the 25.7% attrition or mortality rate decreases the representativeness of the sample. The sample was obtained from one community hospital in the Northeast, and this decreases the representativeness of the sample also.
9. Because the sample is nonrandom, the mortality is high, and the study involved only one setting, the findings could be generalized to the accessible population but probably not the target population. However, the fact that these findings are consistent with an extensive number of other studies in this area increases the generalizability of the findings.

Wright Study

1. The population was African-American women recovering from substance abuse.
2. Sample criteria: "Each participant met the following criteria: over 18 years of age; identified herself as an African American woman; substance free status for at least 1 year; able to participate and engage in interviews of 1 to 2 hours in length; expressed interest in participating in the study; not currently being treated for psychotic disorders; and was able to read and write in the English language. There was no restriction as to the length of substance abuse to enter the study" (Wright, 2003, p. 283).
3. Sample characteristics: "There were 15 participants who ranged from 29 to 49 years of age. With respect to marital status, the majority—eight of the participants—were never married, whereas six were divorced and one currently married. ... All the participants reported an increase in their spirituality since becoming drug free. All participants identified their higher power as God or Jesus Christ. Of the participants, 12 began using substances between the ages of 5 to 12, with all having some form of structured treatment for substance abuse. A majority of the participants reported having past legal problems. With respect to abstinence eight participants reported 7–12 years of drug free status and seven having 15–39 months of substance free status" (Wright, 2003, p. 283).
4. The sample size was 15 participants. No power analysis was used because this is a qualitative study and sample size is determined by factors other than a power analysis (Burns & Grove, 2009).
5. The sample size does seem adequate for this phenomenological study because data saturation was reached with no new themes appearing, and various perspectives of the phenomenon of recovery from substance abuse were obtained. Wright (2003, p. 283) stated that "The number of participants was determined by the number of persons required to permit an in-depth exploration and obtain a clear understanding of the phenomenon of interest from various perspectives. This occurred with 15 participants when data saturation was achieved, with no new themes or essences emerging from the participants and the data were repeating."
6. No sample attrition or mortality is mentioned.
7. The nonprobability network sampling method was used. "Participants were recruited from a women's shelter with the help of a colleague as contact person, from church support groups within the community by the researcher who made church members aware of the study and the search for participants, and through networking, whereby each participant interviewed suggested the name of a potential new participant" (Wright, 2003, p. 283).
8. Representativeness of the sample is not a major focus of qualitative research. The focus is on understanding the specific study subjects and less on their representativeness of a target population. Wright did indicate "the study limitations, however, were the researcher having worked in psychiatry and substance abuse for many years observed a difference in the lives of African American women who had incorporated a spiritual belief in their recover process. Most of the participants were recruited from faith-based women's shelter and church support groups; therefore, it was known that their belief was in God" (Wright, 2003. p. 289). This indicates the subjects in the sample were those with a faith base and are not representative of those women recovering from substance abuse who do not have a faith base.
9. Generalization of findings is not the focus of qualitative research. The focus is on understanding the phenomenon of recovery from substance abuse by African-American women in a selected sample.

Study Settings

1. a. Bindler et al., (2007) used a natural setting of public elementary and middle schools.
2. b. and a. Sethares and Elliott (2004) used a partially controlled setting of a single community hospital where the environment was controlled for the implementation of the treatment and a natural setting of the subjects' homes following discharge.
3. a. Wright (2003) used natural settings of a women's shelter and church community support groups.

CHAPTER 15

Relevant Terms
Levels of Measurement

1. e	5. h
2. d	6. g
3. f	7. c
4. a	8. b

Types of Reliability and Validity for Measurement Methods

1. p	8. q	15. u
2. l	9. s	16. i
3. a	10. g	17. c
4. h	11. f	18. n
5. o	12. b	19. j
6. e	13. d	20. r
7. m	14. k	21. t

Key Ideas

1. trustworthy or accurate
2. true
3. error
4. direct or ratio-level measurement
5. indirect or interval-level measurement
6. 0.80
7. 0.70
8. a. Variations in administration of the measurement procedure
   b. Subjects completing a paper-and-pencil scale accidentally marking the wrong column
   c. Punching the wrong key while entering data into the computer
9. a. A weight scale that reads higher than it should
   b. A thermometer that is not accurately calibrated
   c. Failure to count two exam questions in calculating exam grades
10. a. Norm-referenced testing
    b. Criterion-referenced testing

Making Connections

Error Types

1. b	4. b
2. b	5. a
3. a	

Measurement Levels

1. c	5. a	8. b
2. a	6. b	9. c
3. b	7. c	10. c
4. c		

Sensitivity and Specificity

1.

Diagnostic Test Results	Disease Present	Disease Not Present or Absent
Positive test	a (true positive)	b (false positive)
Negative test	c (false negative)	d (true negative)

2. Formula for sensitivity: $a/(a + c)$ = True positive rate
3. Formula for specificity: $d/(b + d)$ = True negative rate
4. 20 (10%)
5. 30 (15%)
6. Sensitivity = $90\%/(90\% + 15\%)$ = 85.7%
7. Specificity = $85\%/(10\% + 85\%)$ = 89.5%

Puzzles

Word Scramble

"There is no perfect measure."

Secret Message

"Reliability testing needs to be performed on each instrument used in a study."

Crossword Puzzle

Across	Down
1. Collect	2. Equivalence
3. Mail	4. Instrument
6. Measurement	5. Data

10. Rating	7. Reliability
12. Stability	8. True score
13. Rare	9. Age
14. Ratio	11. Precision
16. Scales	12. Score
17. Error	15. Observe
18. Idea	20. Precision
19. Open	23. Interval
21. Place	25. Stress
22. Interview	26. Setting
24. Accuracy	27. Talk
25. Sensitivity	
28. Questionnaire	
29. Likert	
30. Ordinal	
31. Ask	
32. Nominal	

Exercises in Critical Appraisal

1. a. Bindler et al.'s study:

Variable	Method of Measurement	Directness
Fasting glucose	Fasting blood sample (CX 5Delta analyzer)	D
Fasting insulin	Fasting blood sample (Solid-phase radioimmunoassay)	D
Triglycerides	Fasting blood sample (CX 5Delta analyzer)	D
Total cholesterol	Fasting blood sample (CX 5Delta analyzer)	D
HDL-C	Fasting blood sample (CX 5Delta analyzer)	D
LDL-C	Fasting blood sample (Calculated with Friedewald equation)	D
Smoking history	Questionnaire	I
Blood pressure	Blood pressure cuff (average 3 readings)	D
Metabolic cost of activity (MET)	Godin Leisure Time Questionnaire	I
Height	Standard way—Tape measure	D
Weight	Standard way—Scale	D
Triceps skinfold thickness	Standard way	D
Body mass index (BMI)	Calculated weight/height ratio	D
VO_{2max}	Canadian Aerobic Fitness Test	D
Dietary variables	Youth/Adolescent Question (YAQ) (151-item food frequency questionnaire)	I
Health Eating Index (HEI)	24-hour diet recall	I

b. Sethares and Elliott (2004) study:

Variable	Method of Measurement	Directness
Heart failure readmission rates	Counting total number of admissions for HF in each group during the 3-month study interval	D
Quality of life	Minnesota Living with Heart Failure questionnaire	I
Benefits and barriers	Health Beliefs Scales	I

2. a. Physiological measures:

Precision or Accuracy	Information Listed in Study
Blood samples: Precision and accuracy	Blood samples drawn early in morning by licensed phlebotomist, children fasted 10 hours
Blood pressure	No precision or accuracy information
Height, weight, skinfold thickness	No precision or accuracy information
BMI	No precision or accuracy information

b. Questionnaires:

Scale and Type of Reliability or Validity	Values and Indicate Previous Studies or Current Study?
YAQ convergent validity	Correlates well (0.54) with 24-hour diet recall
Smoking Questionnaire	No reliability or validity information
Godin Leisure Time Questionnaire	No reliability or validity information

3. Scales:

Scale and Type of Reliability or Validity	Values and Indicate Previous Studies or Current Study?
Heart Failure Readmission Rates	No reliability or validity information
Minnesota Living with Heart Failure Questionnaire	
Construct validity	$R = 0.80$, $p = 0.01$ (previous studies)
Cronbach alpha on total instrument	0.94 (previous studies)
Cronbach alpha on total instrument	0.87 (current study)
Health Belief Scales	
Reliability of Health Belief Scales	
Benefits of medications subscale: Cronbach alpha	0.87 (previous studies)
Benefits of medications subscale: Cronbach alpha	0.87 (current study)
Barriers of medications subscale: Cronbach alpha	0.91 (previous studies)
Barriers of medications subscale: Cronbach alpha	0.72 (current study)
Benefits of diet subscale: Cronbach alpha	0.84 (previous studies)
Benefits of diet subscale: Cronbach alpha	0.85 (current study)
Barriers of diet subscale: Cronbach alpha	0.69 (previous studies)
Barriers of diet subscale: Cronbach alpha	0.62 (current study)
Benefits of self-monitoring: Cronbach alpha	0.89 (current study)
Barriers of self-monitoring: Cronbach alpha	0.83 (current study)
Validity for Health Belief Scales	
Content validity	81% agreement (previous studies)
Confirmatory factor analysis—BDCS	41% of variance explained (previous studies)
Confirmatory factor analysis—BMCS	50% of variance explained (previous studies)

4. Adequacy of each measure:
   a. This study lacks precision and accuracy information for all physiological measures except for the blood samples. The researchers indicate standard methods were used to measure some of the physiological variables, but the measurement section of the study would have been strengthened by a discussion of precision and accuracy for each physiological measure. It is not possible for reviewers to determine the precision and accuracy of most of the physiological measures with the information provided. The questionnaires in this study lack discussion of reliability and validity except for the YAQ. Thus, there is insufficient information to judge the validity and reliability of these questionnaires.
   b. These authors provide good information on the reliability and validity of their measurement methods, including values from previous studies and from the current study. The values indicate that the measurement methods have good reliability and validity. However, the two *Health Belief* subscales did not meet the expected 0.80 minimum threshold Cronbach's alpha for internal consistency reliability in the current study. No reliability or validity information is provided on heart failure readmission rates; this information may not exist, but the authors could have commented on the validity of their data sources for this information.

CHAPTER 16

Relevant Terms

1. e	5. k	9. h
2. d	6. g	10. a
3. b	7. f	11. j
4. i	8. c	

Key Ideas

1. clinical
2. self-report
3. Direct
4. alter the reading or measurement
5. consistency
6. control
7. higher
8. depth or content
9. reliable
10. Likert scale
11. Visual analogue scale
12. Health and Psychological Instruments (HAPI) Online
13. Delphi technique
14. You may have listed any of the following:
    a. Locate existing instruments.
    b. Evaluate existing instruments for appropriateness.
    c. Evaluate existing instruments performance or reliability and validity.
    d. Assess the readability levels of instruments.
15. construct or develop

Making Connections

1. a	6. c
2. d	7. a
3. a	8. d
4. c	9. b
5. b	10. d

Puzzles

Word Scramble

"In publishing the results of a physiologic study, the measurement technique needs to be described in considerable detail."

Secret Message

"Observational categories should be mutually exclusive."

Exercises in Critical Appraisal

1. Bindler et al., study:
   a. There is no information about by whom or when the fasting insulin measure was developed. The researchers provided specific details about when the blood was drawn (early in the morning), who drew the blood (licensed phlebotomist), and how long the subjects fasted (10 hours). Specifically "insulin was measured by solid-phase radioimmunoassay with the Coat-A-Count Insulin System (Diagnostic Products, Los Angeles, CA)" (p. 297). The range of possible values is not reported. These researchers provided a fairly detailed discussion of the measurement of fasting insulin that promotes accuracy and precision in the measurement process and quality data to address the research questions.
   b. The researchers provide no details about the equipment that was used to measure BP. However, they do provide details on the process for measuring the children's BPs to promote accuracy and precision in the BP data. "BP was measured on the right arm at heart level while the children were sitting; three readings were made with a 5-minute rest in between, and the mean of the three readings was used in the analysis" (Bindler et al., 2007, p. 297). However, the measurement of BP would have been much stronger if the equipment used to obtain the BP readings and information about its calibration were described.
   c. The researchers provided excellent detail on the YAQ, which included the number of items on the questionnaire, use with children ages 8 to 18, the process for determining intake of food, and the calculation of percentage of recommended dietary allowances (RDA) for each nutrient. Bindler et al. (2007, p. 297) described YAQ as follows: "Dietary data were collected by the use of the Youth/Adolescent Question (YAQ). … This 151-item food frequency questionnaire has been used with children from 8 to 18 years and correlates well (0.54) with 24-hour diet recall results. It uses the Statistical Analysis System and calculates means and standard deviations for energy and all nutrients. It collects the data about the intake of food items for days, weeks, and months. The trained nursing students and the dietitian assisted subjects, as needed, with the questionnaire and had a list of foods common to Hispanic and Native American communities to add, as necessary, to individual child forms. Completed questionnaires were returned to YAQ developers at the Harvard School of Public Health for the calculations of the dietary intake of nutrients from the questionnaire and for the calculations of the percentage of recommended dietary allowance (RDA) for each nutrient."
   d. The researchers provided almost no information on the smoking history questionnaire that just "asked if they were current smokers or if they had ever tried smoking" (Bindler et al., 2007, p. 297). Thus, the measurement of the children's smoking history is limited and provides questionable data for analysis.

2. Sethares and Elliott's study:
   a. This rate was calculated by counting the total number of admissions for heart failure in each group during the 3-month study interval divided by the number of patients in the group. Each admission was counted as 1 regardless of the number of days the patient was in the hospital. This measurement method provided minimal understanding of the hospitalization for heart failure.
   b. Minnesota Living with Health Failure (MLHF) questionnaire. Patients with heart failure rate their perception of the extent to which heart failure affects socioeconomic, psychological, and physical aspects of their daily life, using a rating scale of 0 (not at all) to 5 (very much). Scores range from 0 to 105, with higher scores indicating a worse perceived quality of life.
   c. The Health Beliefs Scale was developed by Bennett and colleagues in 1987. The instrument contains three scales based on the Health Beliefs Model: Beliefs about Diet Compliance Scale (12 items), Beliefs about Medication Compliance Scale (12 items), and Beliefs about Self-Monitoring Compliance (18 items), for a total of 42 items. Each scale has two subscales, one of benefits and the other of barriers. The instrument uses Likert-type scale scores from 1 to 5, with 1 being "strongly disagree" and 5 "strongly agree." The benefit subscale and the barrier subscale are scored for each of the three scales.

CHAPTER 17

Relevant Terms

1. f
2. h
3. d
4. e
5. a
6. b
7. g
8. i
9. j
10. c

Key Ideas

1. You might identify any of the following decision points:
   a. Whether potential subjects meet the sampling criteria
   b. Whether a subject understands the information needed to give informed consent
   c. What group the subject will be assigned to during the study
   d. Whether the subject comprehends instructions related to providing data
   e. Whether the subject has provided all of the data needed
2. You might identify any of the following situations that could affect data collection consistency:
   a. Using more than one data collector
   b. Variation in days and hours of data collection
   c. Care recently received or currently being received
   d. Experience of data collectors
   e. Interaction of subject and data collector during the data collection process
   f. Interactions with family and visitors during the data collection process

3. Direct costs of data collection include the following:
   a. Purchase of measurement instruments
   b. Typing and photocopying costs
   c. Printing costs
   d. Postage costs
   e. Travel costs to and from data collection sites
   f. Charges for coding and entering data
   g. Statistical consultation
4. Indirect costs of data collection include the following:
   a. Researcher's time
   b. Meals eaten out
   c. Subjects' time
   d. Health care providers' time
   e. Child care while collecting data
5. Tasks of researchers during data collection:
   a. Selecting subjects
   b. Collecting data in a consistent way
   c. Maintaining research controls indicated by the study design
   d. Protecting study integrity or validity
   e. Solving problems that threaten to disrupt the study

Making Connections

1. Age:
   a. The age ranges are not equal.
   b. There is no category for the age of 18.
   c. The age 45 could be placed in either of two categories (or both).
2. Problems with data coding
   a. Family members with the flu:
      - One item cannot be used to code these data because subjects could mark several family members. This would require a separate item for each family member, with each member having a code of 0 = no or 1 = yes.
      - There is no option for subjects to mark if the information about who had the flu is "unknown" to them. Thus they might guess, and this increases the potential for error.
      - A subject could have more than one of certain relatives, leaving the subject confused about how to respond. For example, a subject may have two children, one of whom had the flu and the other who did not.
      - Family members are defined differently by different people. Does the researcher wish to allow the respondent to self-identify family members, or does the study use a specific definition of family?
   b. Drugs for nausea and vomiting:
      - The number of drugs needing to be coded could be large. The existing plan only includes 3 potential drugs.
      - There is no identified coding scheme for dosage.
      - The dosage matched with the drug would require a separate data item for each dosage and drug combined. If several drugs were used, matching dose with drug could be error-prone.

c. Length of hospital stay:
   - Is a day 24 hours or a calendar day?
   - If the day is measured in hours, will minutes or fractions of hours also be measured?
   - Is the measurement of length of stay, precise and accurate or somewhat arbitrary from one subject to another? Develop a detailed plan for calculation of length of stay including hours and minutes from the initial time and date of admission to the time and date of discharge.
d. Voting:
   - Subjects are likely to respond inconsistently to this form or response set. For example, some subjects might mark yes by placing a checkmark before the word yes, whereas others might mark yes by placing a checkmark after the word yes. There would be no way to determine later what the subject's intent had been. This could increase the error rate during data collection. Putting each of these response options on a separate line would greatly decrease the chance for error.
   - The question does not specify the contest or election of interest.

Puzzles
Word Scramble

"Problems can be perceived either as a frustration or as a challenge."

Secret Message

"If anything can go wrong, it will, and at the worst possible time."

Crossword Puzzle

Across	Down
1. Serendipity	2. Data collection plan
4. Codebook	3. Coding
6. Cleaning data	5. Data collection
7. Mortality	
8. Computerized database	
9. Data coding sheet	

Exercises in Critical Appraisal

1. The Bindler et al. (2007, pp. 296–297) study was conducted to describe serum insulin levels and to investigate their relationships to metabolic syndrome criteria in a multiethnic sample of schoolchildren. These researchers provided a detailed description of data collection in the section of their study titled "Procedures and Instruments":

"Study personnel consisted of a registered nurse/nutrition doctoral student, eight baccalaureate nursing students, a phlebotomist, one dietitian, and one dietetics students. All were trained and evaluated for reliability on measurement and for assistance to children during questionnaire completion. All measurements and questionnaires involving the children were implemented within a single day in the children's schools. …

Parents of children in the study completed a medical family history form (accomplished during the informational evening session, or accomplished and sent later).... All forms were available in English and Spanish languages.

Blood draws were completed in the early morning by the licensed phlebotomist after the children had fasted for at least 10 hours; children were then fed breakfast before completing the remainder of the testing... Insulin was measured by solid-phase radioimmunoassay with the Coat-A-Count Insulin System (Diagnostic Products, Los Angeles, CA)....

Dietary data were collected by the use of the Youth/Adolescent Question (YAQ) (Rockett et al., 1997; Rockett & Colditz, 1997). This 151-item food frequency questionnaire has been used with children from 8 to 18 years and correlated well (0.54) with 24-hour diet recall results. It uses the Statistical Analysis System and calculates means and standard deviations for energy and all nutrients.... In addition, a 24-hour diet recall was completed verbally with each child by a trained dietitian. These results were used to calculate Healthy Eating Index (HEI) scores.... The 10 HEI scores are for grains, vegetables, fruit, milk, meat, total fat, saturated fat, cholesterol, sodium, and variety (Bowman, Lino, Gerrior, & Basiotis, 1998; Kennedy, Ohls, Carlson, & Fleming, 1995; Variyam, Smallwood, & Basiotis, 1998)."

2. Bindler et al., (2007) provided good detail about the measurement methods (questionnaires and physiological measures) and how data were collected with these methods. The consistency of data collection was promoted with the used of highly qualified professionals who were trained for reliability in the data collection process. The forms and questionnaires were in both English and Spanish to increase the understanding of the subjects (both parents and children) and decrease possible errors in the data collected. The accuracy and precision of the physiological methods were discussed in detail. One area of concern is the validity of the dietary information because it was based on recall. The researchers tried to improve the quality of the dietary information by using the YAQ and conducting the 24-hour diet recall through interview with a trained dietitian.

3. Sethares and Elliott's (2004) study provides a detailed discussion of the instruments used and the data collection process in a section titled "Procedures." Two baccalaureate-prepared research nurses enrolled participants, completed the study intervention as outlined in a detailed protocol, and collected data. Hospitalized subjects whose heart failure (HF) had been stabilized were invited to participate in the study. After consent was obtained and subjects were randomly assigned to groups, an interview was conducted to complete the Minnesota Living with Heart Failure (MLHF) questionnaire and to collect demographic data. Subjects in the treatment group were interviewed using the Health Belief Scales to determine areas in which teaching was needed. Additional demographic and medication data were obtained from the medical record and computerized hospital databases. A follow-up visit was made to subjects in the treatment group 7 to 10 days after discharge. Subjects completed the Health Belief Scales. Medication lists were reviewed, and any medication changes were noted. A final follow-up visit was made to treatment subjects 1 month after discharge. Quality-of-life scores were determined, and medications were reviewed for any changes. A telephone call was made to the control subjects by a blinded data collector at 1 month to determine quality-of-life scores using the MLHF questionnaire. "The outcome variable of HF readmission rates was measured by counting the total number of admissions for HF in each group during the 3-month study interval. Each admission counted as 1 number, regardless of the number of days admitted" (Sethares & Elliott, 2004, p. 272).

4. The MLHF is a valid and reliable scale, as documented in the article, and has been used in a variety of other studies. The MLHF had a reliability of 0.87, which was calculated with the Cronbach's alpha for this study. The Health Belief Scale was used to measure the benefits and barriers of taking HF medications, following a sodium-restricted diet and self-monitoring for signs of fluid overload. "Internal consistencies of these 2 subscales were found to be 0.87 for benefits of medications, 0.91 for barriers to medications, 0.84 for benefits of diet, and 0.69 for barriers of diet. Content validity of the tool was found when evaluated by 2 HF experts, with 81% agreement on the content. In this study, internal consistencies of the subscales were 0.80 for benefits of medications, 0.72 for barriers of medications, 0.85 for benefits of diet, 0.62 for barriers of diet, 0.89 for benefits of self-monitoring, and 0.83 for barriers of self-monitoring" (Sethares & Elliott, 2004, p. 273). Confirmatory factor analysis has also been conducted on this scale to evaluate construct validity. The subscale for barriers to diet of the Health Belief Scale has limited reliability, because it is less than 0.70. The other subscales have solid reliability, and the Health Belief Scale has strong reported construct validity.

Overall the study had strong measurement methods; detailed, reliable implementation of the treatment; and consistent collection of the data with trained data collectors.

Going Beyond

Develop a data coding sheet based on one of the quantitative studies in Appendix B, and ask your faculty or a research expert in your clinical agency to review your sheet and give input.

CHAPTER 18

Relevant Terms

Theories, Concepts, Statistics, Parameters, and Practical Aspects of Data Analysis

1. g	4. j	7. k	10. a	13. m
2. i	5. f	8. d	11. n	14. h
3. b	6. e	9. l	12. c	15. o

Distribution of Scores and Shape of Curve

1. c	5. f	9. h	13. i	17. n
2. l	6. d	10. g	14. o	18. r
3. p	7. m	11. k	15. e	
4. j	8. a	12. q	16. b	

Significance and Confirmations

1. e	4. a	7. f	10. g
2. j	5. c	8. b	11. h
3. i	6. d	9. k	

Key Ideas

1. You may have listed any of the following purposes for conducting statistics:
   a. Summarize demographic and study variables.
   b. Explore the meaning of deviations in the data.
   c. Compare or contrast groups descriptively.
   d. Test the proposed relationships in a theoretical model.
   e. Infer that the findings from the sample are indicative of the entire population.
   f. Predict the dependent or outcome variable using one or more independent variables.
   g. Infer from the sample to a theoretical model.
   h. Examine reliability and validity of measurement methods.
   i. Test differences between the experimental and companion groups.
2. a. Preparing the data for analysis.
   b. Describing the sample.
   c. Testing the reliability of measurement.
   d. Performing exploratory analysis of the data.
   e. Performing confirmatory analyses guided by the hypotheses, questions, or objectives.
   f. Post hoc analyses.
3. a. Every datum is cross-checked with the original datum for accuracy.
   b. All identified errors are corrected.
   c. Missing points are identified.
   d. Missing data are entered into the data file.

Making Connections

Categories

1. c	3. c	5. c	7. b
2. c	4. a	6. b	

Significance

1. a
2. b
3. a

Puzzles

Word Scramble

"To be useful, the evidence from data analysis must be carefully examined, organized, and given meaning."

Secret Message

"Researchers can never prove things."

Crossword Puzzle

Across
2. Clinical significance
4. Level of significance
6. Platykurtic
8. Power analysis
10. Normal curve
13. Tails
15. Skewed
16. Generalize
18. Transform
19. Leptokurtic
20. Distribution
22. Sampling error
23. Post hoc analysis
24. Symmetry

Down
1. Relationship
3. Infer
5. Probability theory
7. Kurtosis
9. Degrees of freedom
11. Mesokurtic
12. Statistic
14. Parameter
17. Exploratory
21. Bimodal

CHAPTER 19

Relevant Terms

Statistics That Summarize Data

1. f	4. h	7. g	10. k	13. b
2. c	5. a	8. l	11. e	
3. j	6. m	9. d	12. i	

Statistics That Explore Deviations and Patterns in Data

1. c	4. h	7. g	10. k	13. l
2. j	5. d	8. m	11. o	14. i
3. f	6. n	9. a	12. e	15. b

Key Ideas

1. descriptive
2. frequency distributions
3. ungrouped frequency distributions
4. loss of information or a grouped frequency distribution
5. Percentage distributions
6. Measures of dispersion
7. squaring
8. standard deviation
9. Standardized scores
10. confidence intervals
11. exploratory data analysis
12. scatter plot
13. You may have listed any of the following analysis techniques used to describe the sample:

a. Measures of central tendency such as mode, median, and mean based on the level of measurement of demographic variables.
b. Measures of dispersion such as range and exploratory analyses to identify outliers. Make it as a smooth symmetrical normal cureve.
c. Measures of dispersion such as standard deviation to determine the spread of scores.

d. Use of a scatter plot to determine relationships among variables.

Making Connections

1. Knowledge of risk factors distribution in treatment group

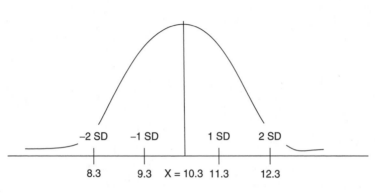

Puzzles

Word Scramble

"Using measures of central tendency to describe the nature of the data obscures the impact of extreme values or of deviations in the data."

Secret Message

"Data analysis begins with descriptive statistics in any study in which the data are numeric, including some qualitative studies."

Crossword Puzzle

Across	Down
1. Sum of squares	2. Standard deviation
5. Inherent variability	3. Scatter plots
6. Variance	4. Ungrouped frequency
9. Dispersion	7. Central tendency
12. Outliers	8. Measurement error
14. Mode	10. Pattern
15. Range	11. Homogeneity
16. Mean	13. Residual analysis
17. Heterogeneity	18. Median
19. Exploratory data analysis	
20. Survival analysis	
21. Difference score	
22. Frequencies	

Exercises in Critical Appraisal

1. The number of subjects in the convenience sample and the percentage of the eligible students represented by the sample; demographic characteristics of the sample: age, gender, ethnicity, the range of the school grades being attended, family history of risk factors, subjects' physical activity measures, smoking history, blood pressure, and measures of body fat/obesity. Table 3 describes the sample using ungrouped frequency distributions and percentage distributions for the nominal level data (such as gender, ethnicity, and family history of risk factors); range for age; and means and standard deviations for the interval/ratio level data (such as blood pressure, height, weight, BMI, and skinfold percentile). Table 4 provides the means and standard deviations of serum measures and dietary intake by ethnic groups. Table 5 provides the frequencies and percentages for the risk factors for metabolic syndrome by ethnic group.

   Indications of exploratory data analysis can be found in the Results section where missing data are identified, and trends are explored in the Discussion and Clinical Implications sections where major findings are highlighted and implications discussed.

   The Bindler et al. (2007) study provides detailed description of the sample and describes the study variables with the results clearly presented in tables. No additional analyses are recommended.

2. Sethares and Elliott (2004) describe the sample size, the number originally recruited, the number who withdrew, and the number who died before the study was completed. A *t*-test was run to compare variable values of subjects who died with those who completed the study. No significant differences were found. Demographic characteristics are presented in Tables 1 and 2. Comparisons of the treatment group and the control group revealed no significant differences. Reliability data are provided on measures used in the study. The authors also report the following discussion of preliminary analyses in their study: "Descriptive statistics were computed on all study variables and examined for the presence of random or systematic missing data, significant skewness, and outliers. Appropriate reliability and validity measures were performed on measurement instruments. Because the outcome variable of heart failure (HF) readmission rates was skewed, the nonparametric Kruskal-Wallis statistic was computed to determine differences in HF readmission rates between the treatment and control groups. The benefits, barriers, and quality of life data were not skewed" (p. 255).

Sethares and Elliott (2004) conducted appropriate descriptive analysis techniques to describe their sample and study variables. These results are clearly presented in tables and narrative in the study. No additional analyses would be recommended.

CHAPTER 20

Relevant Terms

Bivariate Correlational Analysis

1. f	5. r	9. t	13. q	17. l	21. g
2. c	6. e	10. a	14. u	18. o	
3. k	7. n	11. m	15. d	19. j	
4. p	8. i	12. h	16. s	20. b	

Multivariate Correlational Analysis

1. e	5. j	9. i	13. g	17. m
2. b	6. p	10. n	14. k	
3. h	7. a	11. c	15. o	
4. l	8. d	12. q	16. f	

Key Ideas

1. relationships
2. one
3. full range
4. regression line
5. high, low (or low, high)
6. Interval or ratio
7. Phi, Chi square, Contingency coefficient, Cramer's V, or Lambda
8. positive, negative, magnitude or strength
9. ranked
10. correlational matrix
11. Factor analysis
12. $r^2 \times 100$

Making Connections

Macnee and McCabe Study

$r = 0.37$, M
$r = 0.32$, M
$r = 0.46$, M
L < 0.3; M = 0.3–0.5; H > 0.5

Gary and Yarandi Study

1. Principal-factor analysis was used to analyze the study data. Minimum 80% variance criterion and the scree plot were used to determine the optimal number of factors and two factors were identified. These two factors had comparably sized eigen values of 5.35 and 5.53. The first factor included items describing negative feelings, and the author named it the cognitive dimension. The second factor included items describing physical symptoms. This factor was named the somatic-affective domain. The amount of variation in responses to items in the scale explained by the two factors was 89%. The two factors are correlated with $r = 0.57$.

Puzzles

Word Scramble

"Weak correlations may be important when combined with other variables."

Secret Message

"In preparation for correlational analysis, data collection strategies should be planned to maximize the possibility of obtaining the full range of possible values on each variable to be used in the analysis."

Crossword Puzzle

Across	Down
1. Oblique rotation	2. Bivariate
4. Curvilinear relation	3. Positive linear
7. Residual	5. Loading
13. Factor rotation	6. Kendall's Tau
14. Latent	8. Scatter diagram
15. Regression line	9. Factor loading
16. Spurious	10. Scree
17. Eigen values	11. Goodness-of-fit
18. Matrix	12. Homoscedastic
20. Scree test	13. Factor
21. Weighting	16. Strength
	19. Weak

Exercises in Critical Appraisal

1. $r = 0.399^{**}$ was the strongest correlation between insulin and BMI percentile in Table 6. This correlation was significant at 0.01 level indicated by the ** after the correlational value.
2. $r = -0.016$ was the weakest correlation between insulin and VO_{2max} in Table 6. This was a negative relationship as indicated by the minus sign. This correlation was not significant because no * was placed after the correlational value.

3. $r = 0.303^{**}$ for the relationship between insulin and triglycerides.

$$\text{Percentage of variance} = r^2 \times 100 = 0.303^2 \times 100 = 0.092 \times 100 = 9\%$$

This r value is statistically significant at 0.01 level as indicated by the **.

The percentage of variance explained is 9%, which has some but limited clinical importance, because less than 10% of the variance in insulin is explained by triglycerides.

4. $r = -0.071$ for the relationship between insulin and vitamin A.

$$\text{Percentage of variance} = r^2 \times 100 = -0.071^2 \times 100 = 0.0050 \times 100 = 0.5\%$$

This r value is not statistical significant because there is no * after the r value.

The percentage of variance explained is 0.5%, which has no clinical significance, because less than 1% of the variance in insulin is explained by vitamin A. The r value is very close to 0 indicating essentially no relationship between these two variables.

5. Kendall's tau was used to determine the relationships between insulin and the criteria for metabolic syndrome. Bindler et al. (2007, p. 298) found that "Insulin showed highly significant positive correlations with systolic and diastolic BP; weight, BMI, and skinfold percentiles; serum triglycerides and glucose; and triglyceride: HDL and TC: HDL ratios. Furthermore, insulin showed significant positive correlations with having tried smoking, height percentile, and serum TC and LDL-C. It had highly significant negative correlations with total dietary fat and kilocalories per kilogram of weight. It had significant negative correlations with dietary carbohydrate, protein, and total calories, percentage of calories from fat, and serum HDL-C (Table 6)."

Going Beyond

Find an article in one of the nursing research journals, examine the correlational results as suggested, and share your ideas with your faculty or class members.

CHAPTER 21

Relevant Terms
Simple Linear Regression

1. h	5. t	9. g	13. i	17. p	21. l
2. n	6. e	10. s	14. r	18. f	
3. c	7. q	11. a	15. d	19. o	
4. j	8. u	12. k	16. m	20. b	

Multiple Regression

1. c	5. d	9. f	13. h
2. g	6. i	10. l	
3. k	7. a	11. b	
4. e	8. m	12. j	

Key Ideas
1. variance
2. probability
3. causal

4. independent, dependent
5. x (independent variable), y (dependent variable)
6. Method of least squares
7. R
8. variance
9. estimate
10. analysis of variance
11. independent
12. independent
13. generalizability
14. inflated
15. mixture or combination
16. predictive equation
17. group membership
18. Linear discriminant functions (LDFs)

Making Connections
Regression Analysis

1. a. The presence of homoscedasticity equals scatter of values of y above and below the regression line at each value of x (constant variance).
   b. The dependent variable is measured at the interval or ratio level.
   c. The expected value of the residual error is zero.
2. $Y = a + bx$
3. a. Dummy variables
   b. Multiplicative terms
   c. Transformed terms
   d. Interval or ratio level variables

Matching

1. g	3. f	5. a	7. e
2. c	4. b	6. d	8. h

Puzzles
Word Scramble

"The goal of regression analysis is to determine how accurately one can predict the value of a dependent variable based on the value or values of one or more independent variables."

Secret Message

"Discriminant analysis is designed to determine how accurately one can predict the value or values of one or more independent variables."

Crossword Puzzle

Across	Down
1. Horizontal axis	1. Hold out sample
3. Multiplicative term	2. Predictor variable
11. Y intercept	4. Predictive validity
12. Vertical axis	5. Discriminant analysis
13. Bivariate	6. Multiple regression
14. Coefficient R	7. Homoscedasticity
15. Slope	8. Dummy variables
16. Discriminant function	9. Line of best fit
	10. Cross validation

Exercises in Critical Appraisal

1. Research question 4: Which data predict insulin levels in this multiethnic sample of children?

2.

Variable	Level of Measurement
Gender	Nominal
Age	Ratio
Race	Nominal
BMI percentile	Ratio
Glucose	Ratio
Triglycerides	Ratio
HDL-C	Ratio
Systolic BP	Ratio
Diastolic BP	Ratio

3. Multiple linear regression, backward stepwise regression, and binary logistic stepwise regression were used to analyze data in the Bindler et al. (2007). Backward stepwise regression is a more sophisticated procedure used to determine which variables do the best job of predicting insulin levels. Binary logistic stepwise regression results in an *odds ratio*, which in this study indicates that a child with three or more of the risk factors will have a 5.8 times increased chance of having an elevated insulin level than a child who does not have three or more of the indicated risk factors. For more information about backward stepwise regression and binary logistic stepwise regression, see *Statistics for Healthcare Research: A Practical Workbook* by S. K. Grove (2007).

4. Forty-eight percent of the variance in insulin levels is explained by the multiple regression model tested (the model that includes the nine variables listed in question 2).

5. Triglycerides, systolic BP, and race

6. Fifty percent of the variance in insulin levels is explained by the second regression model created by the backward stepwise procedure.

7. a. Significant and predicted

Going Beyond

Discuss the regression analysis results that you found in published studies with your faculty and class members.

CHAPTER 22

Relevant Terms

Contingency Tables

1. e	6. a	11. k	16. q
2. l	7. r	12. p	17. f
3. h	8. g	13. b	18. j
4. o	9. s	14. t	19. n
5. m	10. d	15. i	20. c

t-tests and ANOVA

1. b	6. c	11. t	16. q
2. g	7. p	12. h	17. f
3. l	8. j	13. r	18. m
4. i	9. s	14. d	19. k
5. o	10. e	15. n	20. a

Key Ideas

1. independent
2. dependent
3. contingency tables
4. one entry
5. robust
6. within, between
7. groups
8. regression analysis

Puzzles

Word Scramble

"The *t*-test can be used only one time during analysis to examine data from two samples in a study."

Secret Message

"In many cases, bivariate analysis does not provide a clear picture of the dynamics in the situation."

Crossword Puzzle

Across
1. Statistic
5. Decision theory
8. Significant
11. Power
12. Omit
14. Regression
15. ANOVA
16. Dependent
17. Causal
18. Mean
19. Tail
20. Variance
21. Range
22. Outliers
23. Median
24. Result
25. Inference

Down
2. *t*-test
3. Explanatory
4. Mode
5. Distribution
6. Representative
7. Implications
9. Normal curve
10. Chi square
13. Post hoc

Exercises in Critical Appraisal

1.

Variable	Level of Measurement
Heart failure	
Readmission rate	Interval/ratio

2. a. Intervention group
   b. Control group

3. These two groups are independent. The rationale for the groups being independent is that subjects were randomly assigned to the groups, thus there was no link between the subjects in the intervention group and the control group.

4. Kruskall-Wallis one-way analysis of variance by ranks

5. Kruskall-Wallis is a commonly used technique to compare two or more groups when the data are interval/ratio but do not meet the assumptions for parametric tests. The data in this study were skewed, and therefore a parametric test (i.e. *t*-test or ANOVA) is inappropriate. The interval/ratio data are analyzed as though they are at the ordinal level since the distribution of scores are skewed.

261

6. Results: "HF readmission rate was not significantly related to group assignment in this study (*p.* = .22)" (Sethares & Elliott, 2004, p. 275).
7. b. Nonsignificant
8. As Table IV shows, 12 subjects in the control group were rehospitalized one or more times, whereas 6 subjects in the treatment group were rehospitalized one or more times. Clearly, there was a difference between the two groups, but because of the small sample size (70 subjects), the study did not have sufficient power to detect a statistical difference if there actually is one in the real world. One can reasonably question whether this finding is a type II error. The authors state that "the sample size of 70 for the readmission and quality of life variables was determined through a power analysis with an effect size of 0.35, an alpha of .05, and a power of 0.80" (Sethares & Elliott, 2004. p. 272). This is a medium effect size. Power analysis would have required a sample of 192 subject to have the capacity to identify a small effect. Polit and Sherman (1990) indicated that most nursing intervention studies require the power to test small effect sizes because of crude measures of the dependent variables and the strength of the studies' interventions to create a difference between experimental and control groups.
   Polit, D. F., & Sherman, R. E. (1990). Statistical power in nursing research. *Nursing Research, 39*(6), 365–369.
9.

Variable	Level of Measurement
Quality of life	Individual scale items are ordinal but the total score for quality of life are treated as interval

10. a. Intervention group
    b. Control group
11. The groups are independent
12. Repeated measures ANOVA
13. To compare the quality of life data scores at baseline and 1 month between the treatment and control groups. Because multiple measures were taken of the quality-of-life variable, a repeated measures ANOVA was used to analyze the data.
14. "For within-subjects effects, there were significant differences in quality-of-life measures at the 2 time points (*F* = 35.44, *p* = .000), with both groups reporting improved quality of life at 1 month as expected with a group recruited during hospitalization. The mean quality of life score was 55.5 at baseline and 41.6 at 1 month. The assumption of homogeneity of variance for between-subjects factors was met. There were no significant differences between the group receiving the tailored message intervention and the control group in reported quality of life (*F* = 1.031, *p* = .309). The control group had a mean score of 50.9, and the treatment group had a mean score of 46.2. There was no significant interaction between quality of life and group assigned (*F* = .217, *p* = .575)" (Sethares & Elliott, 2004, p. 275).
15. b. Nonsignificant
16. Intervention subjects would report fewer barriers and more benefits to performing self-care of HF after receiving the tailored message intervention.

Variable	Level of Measurement
Benefits of medications	Individual scale items are ordinal but the total score for benefits of medications are treated as interval
Benefits of diet	Individual scale items are ordinal but the total score for benefits of diet are treated as interval
Benefits of self-monitoring	Individual scale items are ordinal but the total score for benefits of self-moitoring are treated as interval
Barriers of medication	Individual scale items are ordinal but the total score for barriers of medication are treated as interval
Barriers of diet	Individual scale items are ordinal but the total score for barriers of diet are treated as interval
Barriers of self-monitoring	Individual scale items are ordinal but the total score for barriers of self-monitoring are treated as interval

17. a. Intervention group at baseline
    b. Intervention group at 1 week
    c. Intervention group at 1 month
18. Groups are dependent. This is the same group of subjects that is being compared over time, thus the groups are dependent.
19. Within-subjects repeated measures ANOVA
20. "The benefits of medications scores did not change significantly during the study (p = .259). Barriers of medication scores decreased from baseline to the 1-week point (*p* = .000) and significantly decreased from baseline to the 1 month point (*p* = .000). Benefits of diet significantly increased from baseline to 1 week (*p* = .000) and from baseline to 1 month (*p* = .000). The barriers of diet significantly decreased from baseline to 1 week (*p* = .000) and from baseline to 1 month (*p* = .001). The benefits of self-monitoring significantly improved from baseline to 1 week (*p* = .000) and from baseline to 1 month (p = .000). Barriers of self-monitoring decreased significantly from baseline to 1 week (*p* = .002) with further decreases at 1 month" (Sethares & Elliott, 2004, pp. 275–276). Table 5 in the article also includes these results.
21. a. Significant and predicted

Going Beyond

Identify the effectiveness of the interventions in the studies you selected. Examine the process for implementing the intervention or treatment in the study and critically appraise this process. Share your ideas with your faculty.

CHAPTER 23

Relevant Terms
Data Collection in Qualitative Studies

1. e   4. h   7. d   10. a
2. g   5. b   8. i   11. j
3. c   6. k   9. f

Data Management and Reduction (A)

1. e	5. f	9. p	13. n
2. a	6. m	10. d	14. b
3. k	7. c	11. o	15. l
4. h	8. j	12. g	16. i

Data Management and Reduction (B)

1. i	6. p	11. c	16. m
2. d	7. b	12. k	17. g
3. n	8. j	13. h	
4. f	9. e	14. o	
5. l	10. q	15. a	

Qualitative Research Methods

1. e	5. m	9. n	13. b
2. j	6. g	10. k	14. l
3. h	7. o	11. d	15. f
4. a	8. c	12. p	16. i

Qualitative Research Issues

1. d	3. b	5. f	7. i	9. g
2. h	4. j	6. c	8. a	10. e

Key Ideas

1. simultaneously with
2. words, numbers
3. concreteness, abstraction
4. decision rules
5. personality
6. theorizing
7. participants
8.
   a. Complete participation
   b. Participant as observer
   c. Observer as participant
   d. Complete observer
9. You may choose any of the following:
   a. The researcher influences the individuals being studied and, in turn, is influenced by them.
   b. The mere presence of the researcher may alter behavior in the setting.
   c. The researcher's personality is a key factor in conducting the study.
   d. The researcher needs to become closely involved in the subject's experience in order to interpret it.
   e. It is necessary for the researcher to be open to the perceptions of the participants, rather than to attach his or her own meaning to the experience.
   f. Individuals being studied often participate in determining research questions, guiding data collection, and interpreting results.
10. You may choose any of the following:
    a. Coding-developing categories
    b. Reflective remarks
    c. Marginal remarks
    d. Memoing
    e. Developing propositions
11. You may choose any of the following:
    a. Counting
    b. Noting patterns and themes
    c. Seeing plausibility
    d. Clustering
    e. Making metaphors
    f. Splitting variables
    g. Subsuming particulars into the general
    h. Factoring
    i. Noting relationships between variables
    j. Finding intervening variables
    k. Building a logical chain of evidence
    l. Making conceptual and theoretical coherence

Making Connections

1. e	7. c	13. f
2. f	8. d	14. d
3. b	9. a	15. a
4. a	10. b	16. c
5. d	11. c	17. e
6. b	12. e	

Puzzles

Word Scramble

"Analysis requires cross-checking each bit of data with all the other bits of data."

Secret Message

"One important difference between quantitative and qualitative research is the nature of relationships between the researcher and the individuals being studied."

Crossword Puzzle

Across

2. Interpretation
5. Cognitive mapping
9. Segmentation
11. Case study
12. Story
14. Intuiting
15. Data reducing
16. Bracketing
17. Story taker
18. Memoing
19. Explanatory
20. Auditability
21. Coding

Down

1. Reflexivity
3. Premature parsimony
4. Story telling
6. Themes
7. Decision trail
8. Dwelling
10. Participate
13. Triangulation

Exercises in Critical Appraisal

1. The philosophical base of the study is phenomenology.
2. The author used Giorgi's method.
3. Giorgi is a phenomenological methodologist. Clearly the author intentionally selected a phenomenological approach to the study.

4. The researcher was consistent in following the methodology.
5. The author's logic was easy to follow.
6. The author's selection of subjects seemed limited to women who were involved in church activities. The findings may be limited to those who have such connections.
7. The information provides some guidance to those working with substance-abusing women. Their spirituality needs to be included in the treatment plan.

Going Beyond

Select a qualitative study from a journal. Describe the methodology used in this study. Clarify your ideas with your classmates and faculty.

CHAPTER 24

Relevant Terms
Types of Study Results
1. d   4. e
2. c   5. a
3. b

Content Areas of the Discussion Section of a Study
1. e   4. d
2. f   5. c
3. a   6. b

Key Ideas
1. Carefully examined, organized, and given meaning, and both statistical and clinical significance need to be assessed
2. You may choose from the following:
   a. Abstract thinking
   b. Introspection
   c. Reasoning
   d. Intuition
   e. Synthesis
   f. Mathematical logic
   g. Gestalt formation
   h. Forecasting
3. Reexamination of the research plan
4. Adequately measured
5. Consistently
6. You may choose from the following:
   a. How many errors were made in entering the data into the computer?
   b. How many subjects have missing data that could affect statistical analyses?
   c. Were the analyses accurately calculated?
   d. Were statistical assumptions violated?
   e. Were the statistics used appropriate to the data?
7. Amount of variance in the phenomenon
8. The risk of a type II error in relation to the nonsignificant results.
9. Unexpected
10. proves anything
11. Going beyond the data

12. You may list any of the following:
    a. Make an important difference in people's lives.
    b. Have external validity.
    c. Possibly generalize the findings far beyond the study sample so that the findings have the potential to affect large numbers of people.
    d. Go beyond concrete facts to abstractions.
    e. Lead to the generation of theory or revisions in existing theory.
    f. Have implications for one or more disciplines in addition to nursing.
    g. Provide valuable evidence to work toward evidence-based practice.
    h. Provide a basis for solid additional research
13. study sample
14. empirical
15. Many studies
16. framework or theoretical basis

Making Connections
1. c   3. f   5. d
2. a   4. e   6. b

Puzzles
Word Scramble
"Evaluating the research process used in the study, producing meaning from the results, and forecasting the usefulness of the findings, all of which are involved in interpretation, require high-level intellectual processes."

Secret Message
"To be useful, the evidence from data analysis needs to be carefully examined, organized, and given meaning, and both statistical and clinical significance needs to be examined."

Crossword Puzzle

Across	Down
3. Landmark studies	1. Practical significance
7. Evidence	2. Significance
9. Conclusion	3. Generalization
10. Translate	5. Interpretation
11. Implications	6. Findings
	8. Results

Exercises in Critical Appraisal
1. Bindler, Massey, Shultz, Mills, and Short (2007) study findings were as follows:
   - Insulin levels in this study showed large variability, and 20% of the children had high insulin levels.
   - Insulin levels were positively correlated with metabolic syndrome criteria of high blood pressure, high adiposity, high serum triglycerides, and glucose, and low serum HDL-C.
   - Total carbohydrate, protein, and fat intake were negatively related to insulin levels.
   - Dietary intake and insulin levels would be expected to show positive correlations but did not, and maybe the diet recalls did not accurately reflect dietary intake for the children.

- Fiber intake was not a significant correlate with insulin levels, but the relationships was in the direction expected.
- The risk of metabolic syndrome was highest in the Native American female children who had the highest BMI percentiles—a measure of adiposity.
- Race was not a significant factor in predicting insulin variance, but the BMI percentile was highly significant.
- Skinfold percentile, another measure of adiposity, was high among the Native American group.
- Half the Native American children had tried smoking.
- Unexpected finding is that the Hispanic children did not have elevated insulin levels, possibly because they were part of a migrant worker population who had not lived in the United States long.
- Results that contribute to these findings:
  □ The correlates of insulin are presented in Table 6.
  □ The dietary correlates of metabolic syndrome criteria are presented in Table 7.
  □ The linear regression of insulin with metabolic syndrome variables is presented in Table 8.

2. Conclusions: "In summary, this study found significant correlations of insulin with body adiposity, BP, and serum lipid/lipoprotein levels, consistent with the clustering of variables labeled as metabolic syndrome. Furthermore, there were ethnic and gender differences in serum insulin levels, indicating an increased risk for metabolic syndrome among Native Americans, particularly among Native American female children, as compared to Hispanic and Caucasian populations. … In addition, higher insulin levels were related to a lower incidence of meeting the RDAs for dietary nutrients" (Bindler et al., 2007, p. 304).

3. Bindler et al.'s conclusions are warranted by the study results and the findings. In addition, they linked the study findings with those of previous studies.

4. Bindler et al. (2007, p. 303) did identify the limitations of the study: "The present study had several limitations. The sample was a small convenience sample and may not be representative of all populations of Native Americans, Hispanic Americans, and Caucasians. In particular, the Native American and Caucasian samples were small. The children were in an agricultural area of central Washington State and may not reflect urban or other diverse populations. Native American tribes and Hispanics from various geographic locations are not uniform in the incidence of type 2 diabetes and in risk factors; thus, the results cannot be generalized to different tribes or various populations of Hispanics."

5. Bindler et al. (2007, pp. 303–304) had a complete section on "Clinical Implications," and research questions 5 focused on how the study information might be used by pediatric nurses. The researchers developed a table of measures to identify children at risk for metabolic syndrome (see Table 9) to guide nurses and other care providers in clinical settings.

6. The study findings are clinically significant because a growing number of children are eating diets high in carbohydrates and fats and are doing limited physical activities. These behaviors are resulting in an increased incidence of the symptoms of metabolic syndrome in school-age children. So it is important to

determine the criteria that predict metabolic syndrome in children and how these children might be identified and assisted to improve their diet and exercise to decrease their risk for type 2 diabetes and cardiovascular disease in the future.

7. Generalizations: The researchers clearly indicated that because of the study limitations of small sample size, limited group sizes for Native Americans and Caucasians, and rural setting, the findings could not be generalized beyond the sample of this study to the target population (see the response to questions 4).

8. Recommendations for further studies: Bindler et al. (2007, p. 304) indicated "Research efforts need to confirm these findings with larger groups and with Native American tribes and Hispanic samples in a variety of geographic locations. Longitudinal studies would help to demonstrate the persistence of syndrome variables over time with individual children and populations further guiding intervention efforts. … Future research is needed to provide clear guidelines for the identification of insulin resistance and metabolic syndrome in youths to design interventions that decrease the incidence of type 2 diabetes and emergence of cardiovascular disease."

CHAPTER 25

Relevant Terms

1. e	5. a	8. f
2. b	6. c	9. j
3. i	7. g	10. d
4. h		

Key Ideas

1. You may have identified any of the following:
   a. Background and significance of the problem
   b. Problem statement
   c. Statement of the purpose
   d. Presentation of the literature review, empirical and theoretical literature
   e. Discussion of the framework
   f. Identification of research objectives, questions, or hypotheses (if applicable)
   g. Identification of conceptual and operational definitions of variables

2. You may have identified any of the following:
   a. Discussion of the research design
   b. Description of the intervention and intervention protocol (intervention fidelity) if the study had an experimental treatment
   c. Description of the sample
   d. Identification of the study setting
   e. Description of the methods of measurement
   f. Discussion of the data collection process

3. methods

4. a. Discussion of data analysis techniques
   b. Presentation of results

5. bar graphs, line graphs

6. results

7. do

8. meta-analyses, power analysis

9. tables, figures
10. You may have identified any of the following:
    a. Presentation of major study findings
    b. Link of the findings to those of previous studies
    c. Link of the study findings to the study framework
    d. Identification of the study limitations
    e. Identification of conclusions
    f. Generalization of the findings and conclusions
    g. Discussion of the implications for nursing practice
    h. Recommendations for further research
11. framework
12. Implications for practice
13. a. Entry into the site
    b. Selection of participants
    c. Documentation of ethical considerations
    d. Description of the data collection process
14. a. Identification of the phenomenon to be studied
    b. Identification of the aim or purpose of the study
    c. Identification of the study questions
    d. Identification of the qualitative approach used to conduct the study
    e. Discussion of the significance of the study to nursing
    f. Evolution of the study
15. theory, model, culture, event
16. theses, dissertations
17. a. Nurses (clinicians, educators, and researchers)
    b. Other health professionals
    c. Policy makers
    d. Consumers of health care services
18. researchers, educators, and clinicians
19. Internet
20. a. Receiving acceptance as a presenter
    b. Developing a research report
    c. Delivering the report
    d. Responding to questions
21. abstract
22. 5
23. one-to-one or individual
24. a. Basic requirements of the journal
    b. The journal's refereed status
    c. The recent articles published in the journal
25. query letter
26. a. Acceptance of the manuscript as submitted
    b. Acceptance of the manuscript pending minor revisions
    c. Tentative acceptance of the manuscript pending major revisions
    d. Rejection of the manuscript
27. poorly written
28. books; chapters in books
29. duplicate publication
30. reference list

Making Connections

1. a	5. c	8. d
2. b	6. a	9. b
3. d	7. c	10. d
4. a		

Exercises in Critical Appraisal

Bindler, Massey, Shultz, Mills, and Short Study

1. Yes, Bindler et al. (2007) included the four main sections of a research report but also some additional headings:
    a. Introduction (content included but not labeled as such)
    b. Review of Literature
    c. Purpose that included the Operational Definitions
    d. Methods that included headings of Sample, Procedures and Instruments, and Statistical Analysis
    e. Results that included headings of Description of the Sample and Research Question 1, 2, 3, and 4
    f. Discussion
    g. Clinical Implications that included a heading of Research Question 5
    h. Summary
2. This study was published in the *Journal of Pediatric Nursing*, which is read by expert pediatric clinicians, researchers, and educators. The editor of this journal, Dr. Cecily Betz, is a nurse, and the editorial board is also composed of nurses. This journal is probably read mainly by nurses, in particular pediatric nurses; a limited number of other health professionals; and a few consumers.

Sethares and Elliott Study

1. Yes, Sethares and Elliott (2004) covered the main areas of a research report: Introduction, Methods, Results, and Discussion. They also included additional headings that constitute the steps of the research process.
    a. Introduction, Literature Review, Conceptual Framework, Study Purposes and Research Questions, Hypotheses
    b. Methods, Sample, Instruments (heart failure readmission rates, quality of life, benefits and barriers), Procedure, Intervention (treatment subjects; control subjects), Analysis
    c. Results (readmission rates; quality of life; benefits and barriers)
    d. Discussion, Implications
2. This article was published in *Heart & Lung*, a journal read by clinicians in the specialty areas of critical care and medical-surgical nursing. Researchers and educators also read this journal to add to their knowledge base of care provided to patients with complex acute and chronic illnesses. The editor of this journal, Dr. Kathleen Stone, is a nurse, and the section editors and executive editorial board are all nurses. The editorial board includes both nurses and physicians. The journal is probably read mainly by nurses, especially those with an intensive care or medical surgical area of expertise; some physicians; and a limited number of other health professionals. This journal is probably not read by many consumers.

Wright Study

1. Yes, Wright (2003) does include most of the main sections of a research report:
    a. Introduction (provided but not labeled), Purpose

266

b. Methods (Philosophical Perspective, Methodology, Methods, Study Participants, Phenomenological Rigor, Procedure and Data Collection)

c. Findings (includes Results)

d. Discussion, Limitations, Conclusions and Implications

2. This study was published in *Archives of Psychiatric Nursing*, which is read by clinicians, educators, and researchers with a specialty area in psychiatric nursing. The editor of this journal, Dr. Judith Krauss, is a nurse, and the associate editors and editorial board members are all nurses. This journal is probably read mainly by nurses and a limited number of other health professionals, such as counselors, social workers, and psychiatrists, and maybe a few consumers.

CHAPTER 26

Relevant Terms

1. m	6. b	11. h
2. c	7. e	12. f
3. a	8. k	13. l
4. n	9. i	14. j
5. d	10. g	15. o

Key Ideas

1. strengths or merits, weaknesses, meaning, significance

2. You could include any of the following:
   a. What are the major strengths of the study?
   b. What are the major weaknesses of the study?
   c. Are the findings from the study an accurate reflection of reality?
   d. What is the significance of the findings for nursing?
   e. Are the findings consistent with those of previous studies?

3. If you are an undergraduate nursing student, you might critically appraise studies to share the findings with another health care professional. You might read and critically appraise studies to solve a problem in practice or to summarize research in a topic area for use in practice. The synthesized research evidence might be used to develop an evidence-based policy, protocol, or algorithm to the direct care of patients with a particular need or problem. You might critically appraise a proposed study to determine whether it is ethical to conduct in your clinical agency. If you are a student in a master's program, you might do all the previously listed behaviors and also critically appraise studies to use in developing the literature review section of a research proposal. Thus, you would be summarizing the current knowledge base in a selected area as the basis for conducting your own study. If you are a doctoral student, you might conceptually cluster the findings from several studies to determine the current body of knowledge in a selected area to promote evidence-based practice in this area. This synthesis of evidence needs to be published in refereed journals or books. Doctoral students also critically appraise studies to develop a synthesis of current knowledge to provide a basis for developing a research proposal for funding.

4. Select from the following:
   a. Appropriateness of the study for the program planned
   b. Completeness of the research project
   c. Overall quality of the work
   d. Contribution of the study to nursing scholarship
   e. Contribution of the study to nursing theory
   f. Originality of the work (not previously published)
   g. Clarity and completeness of the abstract

5. Select from the following:
   a. Examine the expertise of the researchers.
   b. Critique the entire study.
   c. Address the study's strengths.
   d. Address the study's weaknesses.
   e. Examine the adequacy of the study's logical links.
   f. Evaluate the contribution of the study to nursing knowledge.

6. a. Comprehension
   b. Comparison
   c. Analysis
   d. Evaluation
   e. Conceptual clustering

7. a. Descriptive vividness
   b. Methodological congruence
   c. Analytical preciseness
   d. Theoretical connectedness
   e. Heuristic relevance

Exercises in Critical Appraisal

Conduct a complete critical appraisal of the three studies provided in this study guide. Review the answers for the critical appraisal exercises in Chapters 5 through 11 and Chapters 14 through 24 to assist you in determining the quality of your work for the Bindler et al. (2007) and Sethares and Elliott (2004) studies. Review the answers for the critical appraisal exercises in Chapters 4 through 9, 14 through 17, and 23 to assist you in determining the quality of your work for the Wright (2003) study. Also, ask your instructor to clarify any questions that you might have and to review your work when done.

CHAPTER 27

Relevant Terms

1. l	5. e	9. d
2. b	6. g	10. j
3. i	7. k	11. h
4. a	8. f	12. c

Key Ideas

1. Evidence-based practice promotes desired outcomes for patients, nurses, and health care agencies. Some of these positive outcomes include the following:
   a. Improved quality of care
   b. Improved patient outcomes such as decreased signs and symptoms, improved functional status, improved physical and psychological health, prevention of illnesses, and increased promotion of health through implementation of healthy lifestyles

c. Decreased recovery time

d. Decreased need for health care services

e. Decreased cost of care

f. Improved work environment for nurses with increased productivity

g. Increased access to care by providing different types of health care agencies and services with a variety of health care providers

h. Increased patient satisfaction with care

i. Evidence-based practice important to meet accreditation requirements

j. Evidence-based practice is important for a health care agency to achieve Magnet status

2. You may have identified any of the following:

a. Research journals in nursing and other health care disciplines

b. Clinical journals with a major focus on publishing research articles

c. Evidence-based websites such as the Agency for Healthcare Research and Quality and many others that communicate evidence-based guidelines and reference a variety of research publications

d. Professional nursing meetings and conferences

e. Nursing research conferences

f. Some collaborative groups of nurses and other health professionals that share research findings

g. Study findings reported on television and on the Internet

h. Research findings reported in newspapers and popular journals

3. You may have identified any of the following:

a. Nursing lacks the research evidence for the implementation of evidence-based practice (EBP).

b. There is a concern that research evidence generated based on population data might not transfer to the care of individual patients who respond in unique ways.

c. Best research evidence is currently generated mainly from quantitative, outcomes, and interventions research methodologies, and more work is needed to synthesize qualitative research and determine its contribution to EBP.

d. EBP movement might lead to the development of evidence-based guidelines that provide a "cookbook" approach to health care.

e. Health care agencies and administrators do not provide the resources to support the implementation of EBP by nurses.

4. You may have identified any of the following:

a. EBP requires the synthesis of research evidence from randomized controlled trials, and these types of studies are limited in nursing.

b. Researchers have found limited association between nursing interventions/processes and patient outcomes in acute care settings.

c. There is significant variation in the methods to measure the effect of independent variables (nursing interventions) on patient outcomes.

d. There is a need for additional studies to determine the effectiveness of nursing interventions.

e. There is a need to identify areas where research evidence is needed for practice.

f. Nurses need to be more active in conducting quality syntheses (systematic reviews, meta-analyses, and integrative reviews) of research evidence in selected areas.

g. Most nurses lack the academic preparation to critically analyze and adopt research into practice.

5. a. Immediate use—using research-based intervention in practice exactly as it was developed

b. Reinvention—occurs when the research intervention is modified to meet the needs of a health care agency or nurses within the agency

c. Cognitive change—occurs when nurses incorporate research findings into their knowledge base and use this information to defend a point, write agency protocols or policies, or develop a clinical paper for presentation

6. a. National Guideline Clearinghouse website (www.guideline.gov) that includes integrative reviews of research. This website was initiated by the Agency for Healthcare Research and Quality (AHRQ).

b. Cochrane Collaboration, which includes systematic reviews, meta-analyses, and integrative reviews of research to determine best research evidence in selected practice areas.

c. Meta-analyses of nursing literature (A list of meta-analyses is included on the textbook website.)

d. Integrative reviews of nursing research (A list of integrative reviews of research is included on the textbook website.)

7. a. Phase I: Preparation

b. Phase II: Validation

c. Phase III: Comparative Evaluation/Decision-Making

d. Phase IV: Translation/Application

e. Phase V: Evaluation

8. feasibility, current practice

9. a. Use research evidence in practice now.

b. Consider using research knowledge in practice.

c. Do not use the research findings in practice.

10. Iowa

11. evidence-based guidelines

12. Healthcare Research and Quality (AHRQ)

13. a. American Medical Association (AMA)

b. American Association of Health Plans (AAHP), now called the American's Health Insurance Plans (AHIP)

14. evidence-based practice

15. evidence-based practice for nursing

Making Connections

1. a   4. e

2. d   5. b

3. c

Going Beyond

1. Obtain the answers to these questions by gathering information in the agencies where you have clinical practice this semester. You could also use your worksite and answer these questions to determine how rapidly research evidence might be used in this practice setting.

2. Use the steps of Stetler's Model of Research Utilization to Facilitate Evidence-Based Practice or the Iowa Model of Evidence-Based Practice as outlined in Chapter 27 of your text to assist you in using research knowledge in practice. Seek guidance from your instructor as needed.
3. Use the Grove Model for Implementing Evidence-Based Guidelines in Practice to implement an evidence-based practice guideline from the Agency for Healthcare Research and Quality (www.ahrq.gov). Use Chapter 27 in Burns and Grove textbook as a resource.

CHAPTER 28

Relevant Terms

1. d
2. e
3. c
4. a
5. b

Key Ideas

1. concise, complete
2. a. Developing ideas logically
   b. Determining the depth or detail of the proposal content
   c. Identifying critical points in the proposal
   d. Developing aesthetically appealing copy
3. American Psychological Association
4. a. Introduction
   b. Review of relevant literature
   c. Framework
   d. Methods and procedures
5. You may have identified any of the following aspects of a quasi-experimental or experimental study design:
   a. Describing how the research situation will be structured
   b. Detailing the treatment to be implemented
   c. Describing how the effect of the treatment will be measured
   d. Indicating the variables to be controlled and the methods for controlling them
   e. Identifying uncontrolled extraneous variables and determining their impact on the findings
   f. Describing the methods for assigning subjects to the treatment and comparison or control groups
   g. Describing the strengths and weaknesses of a design
6. institutional review board
7. You may have identified any of the following content areas of the introduction to a qualitative study:
   a. Identify the phenomenon to be studied.
   b. Identify the study aim or purpose.
   c. State the study questions.
   d. Describe the evolution of the study.
   e. Provide a rationale for conducting the study.
   f. Place the study in context historically.
   g. Discuss the researcher's experience with the phenomenon.
   h. Discuss the relevance of the study to nursing.

8. You may have identified any of the following aspects of a preproposal:
   a. Letter of transmittal
   b. Brief introduction of the proposed research project
   c. Personnel for the project
   d. Facilities to be used
   e. Budget
9. a. To ensure that adequate measures are being taken to protect human subjects
   b. To evaluate the impact of conducting the study on the reviewing institution
   c. To generally assess the quality of the study
10. a. How the clinical facility's name is to be used in reporting findings.
    b. Who will present the findings and where they are presented will be determined.
    c. How authorship of publication(s) and possible journals for publication will be determined.
11. funding agency
12. a. What needs to be changed?
    b. Why is the change necessary?
    c. How will the change affect the implementation of the study and the study findings?

Making Connections

1. a
2. b
3. a
4. b
5. b

Going Beyond

1. Review the guidelines and example quantitative research proposal presented in Chapter 28. Think about writing a thesis, which would involve developing and implementing a study under the direction of an expert faculty researcher. Or you might develop a proposal with another student or with a member of a health care agency. Many health care agencies now have nurse researchers on staff who might review your study and assist you in the approval process and the conduct of the study.
2. Meet with the chair of the institutional review board for the agency where you would like to conduct your study. Follow the guidelines provided to obtain approval to conduct your study in that agency. Review the helpful hints in Chapter 28 to assist you in successfully defending your proposed study.

CHAPTER 29

Relevant Terms

1. b	5. c	9. l	12. e
2. g	6. m	10. a	13. h
3. f	7. i	11. j	
4. k	8. d		

Key Ideas

1. increase
2. Scientific credibility or research expertise
3. Small grants
4. Focus their efforts in one area of study
5. program, research
6. Review proposals of others that were funded, know the process for decisions about funding, and review a critique of a funded proposal.
7. small grants
8. foundation directory
9. foundation's guidelines
10. federal government
11. Catalog of Federal Domestic Assistance
12. Contact an official with the government agency early in the planning process to inform the agency of the intent to submit a proposal
13. Federal Register
14. highly competitive
15. a. Identifies the problem of concern
    b. Describes the design of the study
16. study section
17. 1 year
18. Before the first grant has ended

Making Connections

1. You may list any of the following:
   a. Attend grantsmanship courses.
   b. Develop a reference group.
   c. Join research organizations.
   d. Serve on research committees.
   e. Network.
   f. Assist a researcher.
   g. Obtain a mentor.

2. You may list any of the following:
   a. Within the university
   b. Nursing organizations
   c. Local agencies
   d. Private individuals
   e. Clinical agencies

Puzzles

Word Scramble

"Well-designed studies can be expensive."

Secret Message

"The scientific credibility of the profession is related to the quality of studies conducted by its researchers."

Crossword Puzzle

Across

1. Funded research
6. Pink sheet
8. Mentor
9. Requests for proposals
10. Grantsmanship
11. Research grant
12. Request for application

Down

2. Reference group
3. Networking
4. Foundation grant
5. Developmental grant
7. Query letter

Going Beyond

Seek assistance from a faculty member as you review his or her grant(s) and the letter that was received about the funding status of the grant.

Appendix B: Published Studies

Study 1: The Effect of a Tailored Message Intervention on Heart Failure Readmission Rates, Quality of Life, and Benefit and Barrier Beliefs in Persons with Heart Failure

Kristen A. Sethares, RN, PhD, and Kathleen Elliott, BN, MSN, ANP-C, Dartmouth, Massachusetts

Objective: The purpose of this study was to determine the effect of a tailored message intervention on heart failure readmission rates, quality of life, and health beliefs in persons with heart failure (HF).

Design: This randomized control trial provided a tailored message intervention during hospitalization and 1 week and 1 month after discharge.

Theoretic Framework: The organizing framework was the Health Belief Model.

Subjects: Seventy persons with a primary diagnosis of chronic HF were included in the study.

Results: HF readmission rates and quality of life did not significantly differ between the treatment and control groups. Health beliefs, except for benefits of medications, significantly changed from baseline in the treatment group in directions posited by the Health Belief Model.

Conclusions: A tailored message intervention changed the beliefs of the person with HF in regard to the benefits and barriers of taking medications, following a sodium-restricted diet, and self-monitoring for signs of fluid overload. Future research is needed to explore the effect of health belief changes on actual self-care behaviors. (Heart Lung © 2004; 33:249-60.)

From Sethares, K.A. & Elliott, K. (2004). The effect of a tailored message intervention on heart failure readmission rates, quality of life, and benefit and barrier beliefs in persons with heart failure. *Heart & Lung, 33*(4), 249-260. © 2003 Elsevier, Inc. All rights reserved.

INTRODUCTION

Cardiovascular disease, the leading cause of death in the United States today, is one of the most prevalent chronic illnesses of adulthood.[1] A common clinical endpoint of many cardiovascular disorders is heart failure (HF), defined as the inability of the heart to provide the tissues with oxygen at a rate necessary to meet oxidative requirements.[2] The American College of Cardiology/American Heart Association Task Force reports that 4.8 million Americans experience HF, with 550,000 new ases and 50,000 deaths reported annually.[1,3] In 1999, 62,000 Americans were discharged from acute care cilities with a primary diagnosis of HF, the most prevant diagnosis in those aged more than 65 years.

HF is characterized by an unstable course of illness th unpredictable exacerbations and progression of mptoms, often without further damage to the myocarm.[4] Symptoms such as weight gain, edema, dyspnea, fatigue characterize these exacerbations and further t functional status and quality of life.[5,6] Because HF is ronic condition, most lifestyle change is made on an atient basis, necessitating follow-up in the home setto evaluate medication effectiveness, monitor symp, and promote self-care behaviors. However, current ation rates fiscally limit the quantity of nursing care ded in the home. The end result of these combined s is a high cost, reported to be close to 10 billion .[7]

imperative that nurses develop innovative methimprove the self-care behaviors of this population ttempting to decrease costly rehospitalizations. ed message intervention is one proposed alternathis case, education is based on an evaluation of fs of the person with HF concerning perceived nd perceived barriers of performing certain HF ehaviors. In self-care areas with more identifis or less perceived benefits, a tailored message he purpose of this investigation was to deter er the tailored message intervention decreased rates, improved reported quality of life, and efs about perceived benefits and perceived fcare in persons with HF.

LITER. EVIEW

Resear trates that older adults with HF have the hig tal readmission rates, ranging from 29% to l hospitalized adult patient groups, primarily few weeks after discharge.[8–11] As a result, mo ion studies have focused on trying to decreas on rates in this vulnerable population. Inte y teams composed of dietitians, social worke ists, physicians, and nurses have all played a ificantly reducing readmission rates of perso through education, discharge planning, and evaluation.[12–14] Standardized care maps guide disciplinary team efforts in

several studies.[4,15–17] Disease management interventions that include monitoring across the spectrum of care by multidisciplinary teams seek to improve the management of HF through guideline-based surveillance, education, and frequent outpatient follow-up.[15–20] These plans have shown moderate success in decreasing readmission rates and costs in a subset of the population with HF. However, this type of plan fails to account for the activity limitations of some persons with HF and the difficulty of attending frequent outpatient visits because of symptoms brought on by minimal activity. Anderson et al[8] and Elkman et al[21] reported that 29% to 50% of persons with HF have difficulty attending outpatient follow-up appointments because of symptoms during activity that limit function.

Numerous interventions have included some component of telephone follow-up for persons with HF, resulting in reduced readmission rates,[22,23] no change,[21] and significantly increased readmission rates.[24] Although these interventions minimize the need for frequent outpatient follow-up, nurses still managed the care of HF. In most cases, the telephone follow-up was provided by nurses, using standardized algorithms that assessed symptoms and self-care behaviors.[23,25] Follow-up was performed in cases in which persons reported increased symptoms. In these models of care, the frequent followup provided by nurses did not allow the person with HF to develop his or her own ability to initiate follow-up for identified symptoms.

Transitional care models, first described by Brooten and colleagues[26] for low birth weight infants, have also been applied to elderly persons with HF. In this model, advance practice nurses assisted persons with cardiac diagnoses to transition from the hospital to home by providing individualized discharge planning, education, and follow-up for the first 2 weeks at home.[14,27–29] Most of the interventions provided by the advance practice nurses included surveillance of signs and symptoms and health teaching.[30] The use of this model has resulted in significant reductions in readmission rates, cost, and length of time to readmission. However, not all regions of the country have advanced practice nurses with the knowledge and skills necessary to provide these services.

In many of these studies, the efficacy of the educational component of the intervention alone has been less well studied. In those studies that did contain educational interventions, standardized forms and care maps guided the education. Teaching interventions based on clinical guidelines and care maps alone fail to account for the individual characteristics present in the learner.[31–36] Nurses educating persons with HF need to include individualized learning assessments in all plans of care to account for multiple contextual variables present in these individuals. Transfer of knowledge alone is often not sufficient to promote behavior change without some further behavioral support strategies throughout the process, often in the outpatient setting.[37,38] Further, the Joint Commission on Accreditation of Healthcare Organization[39] mandates that individuals must receive education at a level appropriate

272

to their degree of understanding. Nurses are well suited to provide this education because of their knowledge and close interpersonal relationship with persons with HF. The use of a tailored message intervention may reduce the need for reading if the education is verbal and tailored to the specific learning needs of the person with HF.

CONCEPTUAL FRAMEWORK

The Health Belief Model (HBM) provides the organizing framework for the study. In this model, an individual performs a health behavior based on perceived susceptibility, perceived severity, perceived benefits, and perceived barriers to an illness.[40–42] Perceived susceptibility and perceived severity relate to the psychologic components of the model whereby individuals evaluate subjective risk of HF to them. Inherent in the process of psychologic evaluation of risk is both internal moderating factors and external cues to action. Personal factors, including demographics, sociocultural variables, and level of knowledge about HF, are believed to modify the health beliefs of persons with HF.[40] Unlike demographic and sociocultural variables that are stable traits of persons, knowledge is amenable to change. External cues to action are found in the mass media and through contact with health care providers.[43] Severity of illness in the person with HF may be manifest in potentially function-limiting symptoms, such as shortness of breath and fatigue.

Perceived benefits of performing a certain health behavior relate to a subjectively determined course of action that reduces the susceptibility of illness.[40] Kasl[44] reconceptualized susceptibility for chronically ill persons as resusceptibility to exacerbations of the illness. In the case of the person with HF, taking medications or following a low-salt diet may reduce the progression of symptoms and be seen as beneficial. These benefits are weighed against perceived barriers to a certain course of action. Perceived barriers are the potential negative consequences of a certain health behavior. In the population with HF, a barrier to following medication recommendations might be the outcome of frequent urination caused by diuretic therapy. In this case, the person with HF would weigh risks and benefits before making a decision about whether to follow a recommended course of action.

In this study, the tailored message intervention focused on decreasing client-identified barriers to self-care. Individualized teaching by a nurse focused on enhancing the benefits and decreasing the barriers to self-care of a person with HF. Although a person with HF may believe that a certain behavior will decrease HF symptoms, if that action is expensive, time-consuming, or unpleasant, these can serve as barriers to taking that action. If readiness to act is high and barriers to act are low, then self-care action is more likely.[45] The goal of this tailored message intervention was to improve the readiness of the person with HF to perform self-care behaviors by decreasing identified barriers and increasing perceived benefits of action while supporting the individual needs of the person with HF in the process. By changing perceived beliefs related to self-care, it is anticipated that persons with HF will improve self-care behaviors, which may lead to improved quality of life and lower readmission rates.

STUDY PURPOSES AND RESEARCH QUESTIONS

This study determines the efficacy of a tailored message intervention administered during hospital admission and at 1 week and 1 month after discharge on HF readmission rates, reported quality of life, and perceived benefit and barrier beliefs in elderly patients with HF. The times selected for study correspond with times identified in the literature as the period of greatest risk for rehospitalization in elderly patients.[8,27,28] The following research questions are the basis for the study:

1. Do individuals who receive the tailored message intervention have lower HF readmission rates than a control group at 3 months?
2. Do individuals who receive a tailored message intervention report better quality of life at baseline and 1 month after discharge than a control group?
3. What is the effect of the tailored message intervention on the perceived benefit and barrier beliefs of the treatment group at baseline, 1 week, and 1 month?

HYPOTHESES

There were 3 hypotheses for the study. The first 2 hypotheses were that persons who received the intervention would have lower HF readmission rates and report better quality of life. The third hypothesis was that intervention subjects would report fewer barriers and more benefits to performing self-care of HF after receiving the tailored message intervention.

METHODS

A randomized control trial was used to evaluate the effect of a tailored message intervention on HF readmission rates, quality of life, and perceived benefit and barrier beliefs in an elderly sample of subjects with HF. Benefit and barrier scores were measured during initial hospitalization and 1 week and 1 month after discharge in the treatment group. Quality of life scores were obtained in both groups during initial hospitalization and 1 month after hospital discharge. HF readmission rates were measured 3 months after hospital discharge in both groups.

SAMPLE

The sample was drawn from a population of adults with a primary diagnosis of chronic HF who were admitted to 1 community hospital in the Northeast between October 1999 and December 2000. Persons with HF who consented to participate were randomly assigned to the treatment or control group. Criteria for study enrollment included the following: (1) primary diagnosis of either

273

systolic or diastolic HF listed in the medical record, confirmed by the presence of symptoms of HF for 3 months or longer; (2) echocardiography for confirmation of ejection fraction; (3) English speaking; (4) freedom from serious cognitive deficits, as determined by the Mini Mental Status Exam; and (5) anticipated return to a community setting, rather than long-term care. HF stage (New York Heart Association [NYHA]) was determined by asking the subject the current level of activity that precipitated symptoms. The sample size of 70 for the readmission and quality of life variables was determined through a power analysis with an effect size of 0.35, an alpha of .05, and a power of 0.80.[46]

Data were collected by a baccalaureate-prepared research nurse during an interview with 88 subjects hospitalized for HF. Over-recruitment was performed in a sample known to have high attrition rates. Eight subjects withdrew, and 10 subjects were lost from the study because of death before the end of the 3-month follow-up period. A t test was run to compare the 2 groups of patients (those who died within 3 months of discharge and those who survived) on the following measures: age, NYHA class, ejection fraction, comorbidities, educational level, and initial quality of life scores. There were no significant differences on any of the measures between the 2 groups. The final sample consisted of 37 control and 33 treatment subjects. The sample characteristics are shown in Table I.

Table II lists demographic characteristics, presence of visiting nurse follow-up (Visiting Nurse Association), and medication use in the sample. Chi-square analysis demonstrated no significant differences between the treatment and control group on any of the characteristics listed in Table II. The sample size provided adequate power for all outcome variables.

INSTRUMENTS

Heart Failure Readmission Rates
The outcome variable of HF readmission rates was measured by counting the total number of admissions for HF in each group during the 3-month study interval. Each admission counted as 1 number, regardless of the number of days admitted.

Quality of Life
The variable of quality of life was measured with the Minnesota Living with Heart Failure (MLHF) questionnaire.[47] The MLHF is a disease-specific 21-item measure of health-related quality of life. Patients with HF rate their perceptions about how much HF impacts their socioeconomic, psychologic, and physical aspects of daily life, from 0 (not at all) to 5 (very much). Scores on the total instrument range from 0 to 105, with higher scores reflective of worse perceived quality life. Construct validity was demonstrated by significant correlations of MLHF scores with NYHA functional classifications in 83 subjects with HF caused by left ventricular dysfunction ($r = .80$, $P < .01$).[48] Significant correlations were also noted between the MLHF and a single-item measure that rated overall how much HF prevented them from living as they wanted in the past month ($r = .80$, $P < .01$). Internal consistency reliability on the instrument is high, with Cronbach's alpha of 0.94 reported for the total scale.[49] The Cronbach's alpha for the total scale in this study was 0.87.

Benefits and Barriers
The instruments used to measure the benefits and barriers of taking HF medications, following a sodium-restricted diet, and self-monitoring for signs of fluid overload are the Health Belief Scales developed by Bennett and colleagues (personal communication, Susan J. Bennett, RN, DNS, FAAN, 2003).[49,50] The 3 scales are based on the HBM and consist of the Beliefs About Diet Compliance Scale (BDCS), Beliefs About Medication Compliance Scale (BMCS), and Beliefs About Self-Monitoring Compliance Scale (BSMCS). Each scale consists of a benefit and barrier subscale that describes potential benefits or barriers to taking HF medications, following a sodium-restricted diet, or self-monitoring for signs of fluid overload. The BDCS and BMCS each contain 12 items and the BSMCS contains 18 items. The total number of items is 42.

A Likert-type scale is scored from 1 to 5, with 1 corresponding to "strongly disagree" and 5 corresponding to "strongly agree," with the benefit or barrier item presented. The benefit and barrier subscale scores for each of the 3 scales are summed, with a range determined by the number of benefit and barrier items in the subscale. The BDCS has 5 benefit and 7 barrier items. The barrier

Table I Characteristics of the Sample				
	Treatment group (n = 33)		Control group (n = 37)	
	MEAN	SD	MEAN	SD
Age	75.70	12.25	76.84	10.48
NYHA	3.00	0.62	3.00	0.57
EF	41.45	18	38.75	19.5
No. of comorbidities	3.67	2	3.96	2
Education (y)	11	3.71	11	2.24

ATHA, New York Heart Association; EF, ejection fraction.

274

Table II Sample Demographic, Visiting Nurse, and Medication Use Characteristics

	Treatment group (n = 33)		Control group (n = 37)	
	FREQUENCY	%	FREQUENCY	%
Marital status				
Single	6	8.6	7	10
Married	12	17.1	13	18.6
Widowed	13	18.6	14	20
Divorced/separated	2	2.9	3	4.3
Race				
White	31	93.9	33	89.2
Black	2	6.1	4	10.8
Gender				
Female	16	48.5	21	56.8
Male	17	51.5	16	43.2
Medications				
Beta blockers				
Yes	18	54.5	16	43.2
No	15	45.5	21	56.8
ACE inhibitors				
Yes	19	57.6	24	64.9
No	14	42.4	13	35.1
Lasix				
Yes	28	84.8	31	83.8
No	5	15.2	6	16.2
Digoxin				
Yes	15	45.5	14	37.8
No	18	54.5	23	62.2
VNA services				
Yes	17	51.5	17	45.9
No	16	48.5	20	54.1

ACE, Angiotensin-converting enzyme; VNA, Visiting Nurse Association.

scores range from 7 to 35, and the benefit scores range from 5 to 25. The BMCS contains 6 benefit and 6 barrier items, so the scores for both subscales range from 6 to 30. The BSMCS contains 12 barrier questions and 6 benefit questions and scores on benefit questions range from 6 to 30, and barrier scores range from 12 to 60.

Internal consistencies of the BDCS and BMCS subscales were psychometrically evaluated in a convenience sample of 101 clients with HF. Internal consistencies of these 2 subscales were found to be 0.87 for benefits of medications, 0.91 for barriers to medications, 0.84 for benefits of diet, and 0.69 for barriers of diet.[50] Content validity of the tool was found when evaluated by 2 HF experts, with 81% agreement on the content.

In this study, internal consistencies of the subscales were 0.80 for benefits of medications, 0.72 for barriers of medications, 0.85 for benefits of diet, 0.62 for barriers of diet, 0.89 for benefits of self-monitoring, and 0.83 for barriers of self-monitoring. Bennett and colleagues[50] suggest that the barriers to diet subscale score may be slightly less the others because of the heterogeneous nature of that subscale. A con-

firmatory factor analysis was performed on the BDCS and the BMCS in a sample of 234 persons with HF.[51] A 2-factor solution (benefits and barriers) resulted from the analysis (n = 196) of the BMCS items, accounting for 41% of the variance. In the analysis of the BDCS, a similar 2-factor solution (benefits and barriers) emerged that represented 50% of the variance. All but 1 item loaded more than 0.40.

Demographic data were collected with a tool developed by the researchers and obtained during a preliminary chart review and interview while the subject was hospitalized. Additional data were collected on medication changes during each intervention session.

PROCEDURE

Approvals were received from the institutional review board at the community hospital where the study was conducted. Two baccalaureate-prepared research nurses enrolled participants and completed the study intervention as outlined in a detailed protocol. Weekly meetings were

275

held between the coinvestigators and the research nurses to review the protocol, answer any questions, and update the status of data collection. Periodic practice with delivering the intervention according to the protocol was performed during these meetings to prevent treatment drift.

After stabilization of HF, hospitalized subjects were invited to participate in the study, and written informed consent was obtained. After consent, subjects were randomly assigned to groups using the sealed envelope technique.[52] An interview was conducted with subjects by the research nurse during initial hospitalization to obtain relevant demographic data and complete the MLHF tool. Subjects in the treatment group were interviewed using the Health Belief Scales to determine areas in which teaching was needed. Additional demographic and medication data were obtained from the medical record and computerized hospital databases.

In a follow-up visit, 7 to 10 days after hospital discharge, the research nurse who enrolled the subject visited the subject in his or her home and again completed The Health Belief Scales. Medication lists were reviewed, and any medication changes were noted. An analysis of medications was performed to monitor changes in medications that might impact readmission rates. Prior research suggests that readmission may occur because of difficulty adjusting to medication changes.[8] The final follow-up visit took place 1 month after discharge in the subject's home, and the same research nurse again visited the subject. Quality of life scores were determined at the final interview, and medications were reviewed for any changes. A telephone call was made to the control subjects by a blinded data collector at 1 month to determine quality of life scores using the MLHF. The outcome variable of HF readmission rates was obtained through both the hospital computerized database and a telephone call by a blinded data collector to all subjects at 3 months to assess whether they had been readmitted to a hospital other than the initial hospital.

INTERVENTION

Treatment Subjects

Subjects in the treatment group received a tailored message intervention by the same research nurse during hospitalization and 1 week and 1 month after hospital discharge. All subjects assigned to the treatment group received the intervention. The intervention was based on the perceived benefits and barriers to self-care of HF that were identified by persons with HF. An evaluation of health beliefs was performed using the Health Belief Scales. Questions on the Health Belief Scales are divided into benefit and barrier questions based on the HBM definitions of those terms. At each time period, subjects in the treatment group were administered all 3 scales of the Health Belief Scales. Items on the scales were scored, and if the person with HF scored 4 or above on a benefit question or below 3 on a barrier question, then a tailored message was not given. It is presumed that the person with HF already understands the barriers or benefits identified in that question. Subjects who scored outside these parameters received a message tailored to the benefit or barrier item identified in the statement (messages based on those developed by Susan J. Bennett).[49] The messages used in this study were a shortened version of those developed by Susan J. Bennett, but they included the same content. The total time for administration of the tailored message intervention averaged 15 minutes per participant. Written copies of the messages were not given to the participants. Examples of tailored messages used in this study are presented in Table III.

Table III Sample Tailored Messages

DIET	
Benefit question: Salty food is not good for me. Message: Salt is not good for you because salt causes your body to hold more water. When your body holds more water then your heart has to work harder to pump blood through your body.	Barrier question: Food does not taste good on a low-salt diet. Message: After you have followed the low-salt diet a while, you will get used to the taste of the foods. Foods can still be flavored with other spices and also salt substitutes. You can see a dietitian or refer to cookbooks on low-salt cooking.

MEDICATIONS	
Benefit question: If I take my water pills, I will lower my chance of being hospitalized. Message: Taking your pills at the time and in the amount ordered by your doctor will help keep your body from holding extra fluid. Getting rid of this extra fluid will prevent swelling in your body and may make you feel better.	Barrier question: Taking water pills makes it hard to go away from home. Message: Try to take your pills earlier in the day when you are going out so that they will work before you leave the house. Also when you go out be sure to find the bathroom wherever you go.

Reprinted with permission of the author, Dr. Susan J. Bennett.

276

Control Subjects

Subjects in the control group received usual care, which included discharge teaching by a staff nurse on the unit and written educational sheets describing the uses, side effects, and frequency of any ordered medications. In addition, approximately one half of the subjects also received referrals to local visiting nurse agencies. After enrollment, the control subjects were contacted at 1 month by a blinded data collector to evaluate quality of life and at 3 months to evaluate readmission rates.

ANALYSIS

Data were entered into the Statistical Package for Social Sciences 10.0 (SPSS Inc, Chicago, IL), and descriptive statistics were computed on all study variables and examined for the presence of random or systematic missing data, significant skewness, and outliers. Appropriate reliability and validity measures were performed on measurement instruments. Because the outcome variable of HF readmission rates was skewed, the nonparametric Kruskall-Wallis statistic was computed to determine differences in HF readmission rates between the treatment and control groups. The benefits, barriers, and quality of life data were not skewed. Repeated-measures analysis of variance (ANOVA) was performed to compare the quality of life scores at baseline and 1 month between the treatment and control groups. A repeated-measures ANOVA was run on the benefits and barriers scores at 3 time points to determine whether there were significant differences in benefit and barrier beliefs over time. Subjects who withdrew or died before the 3-month follow-up point were excluded from the analyses.

RESULTS

Readmission Rates

A Kruskall-Wallis test was run to answer research question 1. HF readmission rate was not significantly related to group assignment in this study ($P = .22$). As seen in Table IV, 12 subjects in the control group were rehospitalized 1 or more times, whereas 6 subjects in the treatment group were rehospitalized 1 or more times.

Quality of Life

A repeated-measures ANOVA comparing quality of life by group assignment over time was performed to answer research question 2. The assumption of equality of covariance matrices was met. Because Mauchly's test of sphericity was not significant, univariate results are reported.[53] For within-subjects effects, there were significant differences in quality-of-life measures at the 2 time points ($F = 35.44$, $P = .000$), with both groups reporting improved quality of life at 1 month as expected with a group recruited during hospitalization. The mean quality of life score was 55.5 at baseline and 41.6 at 1 month. The assumption of homogeneity of variance for between-subjects factors was met.[53] There were no significant differences between the group receiving the tailored message intervention and the control group in reported quality of life ($F = 1.051$, $P = .309$). The control group had a mean score of 50.9, and the treatment group had a mean score of 46.2. There was no significant interaction between quality of life and group assigned ($F = .317$, $P = .575$).

Benefits and Barriers

To answer research question 3 (Table V), a within-subjects repeated-measures ANOVA was run to compare benefit and barrier scores of diet, medications, and self-monitoring at baseline, 1 week, and 1 month in the group receiving the tailored message intervention (n = 33).

In Table V, the mean scores for benefits of medications, diet, and self-monitoring were lowest at the baseline period and highest at 1 month follow-up. Conversely, the barriers of diet, medications, and self-monitoring were noted to be highest at baseline and lowest at 1 month. Because Mauchly's test of sphericity was significant for all but the benefits of medications data, univariate tests with the Greenhouse-Geisser epsilon correction factor are reported.[53] The benefits of medications scores did not change significantly during the study ($P = .259$). Barriers of medications scores decreased from baseline to the 1-week point ($P = .000$) and significantly decreased from baseline to the 1-month point ($P = .000$). Benefits of diet significantly increased from baseline to 1 week ($P = .000$) and from baseline to 1 month ($P = .000$). The barriers of diet significantly decreased from baseline to

Table IV Heart Failure Readmission Rates by Group			
NUMER OF HF READMISSIONS	**TREATMENT (N = 33)** NO. (%)	**CONTROL (N = 37)** NO. (%)	**TOTAL HF READMISSIONS** NO. (%)
0	27 (82)	25 (68)	52 (74)
1	3 (9)	9 (24)	12 (17)
2	3 (9)	2 (5)	5 (7)
3	0 (0)	1 (3)	1 (1)

Statistical test = Kruskall-Wallis. P = .22. HF, Heart failure.

Table V Changes in Benefits and Barrier Scores Over Time

	BASELINE M (SD)	1 WK M (SD)	1 MO M (SD)	DF	F	P
Benefits of medications	21.2 (3.6)	22 (2.1)	22.2 (3.7)	2	1.381	.259
Barriers of medications	15.5 (4.1)	15.1 (3.8)	13.3 (3.2)	2	12.627	.000*
Benefits of diet	25.2 (5)	28.2 (2.7)	29.7 (3.8)	2	11.890	.000*
Barriers of diet	13.6 (3.6)	11.8 (2.3)	10.4 (3.5)	2	10.145	.001*
Benefits of self-monitoring	19.8 (5.6)	22 (3.9)	23.5 (3.2)	2	10.356	.000*
Barriers of self-monitoring	27.9 (9.3)	23.8 (4.9)	22.4 (5.2)	2	8.897	.002*

Greenhouse-Geisser epsilon correction factor used.

1 week (P = 000) and from baseline to 1 month (P = .001). The benefits of self-monitoring significantly improved from baseline to 1 week (P = .000) and from baseline to 1 month (P = .000). Barriers of self-monitoring decreased significantly from baseline to 1 week (P = .002), with further decreases at 1 month. All changes occurred in the expected theoretic directions.

DISCUSSION

Although overall HF readmission rates between the treatment and control groups did not differ significantly, fewer individuals in the treatment group were readmitted during the 3-month follow-up period (6 vs 12). The 35% of subjects rehospitalized in this study is comparable to rates reported in the literature of 29% to 66% for other samples with HF.[11,54,55] Previous research has demonstrated that persons with HF are frequently readmitted for the same reason as their primary admission because a period of time is required for stabilization of fluid status and adjustment to new medication doses.[8] With shorter lengths of hospital stay, elderly subjects with HF have not had the time to adjust physiologically to altered doses or additional medications. As a result, this population would benefit from more close home monitoring and routine referral for visiting nurse follow-up. In this sample, only slightly more than half of the subjects reported receiving home follow-up (Table II).

This intervention was a tailored message intervention and did not account for the medical management of persons with HF in the study. Clinical practice guidelines recommend the use of angiotensin-converting enzyme (ACE) inhibitors, digoxin, and diuretics in the management of HF and its associated symptoms.[3,56] As seen in this study, approximately half of all subjects were receiving beta-blockers and digoxin, approximately 60% were receiving ACE inhibitors (Table II), and 84% were receiving diuretics. These findings are consistent with those reported in the literature for patterns of use of medications for HF. Luzier and colleagues[57] reported digoxin use in 72%, diuretic use in 86%, and ACE inhibitor use in 67% of 314 subjects with HF. Oka and colleagues[58] reported digoxin use in 70%, ACE inhibitor use in 60%, and diuretic use in 95% of subjects with HF. Doyle et al[59] reported that 60% of subjects with HF were not receiving ACE inhibitors, even when no contraindications were noted, and Kermani et al[60] reported that 48% of 107 subjects with HF were not receiving ACE inhibitors on admission to the hospital. Sneed and colleagues[61] reported comparable rates with 77% receiving ACE inhibitors, 27% receiving beta-blockers, and 77% receiving diuretics in a study of persons with HF (n = 30) in an outpatient clinic. The evidence suggests a pattern of underuse of medications for HF that can lead to poor medical stabilization of the condition and render educational interventions ineffective in reducing rehospitalization rates. Without proper medical stabilization, educational interventions may be ineffective in reducing rehospitalization rates.

The quality of life results in this study are comparable to other studies. In this study, no difference in quality of life scores was noted between the 2 groups at baseline and 1 month. However, significant differences were noted in quality of life at the 1-month follow-up point across both groups. These results indicate that quality of life improved independently of intervention after hospital discharge in both groups. This finding is consistent with other studies that have shown quality of life scores to be lowest in persons with HF during hospitalization and to improve during the discharge period even in a group that does not receive intervention.[62,63] A reduction in symptoms and resulting improvement in functional status because of stabilization of symptoms during hospitalization may account for these changes in this population, because the MHLF is a disease-specific measure of quality of life. It is possible that persons who were lost to follow-up may have reported worse quality of life, so these results must be interpreted with caution.

278

Perhaps the length and dose of intervention can impact the perception of quality of life of the person with HF.[64] In this study, subjects received an intervention consisting of 3 nursing visits, which may have been insufficient to impact quality of life as measured by the MLHF. This finding is supported with previous research indicating that the dose of the intervention can impact specific outcomes of persons with HF. In a secondary analysis of data collected from 7 sites across the United States, it was found that persons with HF who received a more intensive intervention had greater improvement in quality of life scores than those who received a less-intensive intervention. Subjects receiving interventions over a longer period of time or with more components (education, exercise, and medication management) reported significantly improved quality of life.[63] For example, Oka and colleagues[58] reported significant improvements in quality of life scores in a group who received a 3-month exercise intervention (consisting of exercise 3–5 days/week), but a comparable group of control subjects showed no improvements. Perhaps the intensity of this intervention was insufficient to demonstrate statistically significant changes in quality of life in the treatment group.

Although changes in quality of life scores in the treatment group did not reach statistical significance, the treatment group did report greater improvement in quality of life at 1 month than the control group. Prior research suggests that a 5-point change in the quality of life score is clinically significant in persons with HF.[47,59] Because the MLHF was developed as a disease-specific measure of the perception of function and impact of symptoms on function of the person with HF,[47,61] this finding may represent a reduction in symptoms and improved function for both groups. This finding supports other research suggesting that quality of life may be lowest during hospitalization and improve because of stabilization of symptoms resulting in improved function.[63] On the basis of this criterion, the subjects in both groups reported a statistically and clinically significant improvement in quality of life over time.

Perhaps the strongest finding of this study was that the benefit and barrier scores progressed in the expected theoretic directions. This tailored message intervention without written supplementation was able to create significant changes in health beliefs in a small group of persons with HF. Champion and colleagues[65] found that women who received a tailored message intervention that evaluated specific health beliefs (benefits, barriers, and self-efficacy) combined with practice of psychomotor skills needed to perform breast self-examination were more likely to perform the examination and do it correctly. Other theoretically guided tailored message interventions have been successfully used to reduce smoking behaviors, improve mammography screening behaviors, and improve unhealthy dietary behaviors.[66–69]

In each of these studies, subjects received tailored instruction with personalized written reminders based on an evaluation of benefit or barrier beliefs, self-efficacy beliefs, or stage of change. Subjects receiving tailored education in each of these studies reported reading the literature provided, demonstrating correct performance of self-care behaviors, and changing unhealthy dietary behaviors more often then those in the control situations. This suggests that belief patterns can be influenced by education and that perhaps an evaluation of beliefs should be included in any intervention in which behavior change is an outcome.

IMPLICATIONS

The results of this study demonstrate that a tailored message intervention changed the perceived benefit and perceived barrier of self-care of HF beliefs in this population. The psychoeducational focus of the intervention included facets of self-care that are traditionally part of home-based HF education but were tailored to the specific beliefs of the person with HF This reduced redundancy of the education. The messages in this study were easy to deliver, took approximately 15 minutes, and were suitable for delivery by telephone. In this era of cost consciousness, a reduction in the number of nursing visits and minimization of educational redundancy could be useful in the home care setting. This intervention requires testing in a larger sample of persons with HF to determine for whom the intervention would be most effective.

Although changes in benefits and barrier beliefs did occur in this study, the effect of changes on beliefs and actual self-care practice is an important consideration because actual self-care behavior change would be one potential positive outcome. Certainly the impact of other factors such as physicians or nurses providing education to these subjects could have influenced the findings and should be considered in future research. Future research that focuses on the effect of tailored interventions on actual changes in self-care behaviors and the dose of intervention needed to effect these changes would be beneficial.

LIMITATIONS

There were 3 limitations to this study. The first limitation is the lack of measurement of the actual self-care behaviors of this sample. Although beliefs were measured and did change, actual self-care behaviors, including following a low-sodium diet, daily weighing, and taking medication, were not measured. Future study should include these variables to determine whether a change in beliefs translates to actual behavior change. Second, a number of participants were lost to follow-up because of death or withdrawal and therefore were not included in the analysis. The final outcome measure was evaluated 3 months after the intervention was delivered. Some of the subjects lost to follow-up may have had worse outcomes, but these were not evaluated because of loss to follow-up. Finally, health beliefs were not measured in both the treatment and control subjects because of the nature of the intervention. Because the intervention was based on an evaluation of the health beliefs determined by the Health Belief Scales, the authors thought that administering the scales at 3 time points to control subjects was similar to the intervention given to the treatment subjects. Future study should include administration of the scales to both groups for a more accurate comparison of health belief changes over time.

The authors thank Drs. Diane Carroll, Susan Chase, and Ellen Mahoney for thoughtful review of an earlier version of this article. The authors also thank Stacey Just, BSN, RN, and Denise Tailby, BSN, RN, for assistance with data collection. Finally, the authors thank the staff of the PCU and TCU at St Luke's Hospital for assistance with identifying appropriate subjects for the study.

REFERENCES

1. American Heart Association. 2002 *Heart and Stroke Statistical Update*. Dallas: American Heart Association; 2001.
2. Brashers VL. Alterations of cardiovascular function. In: McCance KL, Huether SE, eds. *Pathophysiology*, 4th edition. St Louis: Mosby; 2002. p. 980-1047.
3. Hunt SA, Baker DW, Chin MH, Cinquegrani MP, Ganiats TG, Goldstein S, et al. *ACC/AHA guidelines for the evaluation and management of chronic heart failure in the adult: a report by the American College of Cardiology/American Heart Association Task Force on practice guidelines*. American College of Cardiology website. Available at: http://www.acc.org/clinical/guidelines/failure/hf_index.htm. Accessed February 2. 2003.
4. Barella P, Monica ED. Managing congestive heart failure at home. *AACN Clin Issues* 1998;9:377-88.
5. Carlson B, Riegel B, Moser DK. Self-care abilities of patients with heart failure. *Heart Lung* 2001;30:351-9.
6. Jaarsma T, Abu Saad H, Halfens R, Dracup K. Maintaining the balance: nursing care of patients with chronic heart failure. *Int J Nurs Stud* 1997;34:213-21.
7. Happ MB, Naylor MD, Roe-Prior M. Factors contributing to rehospitalization of elderly patients with heart failure. *J Cardiovasc Nurs* 1997;11:74-84.
8. Anderson MA, Hanson KS, DeVilder NW. Unplanned hospital readmissions: a home care perspective. *Nurs Res* 1999;48: 299-307.
9. Krumholz HM, Parent E, Tu U, Vaccarino V, Wang Y, Radford MI, et al. Readmission after hospitalization for congestive heart failure among Medicare beneficiaries. *Arch Intern Med* 1997;157:99-104.
10. Shipton S. Risk factors associated with multiple hospital readmissions. *Home Care Provid* 1996;1:83-5.
11. Vinson IM, Rich MW, Sperry JC, Shah AS, McNamara T. Early readmission of elderly patients with congestive heart failure. *Heart Lung* 1990;38:1290-5.
12. Rich MW, Beckham V, Wittenberg C, Leen C, Freedland KE, Carney RM. A multidisciplinary intervention to prevent readmission of elderly patients with heart failure. *N Engl J Med* 1995;333:1190-5.
13. Rich MW, Vinson JM, Sperry JC, Shah AS, Spinner LR, Chung MK, et al. Prevention of readmission of elderly patients with congestive heart failure. *Intern Med* 1993;8:585-90.
14. Naylor M, Brooten D, Jones R, Lavizzo-Mourey R, Mezey M, Pauly M. Comprehensive discharge planning for the hospitalized elderly. *Ann Intern Med* 1994;120:999-1006.
15. Roglieri JL, Futterman R, McDonough KL, Malya G, Karwath KR, Bowman D, et al. Disease management interventions to improve outcomes in congestive heart failure. *Am J Manag Care* 1997;3:1831-9.
16. Rauh RA, Schwaubauer NJ, Enger EL, Moran JF. A community hospital-based heart failure program: impact on length of stay, admission and readmission rates and cost. *Am J Manag Care* 1999;5:37-43.
17. Urden LD. Heart failure collaborative care: an integrated partnership to manage quality outcomes. *Outcomes Manag Nurs Pract* 1997;2:64-70.
18. Moser DK. Heart failure management: optimal health delivery programs. In: Fitzpatrick JJ, ed. *Annual review of nursing research volume 18*. New York: Springer Publishing Company; 2000. p. 91-126.
19. Smith LE, Fabri SA, Pai R, Ferry D, Heywood T. Symptomatic improvement and reduced hospitalization for patients attending a cardiomyopathy clinic. *Clin Cardiol* 1997;20:949-54.
20. Welsh C, McCaffery M. Congestive heart failure management: a continuum of care. *J Nurs Care Qual* 1996;10:24-32.
21. Elkman L, Andersson B, Ehnforst M, Mateika B, Perrson B, Fagerberg B. Feasibility of a nurse-monitored, outpatient care programme for elderly patients with moderate-to-severe, chronic heart failure. *Eur Heart J* 1998;19:1254-60.
22. Shah NB, Der E, Ruggeiro C, Heidenreich PA, Massie BM. Prevention of hospitalizations for heart failure with an interactive home monitoring program. *Am Heart J* 1998;135:173-8.
23. Riegel B, Carlson B, Kopp Z, LePetri B, Glaser D, Unger A. Effect of a standardized nurse case-management telephone intervention on resource use in patients with chronic heart failure. *Arch Intern Med* 2002;162:705-12.
24. Weinberger M, Oddone EZ, Henderson WG. Does increased access to primary care reduce hospital readmissions? *N Engl J Med* 1996;334:1441-7.
25. West JA, Miller NH, Parker KM, Senneca D, Ghandour G, Clark M, et al. A comprehensive management system for heart failure improves clinical outcomes and reduces medical resource utilization. *Am J Cardiol* 1997;79:58-63.
26. Brooten D, Kumar S, Brown L, Butts P, Finkler S, Bakewell-Sachs S, et al. A randomized clinical trial of early hospital discharge and home follow-up of very low birthweight infants. *N Engl J Med* 1986;315:834-9.
27. Naylor MD, Brooten D, Campbell R, Jacobsen BS, Mezey MS, Pauly MV, et al. Comprehensive discharge

planning and home follow-up of hospitalized elders: a randomized clinical trial. *JAMA* 1999;281:613-20.

28. Naylor MD, McCauley KM. The effects of a discharge planning and home follow-up intervention on elders hospitalized with common medical and surgical cardiac conditions. *J Cardiovasc Nurs* 1999;14:44-54.

29. Naylor MD. Transitional care of older adults. In: Fitzpatrick JJ, ed. *Annual review of nursing research volume 20*. New York: Springer Publishing Company; 2002. p. 127-47.

30. Brooten D, Youngblut JM, Deatrick J, Naylor M, York R. Patient problems, advanced practice nurse (APN) interventions, time and contacts among five patient groups. *J Nurs Scholarsh* 2003:35:73-9.

31. Agency for Health Care Policy and Research. *Heart failure: evaluation and care of patients with left-ventricular systolic dysfunction* (AHCPR Publication no. 94–0612). Rockville (MD): US Department of Health and Human Services; 1994.

32. Dunbar SB, Jacobsen LH, Deaton C. Heart failure: strategies to enhance patient self-management. *AACN Clin Issues* 1998;9:244-56.

33. Murray PJ. Rehabilitation information and health beliefs of post-coronary patients: do we meet their information needs? *J Adv Nurs* 1989;14:686-93.

34. Richardson HM. The perceptions of Canadian young adults with asthma of their health teaching/learning needs. *J Adv Nurs* 1991;16:447-54.

35. Turton J. Importance of information following myocardial infarction: a study of the self-perceived learning needs of patients and their spouse/partner compared with perceptions of nursing staff. *J Adv Nurs* 1998:27:770-8.

36. Wehby D, Brenner PS. Perceived learning needs of patients with heart failure. *Heart Lung* 1999;28:31-40.

37. Falvo DR. Education evaluation: what are the outcomes? *Adv Ren Replace Ther* 1995;2:227-33.

38. Lee NC, Wasson DR, Anderson MA, Stone S, Gittings JA. A survey of patient education post-discharge. *J Nurs Care Qual* 1998;13:63-70.

39. Joint Commission on Accreditation of Healthcare Organizations. *JCAHO accreditation manual for hospitals*. Oakbrook Terrace (IL): JCAHO; 1997.

40. Becker MH. The Health Belief Model and sick role behavior. In: Becker MH, ed. *The Health Belief Model: personal health behavior*. Thorofare (NJ): Charles Slack; 1974. p. 82-93.

41. Maiman LA, Becker MH. The Health Belief Model: origins and correlates in psychological theory. In: Becker MH, ed. *The Health Belief Model: personal health behavior*. Thorofare (NJ): Charles Slack; 1974. p. 9-26.

42. Leventhal H, Cameron L. Behavioral theories and the problem of compliance. *Patient Educ Couns* 1987;10:117-38.

43. Sheeran P, Abraham C. The Health Belief Model. In: Connor M, Norman P, eds. *Predicting health behavior: research and practice with social cognition models*. Buckingham: Open University Press; 1996. p. 23-61.

44. Kasl SV. The Health Belief Model and behavior related to chronic illness. In: Becker MH, ed. *The Health Belief Model: personal health behavior*. Thorofare (NJ): Charles Slack; 1974. p. 106-27.

45. Rosenstock IM. Historical origins of the Health Belief Model. In: Becker MH, ed. *The Health Belief Model and personal health behavior*. Thorofare (NJ): Charles Slack; 1974. p. 1-9.

46. Bornstein M, Bornstein H, Cohen J. *Power and precision 1.00 (computer software)*. Bethesda (MD): National Institute of Mental Health; 1997.

47. Rector TS, Kubo SH, Cohn JN. Patient self-assessment of their congestive heart failure part 2: content, reliability and validity of a new measure the Minnesota Living with Heart Failure Questionnaire. *Heart Fail* 1987;3:198-209.

48. Rector TS. Cohn JN. Assessment of patient outcome with the Minnesota Living with Heart Failure Questionnaire: reliability and validity during a randomized, double-blind, placebo controlled trial of pimobendan. *Am Heart J* 1992;124:1017-24.

49. Bennett SJ, Hays LM, Embree JL, Arnould M. Heart Messages: a tailored message intervention for improving heart failure outcomes. *J Cardiovasc Nurs* 2000;14:94-105.

50. Bennett SJ, Milgrom LB, Champion V, Huster GA. Beliefs about medication compliance in heart failure: an instrument development study. *Heart Lung* 1997;26:273-9.

51. Bennett SJ, Perkins SM, Forthofer MA, Brater DC, Murray MD. Reliability and validity of the compliance belief scales among patients with heart failure. *Heart Lung* 2001;30:177-85.

52. Jaarsma T, Halfens H, Senten M, AbuSaad HH, Dracup K. Developing a supportive-educative program for patients with advanced heart failure within Orem's general theory of nursing. *Nurs Sci Q* 1998;11:79-85.

53. Munro BH. *Statistical methods for health care research* (4th edition). Philadelphia: Lippincott: 2002.

54. Rich MW, Freedland KE. Effect of DRGs on three-month readmission rates of geriatric patients with heart failure. *Am J Public Health* 1988;78:680-2.

55. Wolinsky FD, Smith DM, Stump TE, Overhage JM, Lubitz NM. The sequelae of hospitalization for congestive heart failure among older adults. *J Am Geriatr Soc* 1997;45:558-63.

56. Williams JF, Bristow MR, Fowler MB, Francis GS, Garson AJ, Gersh B, et al. Guidelines for the evaluation and management of heart failure. Report of the American College of Cardiology/American Heart Association Task Force. *J Am Coll Cardiol* 1995;26:1376-98.

57. Luzier AB, Forrest A, Adelman M, Hawari FI, Izzo JL Jr. Impact of angiotensin-converting enzyme inhibitor underdosing on rehospitalization rates in congestive heart failure. *Am J Cardiol* 1998;15:465-9.

58. Oka RK, Demarco T, Haskell WL, Botvinick E, Dae MW, Bolen K, et al. Impact of a home-based

walking and resistance training program on quality of life in patients with heart failure. *Am J Cardiol* 2000;85:365-9.

59. Doyle JC, Mottram DR, Stubbs H. Prescribing of ACE inhibitors for cardiovascular disorders in general practice. *J Clin Pharm Ther* 1998;23:133-6.

60. Kermani M, Dua A, Gradman AH. Underutilization and clinical benefits of angiotensin-converting enzyme inhibitors with patients with asymptomatic left ventricular dysfunction. *Am J Cardiol* 2000;86:644-8.

61. Sneed NV, Paul S, Michel Y, VanBakel A, Hendrix G. Evaluation of 3 quality of life measurement tools in patients with chronic heart failure. *Heart Lung* 2001;30:332-40.

62. Reidinger MS, Dracup KA, Brecht ML, Padilla G, Sarna L, Ganz P. Quality of life in patients with heart failure: do gender differences exist? *Heart Lung* 2001;30:105-16.

63. Riegel B, Moser DK, Glaser D, Carlson B, Deaton C, Armola R. et al. The Minnesota Living with Heart Failure Questionnaire sensitivity to difference in responsiveness to intervention intensity in a clinical population. *Nurs Res* 2002;51:209-18.

64. Brooten D, Naylor MD. Nurses' effect on changing patient outcomes. *J Nurs Scholarsh* 1995;27:95-9.

65. Champion V, Foster IL, Menon U. Tailoring interventions for health behavior change in breast cancer screening. *Cancer Pract* 1997;5:283-8.

66. Campbell MK, DeVillis B, Strecher VJ, Ammerman AS, DeVillis RF, Sandler RS. Improving dietary behavior: the effectiveness of tailored messages in primary care settings. *Am J Public Health* 1994;84:783-7.

67. Perry CF, Bauer KD. Effect of printed tailored messaging on cancer risk behavior. *Top Clin Nurs* 2001:16:42-52.

68. Skinner CS, Strecher VJ, Hospers H. Physician's recommendations for mammography: do tailored messages make a difference? *Am J Public Health* 1994;84:43-9.

69. Lu ZYJ. Effectiveness of breast self-examination nursing interventions for Taiwanese community target groups. *J Adv Nurs* 2001;34:163-70.

Study 2: A Phenomenological Exploration of Spirituality Among African American Women Recovering from Substance Abuse

VIOLET L. WRIGHT

Spirituality among African American women recovering from substance abuse is a recovery phenomenon: little is known about the individual's experience in this process. The ameliorating effect of spirituality covering a broad range of positive outcomes has been consistent across populations, regardless of gender, race, study design, and religious affiliation. Giorgi's phenomenological method was used to explore and describe the meaning of spirituality of 15 African American women recovering from substance abuse. The findings are described and discussed relative to the state of the science on spirituality. Implications for substance abuse and recovery practitioners are presented. © 2003 Elsevier Inc. All rights reserved.

RECOVERY FROM SUBSTANCE abuse is a recovery phenomenon that is of importance to nursing. Reports in the literature indicate that recovery from substance abuse is a complex multidimensional process that occurs both with and without expert assistance (Prochaska, DiClemente, & Norcross, 1992). Whereas a combination of human, social, and economic costs of substance abuse have led to a plethora of research on topics such as the epidemiology of substance abuse, treatment outcomes such as client functioning, relapse phenomena, and most recently matching individual and treatment characteristics (Murphy, 1993), very little is known about recovery from substance abuse in African American women. Although studies conducted with women have increased within the last decade, those conducted may not be generalizable to African American women (Davis, 1997; Jackson, 1995; Murphy, 1993). It is estimated that women represent at least one-quarter of all who are dependent on various substances (Davis, 1997; Greenfield & Rogers, 1999). The recidivism rate for substance abusers has been reported to be at 90% 12 months after treatment, with most relapse occurring after 3 months (Substance Abuse and Mental Health Services Administration, 1996).

For many African American women recovering from substance abuse, current treatment modalities and self-help groups do not meet their needs (Hooks, 1993; Nelson-Zlupko, Dore, Kauffman, & Kaltenbach, 1996), because mainstream treatment of substance abuse has traditionally been developed and implemented by male providers for male clients (Abbott, 1994; Reed, 1985). Unlike treatment for men, which can be individualistic oriented, women's treatment must be focused within the context of their relationship to others (Finkelstein, 1994). Research suggests that women may benefit from substance abuse programs that include a residential component, as well as gender-specific services (Dempsey & Wenner, 1996; NelsonZlupko, et al., 1996). Spirituality has often been noted in the health care literature to affect recovery (Ellison & Levin, 1998; McNichol, 1996; Sloan, Bagiella, & Powell, 1999).

Although there has been a proliferation of reports in the health care literature substantiating the ameliorating effects of spirituality with a broad range of positive outcomes, only a few have focused on specific spiritually derived strategies as an aid to recovery (Brome, Owens, Allen, & Vevaina, 2000; Ellison & George, 1994: Green, Fullilove & Fullilove, 1997; McMillen, Howard, Nower, & Chung, 2001). It has also become important to articulate the distinction between spirituality and religion. Although some may regard the two as indistinguishable, others believe religion has specific behavioral, social, doctrinal, and denominational characteristics, whereas spirituality is concerned with the transcendent, and addressing ultimate questions about life's meaning (Carson, 1989: McSherry & Draper, 1998; Nagai-Jackobson & Burkhardt, 1989; Reed, 1992). These differences are acknowledged. Undoubtedly, this confusion between spirituality and religion has been a huge roadblock in the understanding of what it means to be human.

An individual's unique spirituality or spiritual "style," is the way he or she seeks to find or create, use, and expand personal meaning in the context of the universe (Thibault, Ellor, and Netting, 1991). Feminist researchers and theologians have suggested that spirituality may be expressed

From Wright, V.L. (2003). A phenomenological exploration of spirituality among African American women recovering from substance abuse. *Archives of Psychiatric Nursing,* 17(4), 173-185. © 2003 Elsevier, Inc. All rights reserved.

differently by women than by men (Anderson & Hopkins, 1991; Reuther, 1992). Turner et al., (1998) concluded that ethnic minority women returned to church after beginning recovery with greater regularity than Anglo women. It is, therefore, possible that the ethnic minority churches may be meeting the needs of recovering women. The need for an Afrocentric approach in the treatment and recovery of substance abuse that would facilitate the strengthening of identity, spirituality, and community has been articulated by several researchers interested in the Afrocentric worldview (Asante, 1988; Belgrave et al., 1994; Brisbane & Womble, 1985). Spirituality is considered to be the cornerstone of activities within the African American community (Jackson, 1995; Scandrett, 1994). Most of these activities are centered around the Black Church. How spirituality might be used in recovery and healing needs to be explored and described in this population.

Since the conception of modern nursing by Nightingale, spirituality has been central to the essence of nursing. In providing holistic care, nursing now addresses spirituality. The concept that the provision for patients' spiritual needs is encompassed within the nurse's role is supported by prolific nursing writers such as Carson (1989) and nurse theorists like Watson (1988), Roy (1984), Neuman (1989), and Reed (1992). Nurses are obligated to care for the whole human being, presupposing that they understand and accept patients' spiritual experiences irrespective of their ways of expressing them. Therefore, the first step is for nurses and other health care professionals to begin their own spiritual journeys. As nurses achieve awareness of their inner selves, they can more readily address the spiritual needs of others by looking beyond the physical and more deeply within, and become aware that there is something sacred that can be witnessed and shared in the midst of life's illness and disease. A phenomenological understanding of all that spirituality may represent to African American women is relevant to the recovery process from substance abuse.

PURPOSE

A qualitative phenomenological research study was designed to explore the essential elements of the lived experience of spirituality among African American women recovering from substance abuse, and to describe the meanings made of this phenomenon by the person experiencing it.

METHODS

Philosophical Perspective

The perspectives of Frankl (1965, 1984) provide the conceptual orientation for this study, whereas direction for data analyses was provided by the procedural steps of Giorgi's (1985) method. Frankl (1984) states that the meaning of life differs from man to man, from day to day, and from hour to hour. Frankl (1984) proposed that the chief dynamic behind the addictive behavior is "existential frustration" created by a vacuum of a perceived meaning in personal existence, and

manifested by the symptom of boredom. The underpinnings of Frankl's work stresses individual's freedom to transcend suffering and find meaning in life regardless of his circumstances. The substance abuser often looks on his existence as meaningless and without purpose. Frankl's (1984) concept of how meaning in life differs from day to day correlates with the philosophies of Alcoholics Anonymous (AA) in their statement about staying sober "one day at a time." Frankl's (1984) work is based on empirical or phenomenological analysis, which was described as the way in which man understands himself, and how he interprets his own existence.

Methodology

Phenomenology was chosen as the methodology for this study, in that it describes the world as it is experienced before any theories being devised to explain it. The aim of phenomenology in nursing research is to describe the experience of others so that those who care for these individuals may be more empathetic and understanding of the person's experience.

Phenomenology seeks meanings from appearances and arrives at essences through intuition and reflection on conscious acts of experiences, leading to ideas, concepts, judgements, and understandings. The core processes included in the phenomenological methodology are epoche or bracketing, phenomenological reduction (intuiting), imaginative variation (analyzing), and synthesis of meanings and essences (describing). Bracketing involves refraining from judgment, abstaining or staying away from the everyday or ordinary way of seeing things. In our natural attitude we tend to hold knowledge judgmentally, we presuppose that what we perceive in nature is actually there and remains there as we perceive it. Giorgi describes this process as setting aside one's own presuppositions or knowledge about a particular phenomenon. Intuiting involves the task of describing in textural language, just what one sees, not only in terms of the external object but also the internal acts of consciousness. The reduction is strictly a methodological move to temporarily strip the world of the multitude of implicit presumptions about its existence as "real" thereby allowing aspects of the world to occur as pure phenomena for consciousness. The term imaginative variation or analyzing means "to arrive at structural descriptions of an experience, the underlying and precipitating factors that account for what is being experienced" (Moustakis, 1994, p. 98). Giorgi refers to this process as the delineation of "meaning units" and that by freely changing aspects or parts of a phenomenon or object one is able to see if the phenomenon remains identifiable or not. Characteristics that describe a phenomenon are imagined or condensed thoroughly by the researcher and those elements that clearly describe and are characteristic of the phenomenon are considered essential. Describing involves the integration of textural language into a unified statement of the essences of the experience of the phenomenon under investigation. It is describing the central characteristics of the phenomenon by using analogy, negation, and metaphor.

METHODS

Within phenomenological methodology, there are several schools of thought, and various methods for collecting and analyzing data (Ornery, 1983; Spiegelberg, 1982). The types of method are closely associated with the philosophical/theoretical perspectives. For this study, Giorgi's (1985) phenomenological method was chosen. Selecting Giorgi was based on three factors: First, for its well-defined method which was influenced by the works of Husserl (1913/1931) and Merleau-Ponty (1962), secondly, the ability to use psychological analysis of interpretation in formulating meaning units with greater clarity, and third, the researcher is able to analyze the descriptions with a special sensitivity to the perspective of his or her discipline. When analyzed from within a disciplinary framework, Giorgi defines the meaning units as the scientific essences. Thus, his method appeared particularly well suited for the exploration of phenomena, which is of concern for psychiatric-mental health and substance abuse and recovery nursing. Giorgi makes clear that it is critical to distinguish between the use of philosophical phenomenology, which is universal and foundational, and the use of the empirical phenomenological approach that seeks to disclose and elucidate the phenomena of behavior as they present themselves.

This study followed the core processes of phenomenology and the four steps outlined in Giorgi's (1985) method, which are as follows: (1) The researcher reads the entire description of the learning situation obtained from the participants to get a sense of the whole statement; (2) next, once a sense of the whole has been grasped, the researcher rereads the same description more slowly with the specific intent of discriminating "meaning units" from within a psychological perspective and with a focus on the phenomenon of interest; (3) once the "meaning units" have been delineated, the researcher then goes through all of the "meaning unit" and expresses the psychological insight contained in them more directly. This is especially true of the meaning units more revelatory of the phenomenon under consideration: (4) finally, the researcher synthesizes the transformed meaning units.

STUDY PARTICIPANTS

The number of participants was determined by the number of persons required to permit an indepth exploration and obtain a clear understanding of the phenomenon of interest from various perspectives. This occurred with 15 participants when data saturation was achieved, with no new themes or essences emerging from the participants and the data were repeating. Participants were recruited froth a women's shelter with the help of a colleague as contact person, from church support groups within the community by the researcher who made church members aware of the study and the search for participants, and through networking, whereby each participant interviewed suggested the name of a potential new participant.

Each participant met the following criteria: over 18 years of age; identified herself as an African American woman; substance free status for at least 1 year; able to participate and engage in interviews of 1 to 2 hours in length; expressed interest in participating in the study; not currently being treated for psychotic disorders; and was able to read and write in the English language. There was no restriction as to the length of substance abuse to enter the study.

There were 15 participants who ranged from 29 to 49 years of age. With respect to marital status, the majority—eight of the participants were never married, whereas six were divorced and one currently married. The participants reported a mixed range of religious affiliation, with all of them considering themselves to be Christians. Seven participants attended religious activities more than once per week. All the participants reported an increase in their spirituality since becoming drug free. All participants identified their higher power as God or Jesus Christ.

Of the participants 12 began using substances between the ages of 5 to 12, with all having some form of structured treatment for substance abuse. A majority of the participants reported having past legal problems. With respect to abstinence eight participants reported 7-12 years of drug free status. and seven having 15-39 months of substance free status.

PHENOMENOLOGICAL RIGOR

Guba (1991) suggests that credibility, dependability, confirmability, and transferability be used to support rigor in qualitative research. Although Giorgi's (1985) phenomenological analysis does not rely on participant review or intersubjective agreement by expert judges, peer debriefing, or returning to participants to validate findings to establish qualitative rigor, some aspects of rigor drawn from Lincoln & Guba's (1985) work were applied to increase trustworthiness of the interpretation. Streubert and Carpenter (1995) states that rigor or trustworthiness in qualitative research can be achieved through the researcher's attention to and confirmation of the information discovered (p. 25). The goal of maintaining rigor is to accurately represent what those who have been studied experience.

Credibility involves activities that increase the probability that credible findings will be produced (Lincoln & Guba, 1985). One of the best ways to establish credibility is through prolonged engagement with the subject matter. For this, Giorgi (1985) considers the process of bracketing, phenomenological reduction, and concern for essences as evidence of reliability and validity. Bracketing in this study was achieved through "journaling" throughout data collection and analysis. Notes regarding beliefs, presuppositions, and past experiences with spirituality and recovery from substance abuse, as well as thoughts after interviews were recorded and discussed with senior researchers. These entries were useful in achieving bracketing and in rendering noninfluential this researcher's prior experiences and presuppositions on the phenomenon. Dependability is met through credibility (Streubert & Carpenter, 1995). Confirmability is the way one documents the findings by leaving an audit trail.

An audit trail is a recording of activities over time. which can be followed by another individual (Streubert & Carpenter, 1995, p. 26). The objective is to clearly illustrate the evidence and thought process that led to the conclusions. The use of journals also serves to establish confirmability. In this study, presenting the data from the beginning where naive meaning units were identified, to clustering, and finally to themes and the essential descriptions achieved this end. Transferability is the probability that the findings of the study have meaning to others in similar situations.

PROCEDURE AND DATA COLLECTION

The participants were contacted in three ways: (1) through a colleague who used a woman's shelter for practice experience and had contact with African American women recovering from substance abuse, (2) from community contacts with church support group members, and (3) through networking. The purpose of the study was explained and informed consent obtained. All participants were interviewed in their homes or the shelter with each interview being audiotaped and lasting from 45 to 90 minutes. Each participant was given a brief introduction regarding the researcher's interest about the phenomenon. The interviews began with the general request: "to describe your experiences, thoughts, perceptions, and feelings of how spirituality contributed to your recovery" followed by a request to "describe an occasion or event during your substance abuse when you decided to use spirituality as a part of your recovery." Neutral probes were then used to elicit fuller description and elaboration of the experience such as "how significant is spirituality in your life?" The researcher encouraged personal perspectives to expand on the descriptions. The recall of painful memories can trigger anxiety and other emotional distress. Therefore, the emotional state of each participant was evaluated throughout the interviews by stopping when the participant was upset and offering support.

Although Giorgi's (1988) phenomenological analysis does not rely on peer debriefing, to establish qualitative rigor, notes were recorded after each interview regarding the process, feelings, and experiences of the researcher elicited by the interview. In this study during each interview the researcher was genuinely interested in participant's experience and listened honestly to their descriptions. This journaling ensured bracketing or the suspension of presuppositions on the part of the researcher. She returned frequently to what she had bracketed (the researcher's knowledge of and belief in God).

FINDINGS

After each interview was transcribed, the researcher carefully listened to the audiotape to ensure accuracy in the transcription. The narrative of each experience was then analyzed according to Giorgi's (1985) phenomenological method. In this study, the researcher read the entire description of the experience and captured the sense of the whole. Each transcript was then read and reread several times in an effort to delineate meaning units as they were conveyed in the participant's words. These are the naive meanings units, and although they are not explicitly stated by the participant they are perceived by the researcher who assumes a psychological attitude towards the concrete examples. Following this approach, the researcher identified 1669 naive meaning units in the transcribed interviews. These naive meaning units were then transformed through the process of reflection and intuitive variation into 631 formulated meaning units or constituents of the essence of spirituality for these recovering women. These essences or themes and supporting theme clusters were then formulated and later discussed in the findings. Five major themes were formulated from the narratives (Table 1). Each of these themes has supporting themes that have been extrapolated from the narratives. A typology of the themes and supporting themes were created. These themes and supporting theme clusters are not exclusive or isolated experiences but represent aspects of the participants' experiences, which sometimes are interwoven or overlap. Two examples of the themes and supporting themes are described in Table 2 to provide the reader with information about activities during the process of formulating naive-meaning units to main themes which emerged as the essence or meaning structure. Each of the themes is presented with supporting verbatims to substantiate the researcher's process in identification of themes and for the reader to grasp a full understanding of the participant's experience.

The absence of spirituality was experienced as abandonment when there was no personal and intimate relationship with God. The absence of spirituality was experienced as abandonment among recovering African American women.

Table 1 Major Meaning Units

MAJOR THEMES FROM THE PARTICIPANTS' NARRATIVES

1. The absence of spirituality was experienced as abandonment when there was no personal and intimate relationship with God.
2. Spirituality was experienced as surrendering when there was a spiritual awakening.
3. The women recovering from substance abuse experienced spirituality as reconnecting when there was recognition, a realignment, and engagement with God, self, and community.
4. Spirituality was experienced as transformation when the women were able to transcend substance abuse and other difficulties and focus on restoration and growth towards new horizons.
5. Spirituality was experienced as maturation when there was attainment of newness in life.

Table 2   Typology of Major Themes, Naïve Units, and Participant's Description

THEMES	MEANING UNITS (MU)	PARTICIPANT'S DESCRIPTION
Example 1: The women recovering from substance experienced the absence of spirituality as abandonment when there was no personal and intimate relationship with God.	MU:1.1. The absence of spirituality was experienced as abandonment when participants recalled feeling as if something was missing from their lives, of being far from God, being in the dark, and being in bondage.	This participant experienced the absence of spirituality as abandonment by stating: "There was something missing before and I didn't know what it was. It was as if I was searching for something. And I had to go through all the hard times to find it. He shown me the light because I was in the dark."
	MU:1.2. The absence of spirituality was experienced as abandonment when the women related feeling alone and saw separation from God and others due to death or other circumstances as contributing factors.	This participant spoke of abandoning her family: "So at that Christmas dinner all my family ganged up on me and confronted me about my drug use... So I left the dinner. I didn't go to any more family gatherings for about 10 years. I abandoned my family... Even though I was clean, I didn't feel happy. I think after I stopped using, this was the loneliest period of my life. I felt alone. Like I had no one in the world."
The women recovering from substance abuse experienced spirituality as surrendering when there was a spiritual awakening.	MU:2.1. The women reporting turning their lives and will over to God, letting go, relinquishing control, and putting the past behind as surrendering.	This woman stated: "...I had to learn how to admit that I really don't have all the answers...I surrendered my know-it-all-ism."
	MU:2.2. The women identified struggling, powerlessness, and a total dependency on God as surrendering.	This woman stated: "When I hit 18 months clean I was struggling and I was crying out to everybody. I was showing up for Bible study, I was showing up for church... I was doing all that I could do, but it wasn't enough. I still didn't have what it took on the inside... I had a dependency. I had been praying to the Lord for dependency. I said Lord I want to be totally dependent on you. So God allowed everything that I had depended on to be gone."

Abandonment was alluded to in all of the narratives; however, the nature of the abandonment varied among the women in this study. The absence of spirituality was experienced as abandonment when participants reported feeling as if something was missing from their lives, of being far from God, and being in the dark. Spirituality was viewed negatively when there was the felt absence of a relationship with God. For these women abandonment was experienced as a lack of intimacy with God, which led to deterioration in fellowship and deepened into darkness. Although they lacked intimacy, they reported that after no longer using substances, realizing that their survival was a result of the unconditional abiding presence of God and that they were the ones who had abandoned God. One participant described her experience of abandonment as follows:

> … Although I was brought up to believe in God. at some point I still feel God failed me and I can't exactly tell where. I don't know if it was after I got married and ended up in an abusive relationship…. For a while I had abandoned God and things in my life were going swell. But what I realize is that He hadn't abandoned me. He was just carrying this fool through so she can realize that

someone was still there for her and you don't have to carry the world on your shoulders…

In addition, the absence of spirituality was also experienced as abandonment when ingrained knowledge of God was overshadowed by substance use. Renewed knowledge, however, resulted in God's illumination within the soul once the substance was removed and was described by one participant as follows:

> When I used substances, I couldn't see; I was blind. When I began not using substances, I could see God. I began to see Him.

Surrendering when there was a spiritual awakening. The lived experience of a spiritual journey begins with surrendering to God or Higher Power and can, therefore, be understood as movement towards spiritual recovery. All of the women in this study identified their belief in God and their Higher Power as referring to God or Jesus Christ. Surrendering allowed them to deal with the pain of their addiction and to hand over their life and addiction to a power greater than themselves. For these women, a spiritual awakening occurred

287

in different ways. Some were able to recall a significant turning point or event in their recovery. One woman stated:

> I can remember very clearly the night my son got killed. He asked me to get some help. I was in the kitchen cooking … and he dropped to his knees and grabbed me and ask me to get some help because he didn't want to see me dead like that. Three hours later the police knocked on my door and said my son is dead… Maybe he was right. That was a real spiritual awakening right there. An omen. I was like why? God took him for me to see, to get myself together…

One of the most genuine dimensions of surrendering for the women occurred when there was sincere repentance, purging the self, and confession. All of them spoke of the decision to turn from selfish desires and seek a higher power. The inward conviction expressed itself in outward actions. And was described by this participant as follows:

> This you have to clean up. Get rid of your old baggage. Cleaning it up. Tell on yourself. That is telling on yourself and telling God. Even though He knows, He has to know that you know what is wrong and right for you: confession. So once you told Him ok, God, I know these things are wrong with me… the lies, the fear. the cheating, the dishonesty…

The women recovering from substance abuse experienced spirituality as reconnecting when there was recognition, a realignment, and engagement with god, self, and community. Participants reported their experience of reconnecting by bringing themselves to God, family, and community honestly and completely; by seeking God's guidance, and being willing to continue to face the truth of who they are, regardless of how threatening or unpleasant their perceptions may be. The spiritual journey for these women was reported to include reconnecting with the community, mainly, through AA, NA, and churches. The most significant reconnecting, however, was with their families. However, they reported that the power of faith communities—the church—provided lasting steadiness and strength for their recovery. All of the women spoke of a nuclear family. A return to the family fold was therefore perceived as reconnecting and a return to their spiritual walk or to normalcy. They were able to begin a new and different kind of learning, a learning that involved openness, honesty, patience, obedience, acceptance, forgiveness, and awareness of sense of self. This woman reported how cut off she was from her family and when reconnection occurred how she became an important part of the family again:

> Me and my husband got back together too… He had written me off … I could spend time with my family… I am sharing with my family and because I dropped all that negative stuff, they are able to hear me now. They are able to connect with what I am feeling.

For some of the women reconnecting was a liberation whereby dormant feelings were able to emerge, as this participant stated:

> I went to rehab and I cried more in those 28 day than I did in my 28 years of life. I was getting honest with myself for the first time. I was brought up in a don't touch, don't talk, don't feel family. So to be able to get in touch with my feelings was something new.

Spiritual reconnection for some of the women was very difficult, but it allowed them to apologize and to be able to move on in their recovery. This participant stated:

> I made apology to my mom. I made amends to my children. I sat down and told them I really. really didn't mean to hurt you. That is who I was then. I was an addict: I can't take none of the years back…

Spirituality was experienced as transformation when participants were able to transcend substance use and other difficulties and focus on restoration and growth towards new horizons. Transformation was experienced when the women described an inward change of something going on inside their hearts. Although some women found it "hard to describe," they were able to impart that there was a communion going on within them at all times with God. Becoming more spiritual had an ameliorating effect on these women and on their recovery, in that they were able to transcend their substance use and be spiritually transformed into God's image and become a vessel or temple and thereby receive all that He has to offer. Spiritual transformation resulted in a change in the women's thinking. The women spoke of this transformation in their thinking as a requirement for recovery. This participant stated:

> My thinking is being transformed now—in a spiritual way. He is working on me inside. Even when I mess up, I don't feel guilty… Yes, no more guilt or shame. I feel worthy now because I've let all that go: I throw all the mess in the garbage can: this was only because of my spirituality. Because of God's love I am trying to transform my thinking and my heart to love and be forgiving…

The lived experience of spirituality for these women was experienced as a life-line in their recovery from substance abuse and as a part of their worldview—their values, customs, and beliefs. In essence spirituality became a part of their everyday life, as this participant stated:

> It is a way of life; is a way of life… I believe that the Creator, whom in AA 1 say Creator, but for real I mean God. Jesus Christ abides in me. So if He abides in me, then he manifest himself through me.

Another participant supported the lived experience of spirituality as part of everyday life as follows:

> When you have a belief in God, spirituality is reflected in everything that you do or say. So for me through all my years of using drugs and alcohol, I was not a spiritual person. That part was not being reflected. Today my spirituality is being reflected in my walk and my talk. To be spiritual you have to nourish your soul, mind, and body. Your body is a temple. I was destroying mine.

Participants were spiritually transformed when they were empowered by hearing the word of God, through their church, and by reading the word of God. They described movement towards wholeness, love, and freedom as empowerment in their spiritual transformation:

> I get more and more empowered with my spirituality. I will pray, read the Bible all I can… I get deeper in touch with my God… My mom gave me a Bible and gave me this little booklet with verse in it. Empowering verses.

One woman described how God used her suffering to teach her and bring her closer to Him and the complex interweaving aspects of her healing process as follows:

> God has different ways of using things to get you where He wants you to be. It is a bad thing if He did that. If God did that, it's a bad thing… but I have learned so much from what happened, most of all I found God.

Spirituality was experienced as maturation when there was attainment of newness in life. Spiritual maturation for these women occurred when there was a constant awareness of the presence of God in their daily lives. The women reported experiencing tremendous relief in knowing God's unconditional love, in knowing that his love for them was utterly real and that prior knowledge of the worst about them could never disillusion Him about them. The women spoke of this time of crossing over from transformation as the integration of all that was learned, and claiming what has happened in their hearts. Spiritual maturation was experienced as the ability to transcend insurmountable difficulties and adversities through faith and hope. Thus healing was not only the result of faith; it also produces faith:

> … Now that I have come to know God … it doesn't matter what adversities come your way; you can still find joy… He will give me the strength to go on, the hope. And the faith to believe that He is there with me. That He hasn't forsaken me.

The study participants described spiritual maturation as freedom. Freedom liberated them from the past and offered an opportunity to explore problems and issues from a fresh perspective.

> It's that freedom … you just don't know. Freedom from the burden. Peace of mind.

For some, spiritual maturation was finding meaning and purpose in their lives.

> You may not know your purpose for tomorrow, but you know the purpose from yesterday is to get to a point of never living that way again … just not doing what you used to do.

And another woman stated:

> Right now the purpose is getting my kids back into my life. I haven't had them for 6 or 7 years during my recovery… I know this was the purpose, to be a mother to these children.

For some participants spiritual maturation was obtained by finding peace.

> Spirituality for me is being able to be in here with faith through all the storms. You know, in hard times, in crazy times. I still have peace… I am at peace now.

In summary, data analysis identified five themes that demonstrated the experiences of the women's spirituality in their recovery from substance abuse, which were clearly articulated in the verbatim transcripts. These themes are not exclusive or isolated experiences but represent aspects of the women's experiences, which sometimes are interwoven or overlap. This was necessary for the researcher to arrive at a plausible comprehensive understanding of the whole phenomenon.

DISCUSSION

Discussion of Findings Relevant to Literature Reviewed

The women spoke of their experience of how they lived in a state of chronic apartness, separated from God and from those who love them. Their attachment to substances usurped God, their desire for love, and their ability to love and trust. The experiences of some of the women caused them to feel that God had not only let them down but that He had set them up. As a result they put God out of their lives. Similar findings were reported (Di Lorenzo, Johnson & Bussey, 2001, and Walant, 1995) as this study, which found that separation between the self and God led to a loss of spirituality and not being able to love, trust, and nurture. It was, however, during their disconnected state that the women were able to achieve insight into their dissatisfying and destructive behavior. Loneliness and isolation are unfortunate realities in the lives of those recovering from substance abuse. The findings of this study revealed that the experience of abandonment was unique for each individual, since the interactions within one's environment are influenced by a variety of factors. As a result, the women experienced abandonment when there was loss of a significant other, or when there was overwhelming feelings of guilt due to their inability to assume roles that were critical to the sense of self and purpose in life. For the women in this study their recovery from substance abuse brought to the surface feelings such as guilt, shame, or inadequacy as a parent. These disclosures support data showing that 74% of child neglect cases involved female caregivers who abused substances (U.S. Department of Health and Human Services, 1999; Woodhouse, 1992). This study supports previous reports that childhood physical and sexual abuse as risk factors for heavy drinking among African American women can be seen as behavior to numb the pain and shame of the abuse. Early childhood trauma precipitated a downhill spiral for the women in that they felt alone and abused, and as their substance abuse escalated, they became isolated from their natural and therapeutic supports.

289

In this study the women's recovery from substance abuse began when they hit rock bottom, struggled and then let go by surrendering and turning their lives over to God. Surrendering contained a message that was directed toward them as they experienced themselves as utterly failing. As Farris (1994) concluded, this failure was projected onto God in such a way that the individual often believed that God sees and judges them as a failure. It was evident that their struggles and suffering had taken their toll spiritually, mentally, and physically as their narratives contained the underlying message that "all guilt will end here" by surrendering. Letting go is a fundamental principle of life. The women in this study recognized that letting go of the past was paramount to their recovery, which is in line with Chopra's (1990) conclusion that to arrive at bliss—this place of peace—one had to let go all the inbuilt words, images, emotions and activities of the mind. By letting go of the past, the women reported they were able to focus on the "now." Many of the women reported that their "know-it-all-ism" and conventional will power alone were not able to help them succeed in their recovery. An important finding in this study was that although surrendering occurred gradually for some participants. many reported having significant events that resulted in their spiritual awakening. The loss of parents. significant other, children, siblings and friends were collectively experienced by all the participants and were the catalyst for many of them surrendering and beginning their spiritual awakening.

All of the study participants recalled having previous knowledge of God some time in their lives before incorporating spirituality into their recovery from substance abuse. The central purpose for reconnecting was to know God again, but this time from a deep spiritual realm. This spiritual reconnection was experienced by going to God in prayer, reading the Bible, and worship. These activities provided them with guidance and strength in their everyday lives. However, they were able to gain extra strength in their spiritual development when they reconnected with families and groups.

The use of community was utilized by all the women in this study, as defined by Eugene (1995) and Villarosa (1994), which was a supportive community or group of people with whom one shares common beliefs and values. Although affiliations with groups such as AA and NA, which were used by some of the women, were supportive, the benefits received from their church-affiliated groups were clearly more strengthening. Some of the women spoke of "the kindred spirit" of the group, as being one in the body of Christ, which therefore made them a family. The comfort and strength received by the women were particularly important in managing the stresses of their everyday lives. Some of the women in this study spoke of "being on trial in AA and NA," some of "slowly weaning themselves away," whereas others had completely stopped using these programs as a support system. Their reasons were varied, with some reporting that these programs were just the building blocks to get them to where they were able to find a God of their own; some felt restricted in their ability to freely give God praise for helping them to overcome their substance use; and some felt that the way the program is structured is hypocritical, in that Bill Wilson received his revelations from God for the 12 steps. which are based on the Bible. The interviewees were able to accept what Kearney (1998) spoke of as the differences of others, working on developing an identity with those of similar beliefs, and forming a community that contributed to healing. The findings of this study also supports the conclusion of Ellison and George (1994) that people's sense of existential isolation are ameliorated by knowing that they are participants in the journey of eternal significance. Through a sense of independence or autonomy, the women were able to see what Ettorre (1992) referred to as their "women-selves" as they recognized and reconnected with their past, present, and future.

Participants experienced transformation as progressive. They revealed that through fellowship with God there was daily spiritual renewal with a deepening knowledge of Him. In this study and in the literature (McMillen, Howard, Nower, and Chung, 2001; Millar and Stermac, 2000), the women spoke of their substance abuse as being a good thing, in that in the process of their substance abuse, God used the very affliction that was responsible for their demise (the old self) to effect an inward renewal and healing that lifted them above the ravishment of their disease.

All of those interviewed reported that healing for them allowed growth, which transformed their thinking. The narratives revealed that there was a spiritual transformation through the act of worshiping, whereby God communicated His presence to them, and when they learned not only to give Him thanks and make a petition, but also to worship Him by giving praise for all that He is. This is in line with Eugene's (1995) conclusion that the Black church can offer healing responses. They also reported that they were transformed by dwelling on God's word, which required devout meditation, serious study, and loyal obedience with a resulting widening grasp of the spiritual principles by which they were to grow and live. Furthermore, they disclosed that they were transformed when they were cleansed from every aspect of wrongdoing through the assurance of God's word that if they walked in obedience to the light that He gives, the blood of Christ would keep on cleansing them despite their tendency to sin. The participants' definitions of spirituality were varied, which supports previous reports of multiple definitions of spirituality in African American women (Mattis, 2000).

Maturation is an integral part of human growth and development. Spiritual maturation was the essence of recovery from substance abuse for the women in that it provided the means by which they were able to do everything. Some authors reported that African American women tend to rely on other African American women for support and that their place of worship is one of the places used in times of crisis instead of conventional counseling with therapists (Scandrett, 1994; Taylor, 2000). Most of the women in this study were single, and the church served as an integral part of their community and as a place for socialization. The literature supports the findings in this study of the women who reported that reading the Bible provided them with a sense of peace and calmness, and for some it was a source of "daily bread," which gave them strength, courage, and guidance (Green, Fullilove, & Fullilove, 1998). The theme of maturation in this study supports the philosophical perspective of Frankl (1984), which guided the study, in that substance abuse was the vehicle of the past that led to a deeper understanding of meaning and purpose in life for these women. When a sense of meaning and purpose in life was not found, these women experienced what Frankl (1984) described as an existential meaning-vacuum. The vacuum was filled with alcohol and drugs.

In summary, an analysis of interviews with 15 African American women supports the literature that recovery from substance abuse is experienced as a multifaceted process involving physical, cognitive, emotional, and psychosocial efforts. Spirituality was experienced as being similarly complex. Although the phenomenon of spirituality has received some recognition for its ameliorating properties in recovery from substance abuse, and in particular among African Americans, there are no exclusive models that address their unique needs and allow for the free expression of self and their spiritual beliefs. As the social and political turmoil continues within the substance abuse and recovery arena, and as a disenfranchised group, African American women recovering from substance abuse will continue to rely on their churches and other "faith-based programs" so that their experiences can be understood for them as a pillar within the recovery process.

LIMITATIONS

In this study, the researcher began with the assumption that all observations are value laden and made every attempt not to impose researcher bias and interpretations on the data. The study limitations, however, were the researcher having worked in psychiatry and substance abuse for many years observed a difference in the lives of African American women who had incorporated a spiritual belief in their recovery process. Most of the participants were recruited from faith-based women's shelters and church support groups; therefore, it was known that their belief was in God. This was bracketed throughout the study and participants were not directly queried about a belief in God or their religious affiliation. General open questions were used to elicit what spirituality meant to the participant.

In addition, Giorgi's (1985) method does not require peer debriefing, discussing emerging themes with study participants, and listening to their feedback to establish rigor; although these activities could help in exposing researcher bias or error. However, journaling was done to enhance self-awareness.

CONCLUSIONS AND IMPLICATIONS

The concept of spirituality is multidimensional with no clear definition. Therefore, conceptual confusion, ambiguity, and scientific skepticism have prevented adequate investigation into its potential healing effects. The lack of a clear and concise definition may in part be preventing even longer recovery for some substance abusers, who may be reluctant to incorporate this concept into their recovery because of its ambiguity. The strength of this concept as it relates to God within this inquiry has also been embraced with caution within the mental health practice and even among strong supporters of the AA model as one of the most effective ways for long-term sobriety despite its saliency. In our zeal to scientifically study, categorize, and measure spirituality, the essence of spirituality may be overlooked.

As a disenfranchised group, the significance of spirituality in the lives of African American women recovering from substance abuse is an important dimension for them to achieve meaning and purpose in their lives. Despite the efforts that have been made to address the unique needs of women in treatment and recovery programs, and in particular the needs of African American women, participants in this inquiry communicated that they experienced resistance when they expressed commitment to religious values and church participation as strategies for their ongoing recovery. Professionals working with these women must become sensitive to the culture of the African American women and integrate their cultural values into the treatment and recovery.

Because nursing espouses holistic care as a central disciplinary tenet and because of its theoretical foundation, nurses are well positioned to contribute to the understanding of the meaning of spirituality in the recovery process for African American women. Spirituality is a strength that nursing and other professionals in substance recovery can no longer afford to ignore. Nurses are called instruments of healing. Nurses, through practice strategies, can enhance the healing process of African American women recovering from substance abuse by providing supportive interventions that enhance their spiritual journey. Nursing is also concerned with human responses to stressors or illnesses. Because spirituality is increasingly being used by many people to ameliorate their pain and suffering and in their recovery, nurses need to be able to identify behaviors that indicate spirituality among these individuals. Nursing assessment and intervention for African American women using spirituality in their recovery should include a holistic approach that includes spiritual care. The power of spirituality as a component of recovery from substance abuse may be lost in a traditional analysis of recovery methods because the sense of having a relationship with or benefiting from, the guidance of a higher power or God may not be captured in standard assessments.

Any activity of life is an opportunity for nurturing the soul when performed with intention and mindfulness. Therefore, Bible study, meditating or walking in the park may provide nurture for the soul and engages one in purpose and meaning. If these are the spiritual aspects of the everyday lifeworld of the African American women recovering from substance abuse, they must be addressed by the mental health/substance abuse and recovery community in clinical practice and research if greater amelioration by spirituality is to be achieved. Only by becoming more knowledgeable about spirituality and the experiences of African American women recovering from substance abuse can nurses become a successful tool in assisting these women in their recovery.

REFERENCES

Abbott, A.A. (1994). A feminist approach to substance abuse treatment and service: Special Issue Women's health and social work, feminist perspectives. *Social Work in Health Care, 19,* 67-83.

Anderson, S.R. & Hopkins, P. (1991). *The feminine face of God.* New York: Bantam Books.

Asante, M.K. (1988). *Afrocentricity.* Trenton, NJ: Africa World.

Belgrave, F.Z., Cherry, V., Cunningham, D., Walwyn, S., Letlaka-Rennert, K., & Phillips, F. (1994). The influence of afrocentric values, self-esteem, and black identity on drug attitudes among African American fifth graders: A preliminary study. *Journal of Black Psychology, 20*(2), 143-156.

Brisbane, F.L., & Womble, M. (1985). Afterthoughts and recommendations. In F.L. Brisbane & M. Womble (Eds.), *Treatment of black alcoholics.* New York: Harworth.

Brome, D.R., Owens, M.D., Allen, K., & Vevaina, T. (2000). An examination of spirituality among African American women in recovery from substance abuse. *Journal of Black Psychology, 26*(4), 470-486.

Carson, V.B. (1989). *Spiritual dimensions of nursing practice.* Philadelphia: W.B. Saunders.

Chopra, D. (1990). *Quantum healing: Exploring the frontiers of mind/body medicine.* New York: Bantam.

Davis, R.E. (1997). Trauma and Addiction Experiences of African American women. *Western Journal of Nursing Research, 19*(4), 442-465.

Dempsey, M.D., & Wenner, A. (1996). Gender-specific treatment for chemically dependent women: A rationale for inclusion of vocational services. *Alcoholism Treatment Quarterly, 14,* 21-30.

DiLorenzo, P., Johnson, R., & Bussey, M. (2001). The role of spirituality in the recovery process. *Child Welfare League of America, 80*(2), 257-273.

Ellison, C.G., & George, L.K. (1994). Religious involvement, social ties, and social support in a southeastern community. *Journal for the Scientific Study of Religion, 33*(1), 46-61.

Ellison, C.G., & Levin, J.S. (1998). The religion-health connection: Evidence, theory, and future directions. *Health Education and Behavior, 25*(6), 700-720.

Ettorre, E. (1992). *Women and substance abuse.* New Brunswick, NJ: Rutgers University Press.

Eugene, T.M. (1995). There is a balm in Gilead: Black women and the Black church as therapeutic agents of a therapeutic community. *Women and Therapy, 16*(2/3), 55-71.

Farris, R.F. (1994). Addiction and dualistic spirituality: Shared visions of God, self, and creation. *Journal of Ministry in Addiction & Recovery, 1*(1), 5-31.

Finkelstein, N. (1994). Treatment issues for alcohol and drug-dependent pregnant and parenting women. *Health & Social Work, 19,* 7-15.

Frankl, V.E. (1965, 1984). *Man's search for meaning.* New York: Simon & Schuster.

Giorgi, A. (1985). *Phenomenology and psychological research.* Pittsburgh, PA: Duquense University Press.

Green, L.L., Fullilove, M.T., & Fullilove, R.E. (1997). Stories of spiritual awakening. The nature of spirituality in recover. *Journal of Substance Abuse Treatment, 15*(4), 325-331.

Greenfield, T.K., & Rogers, J.D. (1999). Who drinks most of the alcohol in the U. S.? The Policy Implications. *Journal of Studies on Alcohol, 60,* 78-89.

Hooks, B. (1993). *Sisters of the yam: black woman and self-recovery.* Boston: South End.

Jackson, M.S. (1995). Afrocentric treatment of African American women and their children in a residential chemical dependency program. *Journal of Black Studies, 26*(1), 17-30.

Kearney, M.H. (1998). Truthful self-nurturing: A grounded formal theory of women's addiction recovery. *Qualitative Health Research, 8*(4), 495-512.

Lincoln, Y.S., & Guba, E.G. (1985). *Naturalistic Inquiry.* Beverly Hills: Sage.

Mattis, J.S. (2000). African American women's definition of spirituality and religiosity. *Journal of Black Psychology, 26*(1), 101-122.

McMillen, C., Howard, M.O., Nower, L., & Chung, S. (2001). Positive by-products of the struggle with chemical dependency. *Journal of Substance Abuse Treatment, 20,* 69-79.

McNichol, T. (1996, April 7). The new faith in medicine. *USA Today,* p. 4.

McSherry, W., & Draper, P. (1998). The debates emerging from the literature surrounding the concept of spirituality as applied to nursing. *Journal of Advanced Nursing, 27,* 683-691.

Merleau-Ponty, M. (1962). *Phenomenology of perception* (C. Smith, Trans.) London: Routledge; Kegan Paul.

Millar, G.M., & Stermac, L. (2000). Substance abuse and childhood maltreatment. Conceptualizing the recovery process. *Journal of Substance Abuse Treatment 19,* 175-182.

Moustakas, C. (1994). *Phenomenological research methods.* Thousand Oaks, CA: Sage.

Murphy, S. (1993). Coping strategies of abstainers from alcohol up to three years post-treatment. *Image: Journal of Nursing Scholarship, 25,* 29-35.

Ngai-Jacobson, M.G., & Burkhardt, M.A. (1989). Spirituality: cornerstone of holistic nursing practice. *Holistic Nursing Practice, 3*(3), 1-26.

Nelson-Zlupko, L., Dore, M.M., Kauffman, E., & Kaltenbach, K. (1996). Women in recovery: Their perceptions of treatment effectiveness. *Journal of Substance Abuse Treatment, 13*(1), 51-59.

Neuman, B. (1982, 1989). *The Neuman systems model: Application to nursing education and practice*. Norwalk, CT: Appleton-Century-Crofts.

Ornery, A. (1983). Phenomenology: A method for nursing research. *Advances in Nursing Science, 5*(2), 49-63.

Prochaska, J.O., DiClemente, C.C., & Norcross, J.C. (1992). In search of how people change: Application to adductive behaviors. *American Psychologist, 47,* 1102-1114.

Reed, P.G. (1985). Drug misuse and dependency in women: The meaning and implications of being considered a special population or minority group. *International Journal of Addictions, 29,* 13-62.

Reed, P.G. (1992). An emerging paradigm for the investigation of spirituality in nursing. *Research in Nursing & Health, 15,* 349-357.

Roy, C. (1984). *Introduction to nursing: An adaptation model* (2nd ed). Englewood Cliffs, NJ: Prentice-Hall.

Ruether, R.R. (1992). Motherearth, and the mega-machine. In C.P. Christ & J. Plaskow (Eds.), *Womanspring rising: A feminist reader in religion.* San Francisco, CA: Harper & Row.

Scandrett, A. Jr. (1994). Religion as a support component in the health behavior of black Americans. *Journal of Religion and Health, 33,* 123-129.

Sloan, R.P., Bagiella, E., & Powell, T. (1999). Religion, spirituality, and medicine. *The Lancet, 353,* 664-67.

Spiegelberg, H. (1982). *The phenomenological movement: A historical introduction.* The Hague: Nijhoff.

Streubert, H.J., & Carpenter, D.R. (1995). *Qualitative research in nursing. Advancing the humanistic imperative.* Philadelphia, PA: Lippincott Company.

Substance Abuse and Mental Health Services Administration (1996). *Advance report number 15. In mental estimates in 1996 national household survey on drug abuse.* Washington, DC: Office of Applied Studies.

Taylor, J.Y. (2000). Sisters of the yam: African American women's healing and self-recovery from intimate male partner violence. *Issues in Mental Health Nursing, 21,* 515-531.

Thibault, J.M., Ellor, J.W., & Netting, F.E. (1991). A conceptual framework for assessing the spiritual functioning and fulfillment of older adults in long-term settings. *Journal of Religious Gerontology, 7,* 29-45.

Turner, N.H., O'Dell, K.J., Weaver, G.D., Ramirez, G.Y., & Turner, G. (1998). Community's role in the promotion of recovery from addiction and prevention of relapse among women: An exploratory study. *Ethnicity and Disease, 8,* 26-35.

U. S. Department of Health and Human Services, Administration of Children, Youth and Families (1999). *Child maltreatment 1997: Reports from the states to the National Child Abuse and Neglect Data System.* Washington DC: U. S. Government Printing Office.

Villarosa, L. (1994). The healing power of spirituality. In L.V. Villarosa (ed.), *Body & soul: The black woman's guide to physical health and emotional well-being.* New York: HarperPerennial.

Walant, K. (1995). *Creating the capacity for attachment: Treating addiction and the alienated self.* Northvale, NJ: Jason Aronson Inc.

Watson, J. (1988). *Nursing: Human science and human care.* Norwalk, CT: Appleton-Century-Crofts.

Woodhouse, L.D. (1992). Women with jagged edges: Voices from a culture of substance abuse. *Qualitative Health Research, 2*(3), 262-281.

Study 3: Metabolic Syndrome in a Multiethnic Sample of School Children: Implications for the Pediatric Nurse

Ruth C. McGillis Bindler, RNC, PhD, Linda K. Massey, RD, PhD, Jill Armstrong Shultz, PhD, Paulette E. Mills, PhD, and Robert Short, PhD

There is lack of translational work that may assist the pediatric nurse in identifying the child who is at risk for metabolic syndrome. Early identification of the syndrome could assist pediatric health care providers in intervening and in lowering child health risks. Fasting serum insulin, metabolic syndrome criteria, and dietary intake were examined in a multiethnic sample of children aged 9–15 years. Forty-seven percent had two or more risk factors for metabolic syndrome, and 28% had three or more risk factors. Insulin levels were negatively correlated with the recommended dietary allowance. A regression model, including gender, age, race, body mass index, serum glucose, high-density lipoprotein cholesterol, triglycerides, and blood pressure, explained 48% of insulin variance. © 2007 Elsevier Inc. All rights reserved.

METABOLIC SYNDROME, ALSO known as dysmetabolic syndrome, syndrome X, or insulin resistance syndrome, is characterized by a group of risk factors and is often a precursor to both diabetes and cardiovascular disease. These risk factors cluster in individuals and populations, both in adults and in youths. The syndrome is typified by a decrease in the number of insulin receptors and in their functional ability at the cellular level (insulin resistance), with resultant hyperinsulinemia and development of type 2 diabetes as the pancreas attempts to compensate. The United States Cholesterol Education Program Adult Treatment Panel III (ATP III) recommended the diagnosis of metabolic syndrome in adults when three of five symptoms are found: high triglyceride levels, low high-density lipoprotein cholesterol (HDL-C), hypertension, obesity (particularly with central adiposity), and fasting glucose > 6.1 mmol/l (110 mg/dl) (National Institutes of Health, 2001). These criteria reflect the major metabolic components of the syndrome, which are abdominal obesity, atherogenic dyslipidemia, increased blood pressure (BP), insulin resistance, proinflammatory state, and prothrombotic state (Grundy, Brewer, Cleeman, Smith, & Lenfant, 2004). Other groups have recommended somewhat different criteria, leading to confusion among clinicians (see Table 1 for a summary of adult criteria recommendations for metabolic syndrome) (Zimmet, Magliano, Matsuzawa, Alberti, & Shaw, 2005).

REVIEW OF LITERATURE

One in four Americans is at risk for developing metabolic syndrome (Ford, Giles, & Dietz, 2002; Roberts, Dunn, Jean, & Lardinois, 2000). Life-style, environment, and genetic component are influential in the syndrome. Lifestyle factors that contribute to the problem are high-saturated-fat and low-fiber diets, stress, and lack of physical activity (Kelley, 2000; Ludwig et al., 1999; Mayer-Davis et al., 1997). The environment promotes metabolic syndrome when there is limited opportunity for daily physical activity or limited access to fresh and nutritious food choices. Lifestyle and environmental factors are closely related, but both may play independent and interactive parts in the emergence of metabolic syndrome. Genetic factors place certain population groups, such as Native Americans and Hispanic Americans, at higher risk for diabetes and insulin resistance (Cruz et al., 2004; Valdez, 2000).

Due to an epidemic in youth obesity and sedentary behaviors, there is an increasing need to describe the factors associated with the development of insulin resistance in youths. For children, only one risk factor, in addition to being overweight, has been suggested as adequate reason to screen for additional clinical abnormalities (Falkner, Hassink, Ross, & Gidding, 2002). Although there is no clear consensus on the criteria for metabolic syndrome in children, on the number of criteria needed for diagnosis,

From the Intercollegiate College of Nursing, Washington State University, Spokane, WA, Food Science and Human Nutrition Department, Washington State University, Spokane, WA, Food Science and Human Nutrition Department, Washington State University, Pullman, WA, Human Development Department, Washington State University, Pullman, WA, and Biostatistics, The Washington Institute, Washington State University, Spokane, WA.
From Bindler, R.C.M., Massey, L.K., Shultz, J.A., Mills, P.E., Short, R. (2007). Metabolic syndrome in a multiethnic sample of school children: Implications for the pediatric nurse. *Journal of Pediatric Nursing, 22*(1), 43-58.

Table 1 Criteria for Metabolic Syndrome, Used in Adults

WORLD HEALTH ORGANIZATION	ATP III	INTERNATIONAL DIABETES FEDERATION
Diabetes mellitus, impaired glucose tolerance, or inclusion in the top quartile of fasting insulin (if nondiabetic), plus two or more of following:	Three or more of following:	Waist circumference > 102 cm for males or > 88 cm for females (or ethnic-specific values), plus two or more of following:
BMI > 30	Waist circumference > 102 cm for males or > 88 cm for females	Triglycerides > 150 mg/dl (1.7 mmol/l) or treatment for this condition
Triglycerides ≥150 mg/dl (1.7 mmol/l) or HDL-C < 35 mg/dl (0.9 mmol/l)	Triglycerides > 150 mg/dl (1.7 mmol/l)	HDL-C < 40 mg/dl (1.03 mmol/l) for males or < 50 mg/dl (1.29 mmol/l) for females, or treatment for this condition
BP ≥140/90 mm Hg or on medication	HDL-C < 40 mg/dl (1.03 mmol/l) for males or < 50 mg/dl (1.29 mmol/l) for females	BP > 130/85 mm Hg or on medication
Albumin ≥20 μg/min or albumin: creatinine ratio ≥30 mg/g	BP > 130/85 mm Hg or on medication	Fasting plasma glucose ≥ 100 mg/dl (5.6 mmol/l) or diagnosed type 2 diabetes mellitus
	Fasting plasma glucose > 110 mg/dl (6.1 mmol/l)	

Note. Data from Zimmet et al. (2005).

or on the differences in criteria at various ages, some researchers have adapted adult metabolic syndrome criteria to the examination of child data. For example, in one analysis, the criteria used to define adolescent metabolic syndrome included fasting triglycerides ≥ 110 mg/dl; HDL-C ≤ 40 mg/dl; fasting glucose ≥ 110 mg/dl; abdominal measurement ≥ 90th percentile for age and gender; and BP ≥ 90th percentile for age, gender, and height (Cook, Weitzman, Auinger, Nguyen, & Dietz, 2003). Another group of researchers defined adolescent metabolic syndrome when three or more of the following criteria were met: fasting triglycerides ≥ 1.1 mmol/l (100 mg/dl); HDL-C < 1.2 mmol/l (45 mg/dl) for male adolescents 15–19 years old and 1.3 mmol/l (50 mg/dl) for all others; fasting glucose > 6.1 mmol/l (110 mg/dl); waist circumference > 75th percentile for age and gender; and systolic BP > 90th percentile for gender, age, and height (de Ferranti et al., 2004). Others have used similar criteria, with differences, including: triglycerides ≥ 90th percentile for age and gender; HDL-C < 10th percentile for age and gender; and impaired glucose tolerance identified by a glucose level of 140–200 mg/dl following a 2-hour postchallenge glucose test (Cruz et al., 2004; Shaibi et al., 2005). Still another group of researchers has used a body mass index (BMI) z score ≥ 2.0; fasting glucose > 140 mg/dl (7.8 mmol/l); triglycerides > 95th percentile; HDL < 5th percentile; and BP > 95th percentile for age and gender (Weiss et al., 2004). Age ranges vary in the studies; thus, no findings and age-specific criteria have been developed. It has been noted that there is as yet no agreement about

the criteria for the overall assessment and treatment of metabolic syndrome in children and adolescents (Golley, Magarey, Steinbeck, Baur, & Daniels, 2006; Steinberger & Daniels, 2003) (see Table 2 for a summary of metabolic syndrome criteria for childhood, as applied by various researchers).

Although it is unclear exactly which criteria should be used to identify metabolic syndrome in children and adolescents, a rapid rise in the prevalence of obesity, abdominal girth, and type 2 diabetes in youths necessitates attention to the issue. One study applied the same 1999–2000 criteria for metabolic syndrome (those described in Cook et al., 2003) to the National Health and Nutrition Examination Survey (NHANES) data for 1988–1992 and found that the rate of the syndrome, defined by the presence of three criteria, increased from 4.2% to 6.4% in that short span of years (Duncan, Li, & Zhou, 2004). The increase in obesity and type 2 diabetes creates the urgent need for research that will assist in the establishment of universal criteria for metabolic syndrome in children (Molnar, 2004). Pediatric nurses are often unfamiliar with metabolic syndrome and need solid research and evidence-based recommendations to apply what is known about this condition to their work with children in a variety of settings.

Few studies have described metabolic syndrome or the marker of insulin in children, and even fewer have examined childhood ethnic differences in risks. A clustering of syndrome variables in children, including high serum triglycerides, low HDL-C, and high glucose,

Table 2　Criteria for Metabolic Syndrome, Used in Children

CRITERIA	DATA FROM COOK ET AL. (2003)	DATA FROM DE FERRANTI ET AL. (2004)	DATA FROM CRUZ ET AL. (2004)	DATA FROM WEISS ET AL. (2004)	PRESENT STUDY
Triglycerides	≥ 110 mg/dl (1.24 mmol/l)	≥ 100 mg/dl (1.1 mmol/l)	≥ 90th percentile	> 95th percentile	≥ 110 mg/dl (1.24 mmol/l)
HDL-C	≤ 40 mg/dl (1.03 mmol/l)	< 45 mg/dl (1.2 mmol/l) for males 15–19 years and < 50 mg/dl (1.3 mmol/l) for all others	< 10th percentile	< 5th percentile	≤ 40 mg/dl (1.03 mmol/l)
Glucose	≥ 110 mg/dl (6.1 mmol/l) for fasting level	> 110 mg/dl (6.1 mmol/l) for fasting level	140–200 mg/dl (7.8–11.1 mmol/l) following a 2-hour postchallenge glucose test	> 140 mg/dl (7.8 mmol/l) for fasting level	≥ 110 mg/dl (6.1 mmol/l) for fasting level
Adiposity	≥ 90th percentile for abdominal measurement	> 75th percentile for abdominal measurement	≥ 90th percentile for abdominal measurement	BMI z-score ≥ 2.0	≥ 85th percentile for BMI
BP	≥ 90th percentile	≥ 90th percentile	≥ 90th percentile	≥ 95th percentile	≥ 90th percentile

adiposity, and high BP, was found to explain 55% of serum insulin variance (Srinivasan, Myers, & Berenson, 1999). Impaired fasting glucose and type 2 diabetes have been identified in children using data from national health surveys (Fagot-Campagna, Saaddine, Flegal, & Beckles, 2001). Insulin was an independent predictor of triglycerides in obese children (Valle et al., 2002).

Most research studies on ethnic variations and metabolic syndrome have included only Black and White children. The Bogalusa Heart Study has studied Black and White children, noting the persistence of elevated insulin levels from childhood into adulthood in all children (Bao, Srinivasan, & Berenson, 1996; Chen et al., 2000), higher triglyceride and insulin levels in Black children than in White children (Chen, Srinivasan, Elkasabany, & Berenson, 1999), and higher dyslipidemia and higher insulin secretion in White obese adolescents than in Black obese adolescents, with low insulin sensitivity in both groups (Bacha, Saad, Gungor, Janosky, & Arslanian, 2003). In other studies, Black children showed greater insulin resistance than White children, even after adjustment for body composition, social class, and dietary intake patterns (Lindquist, Gower, & Goran, 2000). Furthermore, obesity, greater visceral fat, and Black ethnicity were identified as negative and independent health risks (Gower, Nagy, & Goran, 1999). The incidence of hyperinsulinemia in a sample of overweight Black and White 11- to 18-year-olds was 30%; hyperinsulinemic children had significantly higher BMI, total cholesterol (TC), low-density

lipoprotein (LDL), triglycerides, glucose, and insulin: glucose ratio (Sullivan et al., 2004).

Native American/Alaskan Native/First Nation and Hispanic children are at-risk ethnic groups needing further delineation of factors related to metabolic syndrome. Although there are a limited number of studies focusing on ethnic minority groups, the data available demonstrate an increased incidence of risk factors in these groups. In Canadian First Nation children, fasting insulin and glucose levels were associated with BMI percentile (Young, Dean, Flett, & Wood-Steinman, 2000). An analysis of studies on type 2 diabetes in children reported that disease incidence among North American Indians varied from 2.3/1,000 for Canadian Cree and Ojibway to 4.5/1,000 for all U.S. American Indians, to 50.9/1,000 for Pima Indians in the southwest United States (Fagot-Campagna et al., 2000). In one analysis of health records in Montana and Wyoming Indian Health Service facilities, > 50% of cases of diabetes in youths were type 2 (Harwell et al., 2001).

Hispanic children have a higher incidence of overweight and hypertension than White, Black, and Asian children (Sorof, Lai, Turner, Poffenbarger, & Portman, 2004). In addition, the prevalence of impaired glucose tolerance (a precursor to metabolic syndrome and type 2 diabetes) was 17.8% among Hispanic adolescents, as compared with 7% in all ethnic groups (Williams et al., 2002). Although Hispanics in the United States come from many different countries and may have different risk factors, a major group originated from Mexico, and

297

several studies have been carried out with Hispanics of Mexican origin. Mexican American children have a high rate of obesity (27% for female children and 23% for male children) (Suminski, Poston, & Foreyt, 1999), and 45% of new cases of diabetes in Mexican American youths are type 2 (Neufeld, Raffel, Landon, Dhen, & Vadheim, 1998). Analysis of NHANES data for 1999–2000 demonstrates the increasing problem of overweight in Mexican American children because 22.7% of 2- to 5-year-olds, 39.3% of 6- to 11-year-olds, and 43.8% of 12- to 19-year-olds were overweight or were at risk for overweight (Ogden, Flegal, Carroll, & Johnson, 2002). Mexican American adults 20 years and older demonstrate a higher incidence of metabolic syndrome (31.9%) than Whites (23.8%) (Ford et al., 2002).

Many of the criteria for metabolic syndrome are related to dietary intake, and ethnicity may play a part in food choices. High levels of dietary fat intake have been identified in Black youth as compared with other ethnic groups (Lindquist et al., 2000; Weigensberg et al., 2005). However, in a study comparing the dietary intake of White and Native American children in Oklahoma, a high rate of low-nutrient-dense and high-fat foods was ingested by both groups with no significant differences by ethnicity (Stroehla, Malcoe, & Velie, 2005). A study of Hispanic and non-Hispanic toddlers found that intakes at meals and snacks were not significantly different between the two groups (Ziegler, Hanson, Ponza, Novak, & Hendricks, 2006).

Children, in general, and those from Native American and Hispanic groups, in particular, are underrepresented in diabetes and cardiovascular disease origins research. There is scant application of identification methods for metabolic syndrome in the nursing literature. More information is needed to establish the contribution of various characteristics to insulin resistance in children, and translational research is needed so that findings can be applied by nurses and other health professionals in pediatric settings. Descriptive data about children, particularly from disparate ethnic groups, will help to identify children at highest risk so that appropriate interventions can be identified. Clear guidelines for nurses will assist in applying findings about metabolic syndrome to pediatric settings with youths.

PURPOSE

The purpose of this study was to describe serum insulin levels and to investigate their relationships to metabolic syndrome criteria in a multiethnic sample of school children. Furthermore, analysis of results of dietary recall with the criteria for metabolic syndrome was performed to draw conclusions about the usefulness of dietary intake history. Descriptive data, including demographics, physical measurements, dietary intakes, and physical activity characteristics, were analyzed for within-group differences. Specific assessments and referral criteria for nursing practice were developed using the results. The specific research questions were as follows:

1. What are the fasting serum insulin levels in a multiethnic sample of school children in central Washington State?
2. What are the relationships between insulin levels and the criteria for metabolic syndrome in a multiethnic sample of children in central Washington State? See operational definition of metabolic syndrome criteria below.
3. What are the relationships between reported dietary intake and metabolic syndrome criteria?
4. Which data predict insulin levels in this multiethnic sample of children?
5. How can the information learned in this study be used by pediatric nurses in clinical settings?

Operational Definitions

1. In this study, the criteria for metabolic syndrome were selected from those most often used in other studies. These include the following:
   a. High triglycerides, ≥ 1.24 mmol/l (110 mg/dl)
   b. Low HDL-C, ≤ 1.03 mmol/l (40 mg/dl)
   c. Hypertension, $\geq$ 90th percentile considering age, gender, and height percentile
   d. Overweight, $\geq$ 85th percentile BMI considering age, gender, height, and weight
   e. Elevated fasting glucose, ≥ 6.1 mmol/l (110 mg/dl)
   f. Elevated fasting insulin, $\geq 15 \mu$U/ml
2. Borderline high fasting insulin, $\geq 15–20$ AU/ml; high fasting insulin, $> 20 \mu$U/ml.

METHODS

Sample

The convenience sample consisted of 100 children (representing approximately 15% of eligible students) attending fourth to eighth grades at public elementary and middle schools in a predominantly agricultural area of central Washington State. Parents received a flyer about the study (written in English and Spanish languages), which was sent home from school through the children. They could elect to attend an informational program (conducted in both English and Spanish languages) in school one evening. If they signed a consent, their children were informed about the study and could choose whether to sign an assent and participate. Only children with no identified illnesses or medications were included because blood draws and exercise tests were to be performed. Participants who spoke English or Spanish were eligible. Children could select a small gift from a basket at the end of data collection. The protocol was approved by the Institutional Review Boards of Spokane, Washington, and Washington State University, and the school board of the district where the study was conducted.

Procedures and Instruments

Study personnel consisted of a registered nurse/nutrition doctoral student, eight baccalaureate nursing students, a phlebotomist, one dietitian, and one dietetics student. All were trained and evaluated for reliability on measurement and for assistance to children during questionnaire completion. All measurements and questionnaires involving the children were implemented within a single day in the children's schools. Data were collected in large rooms at the schools and separated into stations for testing. The phlebotomist completed serum venous blood draws on the children. The children's body measurements, BP, and exercise tests were completed by the nurse and nursing students. All diet recalls and questionnaires were completed with the children by the dietitian and by the dietetics student.

Parents of children in the study completed a medical family history form (accomplished during the informational evening session, or accomplished and sent later) developed by the Make Early Diagnoses–Prevent Early Deaths Program at the University of Utah. This questionnaire asked about early cardiovascular disease, diabetes, overweight, and hypertension among parents, siblings, grandparents, aunts, and uncles of the children. Parents were also asked to identify to which ethnic groups their children belonged. All forms were available in English and Spanish languages.

Blood draws were completed in the early morning by the licensed phlebotomist after the children had fasted for at least 10 hours; children were then fed breakfast before completing the remainder of the testing. Fasting blood samples were tested for glucose, TC, HDL-C, and triglycerides using the Beckman CX 5Delta analyzer, and low-density lipoprotein cholesterol (LDL-C) was calculated by applying the Friedewald equation [(TC − HDL-C) − triglycerides / 5]. Insulin was measured by solid-phase radioimmunoassay with the Coat-A-Count Insulin System (Diagnostic Products, Los Angeles, CA).

The smoking history of the children was collected on a questionnaire that asked if they were current smokers or if they had ever tried smoking. BP was measured on the right arm at heart level while the children were sitting; three readings were made with a 5-minute rest in between, and the mean of the three readings was used in the analysis. Percentile analysis was performed using grids from the National Heart, Lung, and Blood Institute (2004) that take into account height percentile, age, and gender. Metabolic-cost-of-activity (MET) scores were calculated from the children's reported history of weekly physical activity on the Godin Leisure Time Questionnaire (Godin & Shephard, 1985; Kriska & Casperson, 1997). Physical measurements of height, weight, triceps skinfold thickness, and the Canadian Aerobic Fitness Test (to calculate VO_{2max}) were obtained in uniform and recommended ways. BMI was calculated as weight: height ratio (kg/m^2); percentiles for height, weight, triceps skinfold, and BMI were obtained from the National Center for Health Statistics growth grids (Centers for Disease Control and Prevention, 2000). Because no measure of central adiposity was completed, BMI $\geq$ 85th percentile was used as the obesity criterion for metabolic syndrome in this sample.

Dietary data were collected by the use of the Youth/Adolescent Question (YAQ) (Rockett et al., 1997; Rockett & Colditz, 1997). This 151-item food frequency questionnaire has been used with children from 8 to 18 years and correlates well (0.54) with 24-hour diet recall results. It uses the Statistical Analysis System and calculates means and standard deviations for energy and all nutrients. It collects data about the intake of food items for days, weeks, and months. The trained nursing students and the dietitian assisted subjects, as needed, with the questionnaire and had a list of foods common to Hispanic and Native American communities to add, as necessary, to individual child forms. Completed questionnaires were returned to YAQ developers at the Harvard School of Public Health for the calculation of the dietary intake of nutrients from the questionnaire and for the calculation of the percentage of recommended dietary allowance (RDA) for each nutrient.

In addition, a 24-hour diet recall was completed verbally with each child by a trained dietitian. These results were used to calculate Healthy Eating Index (HEI) scores. The HEI was designed by the United States Department of Agriculture to measure how the diets of Americans conform to dietary guidelines. It provides a score from 0 = *low* to 10 = *high* for 10 components of the diet. Each of the scores is then added for a composite score, with a total possible score of 100. The 10 HEI scores are for grains, vegetables, fruit, milk, meat, total fat, saturated fat, cholesterol, sodium, and variety (Bowman, Lino, Gerrior, & Basiotis, 1998; Kennedy, Ohls, Carlson, & Fleming, 1995; Variyam, Smallwood, & Basiotis, 1998).

Statistical Analysis

Statistical analyses were carried out using the Statistical Package for the Social Sciences (SPSS), version 12.0. Each variable was examined for skewness, and the mean and standard deviation were described. Chi-square test was used to test categorical data, and one-way analysis of variance was used to test continuous variables. The probability levels of .05 and .01 were considered significant and highly significant, respectively. Kendall's τ was used to assess correlations between variables. Stepwise linear regression was used to explore the variables that were influential in explaining insulin variance. An odds ratio for meeting at least three risk criteria on the dichotomized insulin variable was computed using binary logistic regression.

RESULTS

Description of the Sample

The age range of the sample was 9–15 years (M = 12 years). The sample included 52 boys and 48 girls. Sixty-four (64%) claimed to be purely Hispanic, 15 (15%) claimed to be purely Native American, and 9 (9%) claimed to be purely Caucasian. Twelve (12%) additional subjects claimed to have mixed-race ethnic heritage. All Hispanic children had Mexico as origin of the family and were employed in farming or food processing industries. There were no significant

299

differences among ethnic groups regarding age or gender; reported family history of cardiovascular disease, diabetes, overweight, or smoking; physical activity; weight percentiles; BMI percentiles; or triceps skinfold percentiles. Table 3 shows the demographic data and physical measurements of the total sample and of the ethnic subsample (those children identifying with just one major ethnic group). Blood samples were not obtained on two children; thus, serum analysis was completed on 98 children. The 98 children who had blood drawn are included in this analysis (referred to as the total sample); when race differences are examined, calculations are reported on the 86 children who listed just one ethnic group in their demographic profile and had a successful serum blood draw (referred to as ethnic subsample). Further characteristics of the study participants have been previously described (Bindler, Massey, Shultz, Mills, & Short, 2004).

There was a highly significant difference among ethnic groups regarding child smoking history, with a higher frequency of "having tried smoking" reported by Native American children. Significant differences in mean systolic BP and mean diastolic BP were found, with Caucasians having the highest pressures (116/75 mm Hg), followed by Native Americans (113/73 mm Hg), and with Hispanics having the lowest BPs (108/67 mm Hg). Although there were no group differences for weight and BMI percentiles, there was a significant difference among the groups in mean height percentile, with the Caucasians being taller ($M = 81$st percentile) than either the Native American group ($M = 55$th percentile) or the Hispanic group ($M = 54$th percentile). Dietary analysis showed no significant differences among ethnic groups in terms of carbohydrate, protein, fat, calorie, sucrose, or fiber intakes. Likewise, there were no differences among groups in the percentage of calories from fat and the kilocalories of intake per kilogram of weight (Table 4).

The mean fasting glucose was 4.75 mmol/l (85.8 mg/dl), and all but four children had a value below 5.5 mmol/l (100 mg/dl), with no significant differences among ethnic groups. Those with serum glucose above 5.5 mmol/l had values ranging from 5.66 to 6.00 mmol/l. No children had glucose above 6.1 mmol/l (110 mg/dl).

Research Question 1: What Are the Fasting Serum Insulin Levels in a Multiethnic Sample of School Children in Central Washington State?

The mean insulin value was 10.2 µU/ml, with significant differences found among ethnic groups (Native Americans > Caucasians > Hispanics). Eighty percent ($n = 78$) had normal insulin levels (< 15 µU/l), whereas 7% ($n = 7$) had borderline high levels (15–20 µU/l) and 13% ($n = 13$) had high levels (> 20 µU/l).

Research Question 2: What Are the Relationships Between Insulin Levels and the Criteria for Metabolic Syndrome in a Multiethnic Sample of Children in Central Washington State?

Fifty-one children (51%) had BMI ≥ 85th percentile; 20 (20%) had triglycerides above 1.24 mmol/l (110 mg/dl);

24 (24%) had HDL-C ≤ 1.03 mmol/l (40 mg/dl); 14 (14%) had systolic BP ≥ 90th percentile; 24 (24%) had diastolic BP ≥ 90th percentile; and 31 (31%) had either systolic BP or diastolic BP ≥ 90th percentile for height, age, and gender.

Only two children in this convenience sample had no risk factors for metabolic syndrome. Forty-seven (47%) had two factors, 28 (28%) had three factors, and 4 (4%) had four metabolic syndrome factors. The most common risk factor displayed was increased BMI percentile, with high BP being the next most common factor shown (Table 5).

Significant positive relationships were found between insulin and increasing age ($F = 6.164$, $p = .015$, $df = 1,79$), between insulin and female gender ($F = 3.972$, $p = .050$, $df = 1,79$), and between insulin and Native American race ($F = 3.372$, $p = .039$, $df = 2,79$). Female Native American children had the highest mean insulin levels (17.9 µU/ml), where as Hispanic male children had the lowest mean values (6.6 µU/ml) (Figure 1). Although 6 of 9 (67%) Caucasian children and 54 of 63 (86%) Hispanic children had normal insulin levels, only 8 of 14 (57%) Native American children had normal insulin values. All of the Native American children with elevated insulin levels were in the highest category (> 20 µU/l).

Insulin showed highly significant positive correlations with systolic and diastolic BP; weight, BMI, and skinfold percentiles; serum triglycerides and glucose; and triglyceride:HDL and TC:HDL ratios. Furthermore, insulin showed significant height percentile, and serum TC and LDL-C. It had highly significant negative correlations with total dietary fat and kilocalories per kilogram of weight. It had significant negative correlations with dietary carbohydrate, protein, total calories, percentage of calories from fat, and serum HDL-C (Table 6). Insulin resistance index (IRI) was calculated using the model fasting insulin (µU/ml) × fasting glucose (mmol/l) / 22.5. Because the relational statistics for IRI as the outcome variable were nearly the same as those using insulin as the outcome variable, only the findings using insulin are reported.

Research Question 3: What Are the Relationships Between Reported Dietary Intake and Metabolic Syndrome Criteria?

The results of both the HEI obtained by an analysis of 24-hour diet recalls and the dietary nutrient intakes obtained by a food frequency questionnaire were examined by correlations with the risk factors for metabolic syndrome (Table 7). There were two major findings from this analysis.

First, there were many significant negative relationships between serum insulin and the percentage of RDA for nutrients, suggesting that when dietary recalls identify several nutrients not ingested at the recommended level, children may be at risk for insulin resistance and metabolic syndrome.

Second, a lower fat intake of the recommended types of fats, such as monounsaturated, polyunsaturated, and omega 3 fatty acids, is related to a higher incidence of metabolic risk. The reason for several negative correlations between the reported intake of calories per kilogram

300

Table 3 Demographics and Physical Measures, by Ethnic Group

VARIABLES	TOTAL SAMPLE (N = 100)	ETHNIC SUBSAMPLE (N = 88)	NATIVE AMERICAN (N = 15)	HISPANIC (N = 64)	CAUCASIAN (N = 9)	ρ
Gender						
Male	52 (52%)	43 (49%)	7 (47%)	30 (47%)	6 (67%)	.529
Female	48 (48%)	45 (51%)	8 (53%)	34 (53%)	3 (33%)	
Age (years)	11.8 ± 1.6	11.9 ± 1.5	12.4 ± 1.6	11.8 ± 1.5	11.3 ± 1.5	.183
Range	9–15	9–15	9–14	9–15	9–13	
Family history						
Cardiovascular disease	52 (52%)	42 (48%)	5 (33%)	31 (48%)	6 (67%)	.279
Diabetes	28 (28%)	24 (27%)	4 (27%)	19 (30%)	1 (11%)	.503
Over-weight	53 (53%)	43 (49%)	6 (40%)	32 (50%)	5 (56%)	.717
Smoking	74 (74%)	63 (72%)	11 (73%)	43 (67%)	9 (100%)	.122
Physical activity						
VO_{2max} (<Avg / Avg / >Avg)	35 (35%) / 32 (32%) / 33 (33%)	30 (34%) / 29 (33%) / 29 (33%)	6 (40%) / 3 (20%) / 6 (40%)	20 (31%) / 22 (34%) / 22 (34%)	4 (44%) / 4 (44%) / 1 (11%)	.506
MET score	57 ± 25.0	56.0 ± 25.0	52.2 ± 24.3	54.3 ± 23.8	73.8 ± 30.4	.074
Smoking history (+)	20 (20%)	17 (19.3%)	8 (53%)	8 (13%)	1 (11%)	.001**
$\bar{x}$ Systolic BP (mm Hg)	109.2 ± 9.8	109.4 ± 10.0	112.6 ± 10.2	107.7 ± 9.6	116.4 ± 8.8	.017*
$\bar{x}$ Diastolic BP (mm Hg)	68.7 ± 11.6	68.8 ± 12.2	73.1 ± 9.3	66.8 ± 12.6	75.4 ± 9.7	.040*
$\bar{x}$ Height percentile	58.4 ± 29.5	57 ± 30	55 ± 29	54 ± 30	81 ± 15	.035**
$\bar{x}$ Weight percentile	71.1 ± 29.2	70 ± 30	82 ± 25	65 ± 31	81 ± 26	.074
$\bar{x}$ BMI percentile	75.6 ± 25.2	74 ± 26	84 ± 27	72 ± 26	75 ± 27	.283
$\bar{x}$ Skinfold percentile	66.0 ± 28.7	65 ± 30	78 ± 28	62 ± 29	62 ± 38	.169

Notes. Statistics are frequencies (%) and means ± standard deviations. ρ is from one-way analysis of variance. Avg = average.
*Significant at the .05 level (two-tailed test).
**Significant at the .01 level (two-tailed test).

Table 4   Mean Serum Measures and Dietary Intake, by Ethnic Group

VARIABLES	TOTAL SAMPLE	ETHNIC SUBSAMPLE	SUBGROUPS			ρ
			NATIVE AMERICAN	HISPANIC	CAUCASIAN	
Serum	$N = 98$	$n = 86$	$n = 15$	$n = 62$	$n = 9$	
TC (mmol/l)	4.30 ± 0.64	4.28 ± 0.66	4.25 ± 0.60	4.31 ± 0.68	4.09 ± 0.65	.626
LDL-C (mmol/l)	2.60 ± 0.58	2.60 ± 0.60	2.43 ± 0.61	2.64 ± 0.57	2.52 ± 0.67	.462
HDL-C (mmol/l)	1.27 ± 0.26	1.25 ± 0.27	1.33 ± 0.29	1.25 ± 0.26	1.17 ± 0.31	.391
Triglycerides (mmol/l)	0.93 ± 0.56	0.94 ± 0.57	1.07 ± 0.60	0.92 ± 0.59	0.85 ± 0.40	.617
Glucose (mmol/l)	4.75 ± 0.44	4.76 ± 0.45	4.87 ± 0.55	4.73 ± 0.45	4.82 ± 0.21	.530
Insulin (µU/ml)	10.2 ± 7.2	10.3 ± 7.28	14.3 ± 9.9	9.2 ± 5.7	12.0 ± 10.4	.043*
Dietary	$N = 100$	$N = 88$	$N = 15$	$N = 64$	$N = 9$	
Carbohydrate (g)	313.9 ± 236.4	308.0 ± 235.6	235.4 ± 359.1	335.2 ± 208.8	234.7 ± 112.6	.208
Protein (g)	80.1 ± 56.5	78.2 ± 53.9	78.3 ± 86.9	79.1 ± 47.1	71.0 ± 28.3	.916
Total fat (g)	79.3 ± 56.0	78.3 ± 55.6	75.2 ± 83.5	79.6 ± 50.9	73.5 ± 30.5	.929
Saturated fat (g)	28.4 ± 19.0	28.1 ± 18.8	26.4 ± 25.7	28.4 ± 17.9	28.6 ± 12.3	.929
Polyunsaturated fat (g)	14.4 ± 11.3	14.3 ± 11.4	13.6 ± 17.4	14.7 ± 10.3	12.6 ± 6.4	.846
Calories from fat (%)	31.1 ± 5.4	31 ± 6.0	31 ± 6.2	31 ± 5.0	37 ± 6.1	.876
Calories (kcal)	$2,306 \pm 1,565$	$2,218 \pm 2,350$	$2,218 \pm 2,351$	$2,343 \pm 1,398$	$1,859 \pm 786$	.141
Calories/weight (kcal/kg)	50.1 ± 38.7	41.5 ± 46.7	41.5 ± 46.7	52.8 ± 38.8	38.1 ± 18.1	.111
Sucrose (g)	67.5 ± 47.6	68.0 ± 48.2	63.7 ± 65.6	72.3 ± 45.9	44.6 ± 21.0	.257
Fiber (g)	19.1 ± 14.1	18.5 ± 13.5	18.2 ± 19.0	19.5 ± 12.4	12.4 ± 9.2	.342

*Significant at the .05 level (two-tailed test).

Table 5   Incidence of Risk Factors for Metabolic Syndrome

RISK FACTORS	NATIVE AMERICAN	HISPANIC	CAUCASIAN	MIXED RACE
BP > 90th percentile	5 (33%) ($n = 15$)	21 (33%) ($n = 64$)	4 (44%) ($n = 9$)	1 (8%) ($n = 12$)
BMI > 85th percentile	10 (67%) ($n = 15$)	29 (45%) ($n = 64$)	5 (56%) ($n = 9$)	7 (58%) ($n = 12$)
Triglycerides ≥ 110 mg/dl	3 (20%) ($n = 14$)	13 (20%) ($n = 63$)	2 (22%) ($n = 9$)	2 (17%) ($n = 12$)
HDL < 40 mg/dl	1 (7%) ($n = 14$)	15 (24%) ($n = 63$)	3 (33%) ($n = 9$)	1 (8%) ($n = 12$)
Glucose > 100 mg/dl	0	0	0	

Note. Variation in n among variables reflects two children from whom blood could not be obtained.

and the incidence of metabolic syndrome criteria is unclear and may relate to the lack of reliability of dietary recall, especially among child reporters.

Research Question 4: Which Data Predict Insulin Levels in This Multiethnic Sample of Children?

A regression model that included gender, age, race, BMI percentile, serum glucose, HDL-C, triglycerides, systolic BP, and diastolic BP was tested and found to explain 48% of the variance in insulin. Triglycerides, systolic BP, and race were removed in a backward stepwise procedure, with the resulting model explaining 50% of insulin variance (Table 8). Using binary logistic stepwise regression, the odds ratio for having elevated insulin was 5.8 (95% confidence interval = 1.5–22.1) when three or more risk factors were present.

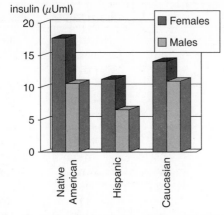

Glucose mean = 85.8 mg/dl
Insulin mean = 10.3 μU/ml (range 2–32)

insulin (μUml)

Figure 1. Serum insulin levels, by ethnic group and gender.

Table 6   Correlates of Insulin

VARIABLES	KENDALL'S τ	ρ
Age	.265**	.001
Sex	−.306**	.001
Family history		
Cardiovascular disease	.129	.149
Diabetes	.128	.153
Overweight	−.045	.613
VO$_{2max}$	−.016	.852
MET score	−.027	.720
Smoking history	.206*	.021
Systolic BP	.345**	< .001
Diastolic BP	.311**	< .001
Height percentile	.198*	.012
Weight percentile	.396**	< .001
BMI percentile	.399**	< .001
Skinfold percentile	.392**	< .001
Serum		
TC	.157*	.034
LDL-C	.163*	.028
HDL-C	−.216**	.004
Triglycerides	.303**	.001
Glucose	.246**	.007

*Correlation is significant at the .05 level.
**Correlation is significant at the .01 level.

DISCUSSION

In this study, the most commonly used criteria were adapted from adults and from various recommendations for the application of criteria to child populations. Insulin levels in this study showed large variability, and 20% of children had borderline or high insulin levels. Consistent with other studies, insulin levels showed a positive correlation with criteria for metabolic syndrome, including high BP, high adiposity (measured in this study by BMI percentiles), high serum triglycerides and glucose, and low serum HDL-C. The odds ratio of having elevated insulin when three risk criteria were present was nearly six times that seen in children without this combination of risk factors.

Total carbohydrate, protein, and fat intake showed negative associations with insulin, as did kilocalories consumed per kilogram. The latter factor was not correlated with MET scores or VO$_{2max}$—the two measures of physical activity used. These findings were unexpected. Intake and insulin levels, particularly at kilocalories per kilogram, would be expected to show positive correlations. Perhaps the diet recalls did not accurately reflect dietary intake for the children—a common problem with this method of nutritional analysis. Negative correlations between RDAs for many nutrients and serum insulin levels suggested that diet histories can be used to identify children with aberrant insulin levels. Interventions to target RDAs are appropriate to improve the general dietary and metabolic profile.

Although fiber intake was not a significant correlate with insulin, its levels and trends were in the direction expected. Children at the ages used in the study should have a daily dietary fiber intake of 26 g (female children) to 38 g (male children) (Food and Nutrition Board, 2002); the mean for this sample was 19.1 g. A pattern of low fiber, high fat, and total energy intake in insulin resistance, along with characteristic lipid profiles, has been identified by researchers working with young adults (Ludwig et al., 1999; Van Horn, 1997).

Although the criteria for metabolic syndrome were demonstrated across ethnic groups in this study, the risk of the syndrome appeared to be highest in the Native American female children in the sample. It was notable that the Native American children had the highest BMI percentiles—a measure of adiposity. Regression analysis found that race was not a significant factor in insulin variance, but that BMI percentile was highly significant. In addition, mean skinfold percentile, another measure of adiposity, was high among the Native American group. This is consistent with the Bogalusa Heart Study findings that obesity was linked to the development of hyperinsulinemia (Srinivasan et al., 1999) and with studies linking childhood obesity to insulin resistance syndrome (Weiss et al., 2004). Perhaps high weight and BMI percentiles in Native Americans in this study, in comparison with their more average height percentiles, place them at greater risk for insulin resistance. However, the food frequency questionnaire did not identify a total caloric intake greater than those in the other ethnic groups studied.

Another factor of potential importance is that about half of the Native American children had tried smoking. Although not directly associated with insulin resistance,

VAR	SYSTOLIC BP > 90th PERCENTILE	DIASTOLIC BP > 90th PERCENTILE	BMI (%))	GLUCOSE	HDL	TRIGLYCERIDES	INSULIN
HEI	−.084	−.071	−.116	−.012	.022	.043	.021
HEI	−.083	.007	−.070	.052	−.014	.040	.037
HEI I	−.090	.071	−.075	−.009	−.036	.073	.072
HEI N	.070	−.078	−.057	−.021	−.103	−.025	−.098
HEI M	.066	.007	−.017	.047	−.024	−.004	.050
HEI Fa	−.089	.112	−.002	−.163*	−.069	.168*	−.051
HEI Sa	−.063	.059	.049	−.062	.015	.200**	.019
HEI Ch	.035	.201*	.017	−.012	.012	.182*	−.048
HEI Sod	−.023	−.012	0.61	−.074	−.005	−.057	−.082
HEI Var	−.148	−.034	−.067	−.037	.099	−.100	−.065
HEI Total	−.065	.088	−.026	−.064	−.055	.164*	−.019
Calories	−.169*	−.192*	−.153*	−.060	.105	−.130	−.209**
Protein	−.152	−.172	−.139	−.045	.139*	−.161*	−.226**
Carbs	−.166*	−.226	−.149*	−.071	.084	−.088	−.197**
Cal/kg	−.256**	−.263**	−.351**	−.103	.197**	−.203**	−.360**
Fat	−.165*	−.173*	−.187**	−.018	.156*	−.200**	−.253**
SatFat	−.131	−.154	−.182*	.009	.126	−.194**	−.223**
MonoFat	−.172*	−.176*	−.183*	−.025	.169*	−.218**	−.258**
PolyFat	−.165*	−.170*	−.158*	−.018	.155*	−.188**	−.270**
Omega 3	−.172*	−.203*	−.149*	−.005	.266**	−.153*	−.215*
Chol	−.179*	−.188*	−.156*	−.008	.133	−.185**	−.236**
Fiber	−.129	−.132	−.072	−.026	.087	−.064	−.026
Ca (% RDA)	−.057	−.104	−.059	.017	.070	−.081	−.146*
Fe (% RDA)	−.129	−.132	−.072	−.064	.108	−.088	−.233**
Vitamin C (% RDA)	−.072	−.133	−.060	−.014	.064	−.039	−.129
Vitamin B1 (% RDA)	−.106	−.109	−.087	−.038	.072	−.076	−.186**
Vitamin B2 (% RDA)	−.103	−.126	−.071	−.030	.094	−.086	−.165*
Niacin (% RDA)	−.147	−.093	−.103	−.079	.101	−.108	−.209**
Vitamin B6 (% RDA)	−.117	−.121	−.050	−.040	.070	−.081	−.187**
Folate (% RDA)	.106	−.091	−.053	−.029	.028	−.048	−.143*
Vitamin B12 (% RDA)	106	−.101	−.033	.084	.147*	−.109	−.145*
Vitamin A (% RDA)	)41	−.109	.066	.015	.006	.037	−.071
Vitamin D (% RDA)	)14	−.115	−.043	.050	.091	−.069	−.160*
Vitamin E (% RDA)	)5	−.049	−.049	.044	.047	−.042	−.152*

**Correlation is significant a   )5 level.
*Correlation is significant at   1 level.

Table 8 Linear Regression of Insulin With Metabolic Syndrome Variables

VARIABLES	β COEFFICIENT	t	ρ
Regression I			
Gender	−3.535	−3.010	.004
Age	.983	2.434	.017
Race	−.586	−.494	.622
BMI percentile	9.409E−02	3.368	.001
Glucose	.275	3.480	.001
Triglycerides	5.566E−03	.409	.684
HDL-C	−.137	−2.136	.036
Systolic BP	−4.493E−02	−4.68	.641
Diastolic BP	.109	1.543	.127
Adjusted R^2 = .484, $\rho \leq$ .001			
Regression II			
Gender	−3.702	−3.270	.002
Age	1.039	2.699	.009
BMI percentile	9.415E−02	3.810	.000
Glucose	.258	3.570	.001
HDL-C	−.137	−2.382	.020
Diastolic BP	8.808E−02	1.596	.115
Adjusted R^2 = .499, $\rho \leq$ .001			

if this behavior persists into adulthood, it is clearly an additional risk in both diabetes and cardiovascular disease. One study has found a positive association of metabolic syndrome criteria with tobacco exposure and serum cotinine levels in adolescents (Weitzman et al., 2006).

It would have been expected that the Hispanic sample subjects would have a high incidence of elevated insulin and would display a high risk perhaps because the study was performed in a farming area where many from among the Hispanic population were migrant workers who had not lived in the United States for long. In addition, the town was small and had only one fastfood restaurant. Eating out was not a common occurrence for most migrant families. This demonstrated that ethnic variations found in other studies should be explored within specific communities. Assumptions should not be made about a particular sample or population based on national findings or on the results of other studies in diverse geographic areas. Such considerations are important in light of findings that racial and ethnic minorities tend to receive a lower quality of health care than nonminorities and that differences in certain disease risk may be present (National Academy of Sciences, 2002).

The present study had several limitations. The sample was a small convenience sample and may not be representative of all populations of Native Americans, Hispanic Americans, and Caucasians. In particular, the Native American and Caucasian samples were small. The children were in an agricultural area of central Washington State and may not reflect urban or other diverse populations. Native American tribes and Hispanics from various geographic locations are not uniform in the incidence of

type 2 diabetes and in risk factors; thus, the results cannot be generalized to different tribes or various populations of Hispanics. In spite of being a conv_____ce sample, finding no significant differences among _____ members in the intake of essential nutrients supp_____ representativeness of the sample. Future studies _____d to enhanced knowledge by adding measures of _____ adiposity and puberty staging to collection proced_____

CLINICAL IMPLICATIONS

A major problem in the application of _____ on metabolic syndrome by nurses in various s_____s the lack of a clear definition of criteria that sign_____ yndrome. A variety of cutoff points for criteria, s_____ erum triglycerides, HDL-C, and glucose, has bee_____ both in adults (Table 1) and in children (Table 2). _____ onsidering children, the use of different definitions _____ etabolic syndrome leads to confusion. For example, _____ dy that contrasted the prevalence of metabolic syndr_____ 1,513 Black, White, and Hispanic adolescents using _____ Health Organization versus U.S. National Cholestero_____ cation Program ATP III definitions, the incidence wa_____ versus 4.2%, respectively, when using the differe_____ iteria (Goodman, Daniels, Morrison, Huang, & Dolan_____). In a study of 99 children, the percentage of children _____ sed with metabolic syndrome varied from 0–4% to _____0%, depending on which set of six criteria was used (_____ y et al., 2006). Nurses in schools, offices, and other set_____ are justifiably confused about which children should b_____ tified as at-risk and in need of further referral.

Research Question 5: How Can the Informat____ Learned in This Study Be Used by Pediatric Nurses in Clinical Settings?

Although specific guidelines to identify insulin resis____e in children are not available, some information is clea____ application to clinical settings is possible. The clust____ of variables seen in many children makes identificatio____ metabolic syndrome easier in clinical situations. Se____ criteria of the syndrome are routinely measured in c____ health care visits. This study demonstrated that evalua____ of common data such as BMI and BP provides crit____ information, and it therefore supports the recommen____ tions of other pediatric nurses (Hardy, Harrell, & B____ 2004; Yensel, Preud'Homme, & Curry, 2004). Heig____ weight, BMI, and BP are commonly assessed, but caref____ analysis of results is not always performed. BMI and B____ must be measured on each child, and percentiles must ____ determined. This practice can be integrated into all chil____ health care settings, such as clinics, schools, well-chil____ visits, episodic illness care, and hospitalization.

Information gained from BMI and BP can be expanded____ on in at-risk children by referring them for the measurement of serum lipids, glucose, and insulin. Triglycerides, HDL-C, and glucose results should be examined where they have been obtained, such as in office or clinic settings. When this total profile is available, an abnormality in three of five assessment criteria (BMI, BP, triglycerides, HDL-C, and glucose) necessitates referral for further data gathering and intervention. In addition, the nurse should be alert to a family history of cardiovascular disease and diabetes, and for membership in high-risk ethnic groups such as Native Americans/Alaskan Natives, Hispanics, and Pacific Islanders. These may be considered additional risk factors, especially when serum levels of lipids and glucose are not available.

Dietary analysis is a supplementary tool that can be used by pediatric nurses in some settings. Although there may not be time to complete recalls in all situations, it may be possible to have families write down the child's 24-hour intake, do a quick check or analyze the diet, and contact the family later with specific suggestions. The child who does not meet a variety of RDAs should be targeted for dietary teaching, particularly if BMI and BP also show abnormalities.

Diabetes and cardiovascular disease pose continuing public health problems for our population and, in particular, for the minority groups represented in this study. The rates of type 2 diabetes have risen, particularly in the ethnic groups studied here and among children. Although glucose levels are commonly believed to be definitive for diabetes, they may not indicate a prediabetes or an insulin-resistant state. A key finding of this study is that, even when fasting glucose levels are normal, insulin may be increased and can indicate a pattern of insulin resistance. Furthermore, baseline insulin in childhood has been linked to hypertriglyceridemia at 6-year follow-up (Raitakari et al., 1995). The presence of three or more metabolic syndrome risk factor criteria in this study was highly suggestive of elevated insulin and may guide nurses and other care providers in clinical settings to establish a definitive set of interventions designed to lower risk in these children, even when serum insulin levels are not available (see Table 9).

SUMMARY

In summary, this study found significant correlations of insulin with body adiposity, BP, and serum lipid/lipoprotein levels, consistent with the clustering of variables labeled as metabolic syndrome. Furthermore, there were ethnic and gender differences in serum insulin levels, indicating an increased risk of metabolic syndrome among Native Americans, particularly among Native American female children, as compared to Hispanic and Caucasian populations. Research efforts need to confirm these findings with larger groups and with Native American tribes and Hispanic samples in a variety of geographic locations. Longitudinal studies would help to demonstrate the persistence of syndrome variables over time with individual children and populations, further guiding intervention efforts. In addition, higher insulin levels were related to a lower incidence of meeting the RDAs for dietary nutrients. Future research is needed to provide clear guidelines for the identification of insulin resistance and metabolic syndrome in youths to design interventions that decrease the incidence of type 2 diabetes and the emergence of cardiovascular disease (Cruz & Goran, 2004). At this time, it is known that overweight is a critical risk factor that is associated with insulin resistance, dyslipidemia, and BP elevations (Steinberger, 2003). Therefore, nurses must be certain that height and weight are measured on all children and that the results are analyzed for BMI and placed on appropriate growth charts. Accurate BP measurement is needed, with the use of grids for analysis, to determine those above the 90th and 95th percentiles. Weight elevations should signal the need for careful further assessment for other risk factors, such as family history, smoking, failure to meet RDAs in dietary intake, physical inactivity, abnormal lipid levels, and, in some cases, abnormal glucose and insulin levels. Pediatric nurses are critically important in the early identification of a cascade of health risk factors, which begins with overweight, continues through elevated BP and other characteristics, and becomes metabolic syndrome and, subsequently, type 2 diabetes.

Table 9   Measures to Identify Children at Risk for Metabolic Syndrome

Schools, clinics, and other community settings:
1. Measure height and weight. Compute percentiles. Compute BMI and BMI percentile. Consider children at $\geq$ 85th percentile to be at risk and children at $\geq$ 95th percentile to be at high risk.
2. Measure BP. Use charts to evaluate percentile. Consider children at $\geq$ 90th percentile to be at risk and children at $\geq$ 95th percentile to be at high risk.
3. Complete dietary recall and analyze diet for deficiencies and excesses. Consider that multiple differences from RDAs may be indicative of abnormal insulin levels.
4. Consider family history of diabetes, overweight, hypertension, and cardiovascular disease as risk factors.
5. Refer to health care provider for additional assessment when more than one risk is observed.
6. Intervene to improve diet and physical activity for children with risks. Provide family and child with resources to lower risks.

Pediatric offices:
1. When the child is overweight and has another risk factor, recommend fasting serum analysis for glucose and lipids/lipoproteins.
2. Plan an intervention program to lower the risks identified. Reevaluate the child's risk at least annually.

ACKNOWLEDGMENTS

The support of the Society for Pediatric Nurses, the Delta Chi Chapter-at-Large of Sigma Theta Tau International, the Intercollegiate College of Nursing/Washington State University College of Nursing Carl M. Hansen Research Fund, the Glen King Fellowship in Nutrition at the Washington State University, The Heart Institute of Spokane, and the Westcoast Hospitality is gratefully acknowledged.

REFERENCES

Bacha, F., Saad, R., Gungor, N., Janosky, J., & Arslanian, S.A. (2003). Obesity, regional fat distribution, and syndrome X in obese black versus white adolescents: Race differential in diabetogenic and atherogenic risk factors. *The Journal of Clinical Endocrinology and Metabolism, 88,* 2534-2540.

Bao, W., Srinivasan, S.R., & Berenson, G.S. (1996). Persistent elevation of plasma insulin levels is associated with increased cardiovascular risk in children and young adults. *Circulation, 93,* 54-59.

Bindler, R.C., Massey, L.K., Shultz, J.A., Mills, P.E., & Short, R. (2004). Homocysteine in a multi-ethnic sample of school-age children. *Journal of Pediatric Endocrinology and Metabolism, 17,* 327-337.

Bowman, S.A., Lino, M., Gerrior, S.A., & Basiotis, P.P. (1998). The health eating index: 1994-1996. Washington, DC: U.S. Department of Agriculture, Center for Nutrition Policy and Promotion CNPP-5.

Centers for Disease Control and Prevention. (2000). CDC growth charts: United States. Available from http://www.cdc.gov/growthcharts/.

Chen, W., Bao, W., Begum, S., Elkasabany, A., Srinivasan, S.R., & Berenson, G.S. (2000). Age-related patterns of the clustering of cardiovascular risk variables of syndrome X from childhood to young adulthood in a population made up of black and white subjects. The Bogalusa Heart Study. *Diabetes, 49,* 1042-1048.

Chen, W., Srinivasan, S.R., Elkasabany, A., & Berenson, G.S. (1999). Cardiovascular risk factors clustering features of insulin resistance syndrome (syndrome X) in a biracial (black–white) population of children, adolescents, and young adults. *American Journal of Epidemiology, 150,* 667-674.

Cook, S., Weitzman, M., Auinger, P., Nguyen, M., & Dietz, W.H. (2003). Prevalence of a metabolic syndrome phenotype in adolescents. *Archives of Pediatric and Adolescent Medicine, 157,* 821-827.

Cruz, M.L., & Goran, M.I. (2004). The metabolic syndrome in children and adolescents. *Current Diabetes Reports,* 4, 53-62.

Cruz, M.L., Weigensberg, M.J., Huang, T.T.K., Ball, G., Shabi, G.Q., & Goran, J.I. (2004). The metabolic syndrome in overweight Hispanic youth and the role of insulin sensitivity. *Journal of Clinical Endocrinology and Metabolism, 89,* 108-113.

de Ferranti, S.D., Gauvreau, K., Ludwig, D.S., Neufeld, E.J., Newburger, J.W., & Rifai, N. (2004). Prevalence of the metabolic syndrome in American adolescents: Findings for the Third National Health and Nutrition Examination Survey. *Circulation, 110,* 2494-2497.

Duncan, G.E., Li, S.J., & Zhou, X.H. (2004). Prevalence and trends of a metabolic syndrome phenotype among U.S. adolescents, 1999-2000. *Diabetes Care, 27,* 2438-2443.

Fagot-Campagna, A., Pettitt, D.J., Engelgau, M.M., Burrows, N.R., Geiss, L.S., Valdez, R., et al. (2000). Type 2 diabetes among North American children and adolescents: An epidemiologic review and a public health perspective. *Journal of Pediatrics, 136,* 664-672.

Fagot-Campagna, A., Saaddine, J.B., Flegal, K.M., & Beckles, G.L.A. (2001). Diabetes, impaired fasting glucose, and elevated HbA1c in U.S. adolescents: The Third National Health and Nutrition Examination Survey. *Diabetes Care, 24,* 834-837.

Falkner, B., Hassink, S., Ross, J., & Gidding, S. (2002). Dysmetabolic syndrome: Multiple risk factors for premature adult disease in an adolescent girl. *Pediatrics, 110,* e 14 [Retrieved from http://pediatrics.aappublications.org/cgi/content/full/110/1/e14].

Food and Nutrition Board, Institute of Medicine. (2002). Dietary reference intakes for energy, carbohydrates, fiber, fat, fatty acids, cholesterol, protein, and amino acids (macronutrients). Washington, DC: National Academy Press.

Ford, E.S., Giles, W.H., & Dietz, W.H. (2002). Prevalence of the metabolic syndrome among US adults: Findings from the Third National Health and Nutrition Examination Survey. *The Journal of the American Medical Association, 287,* 356-359.

Godin, G., & Shephard, R.J. (1985). A simple method to assess exercise behavior in the community. *Canadian Journal of Applied Sports Science, 10,* 141-146.

Golley, R.K., Magarey, A.M., Steinbeck, K.S., Baur, L.A., & Daniels, L.A. (2006). Comparison of metabolic syndrome prevalence using six different definitions in overweight prepubertal children enrolled in a weight management study. *International Journal of Obesity, 30,* 853-860.

Goodman, E., Daniels, S.R., Morrison, J.A., Huang, B., & Dolan, L.M. (2004). Contrasting prevalence of and demographic disparities in the World Health Organization and National Cholesterol Education Program Adult Treatment Panel III definitions of metabolic syndrome among adolescents. *Journal of Pediatrics, 145,* 445-451.

Gower, B.A., Nagy, T.R., & Goran, M.I. (1999). Visceral fat, insulin sensitivity, and lipids in prepubertal children. *Diabetes, 48,* 1515-1521.

Grundy, S.M., Brewer, H.B., Cleeman, J.I., Smith, S.C., & Lenfant, C. (2004). Definition of metabolic syndrome: Report of the National Heart, Lung, and Blood Institute/American Heart Association conference on scientific issues related to definition. *Circulation, 109,* 433- 438.

Hardy, L.R., Harrell, J.S., & Bell, R.A. (2004). Overweight in children: Definitions, measurements, confounding factors, and health consequences. *Journal of Pediatric Nursing, 19,* 376-384.

Harwell, T.S., McDowall, J.M., Moore, K., Fagot-Campagna, A., Helgerson, S.D., & Gohdes, D. (2001). Establishing surveillance for diabetes in American Indian youth. *Diabetes Care, 24,* 1029-1032.

Kelley, D.E. (2000). Overview: What is insulin resistance? *Nutrition Reviews, 58,* S2- S3.

307

Kennedy, E.T., Ohls, J., Carlson, S., & Fleming, K. (1995). The healthy eating index: Design and applications. *Journal of the American Dietetic Association, 95,* 1103-1111.

Kriska, A.M., & Casperson, C.J. (1997). Introduction to a collection of physical activity questionnaires. *Journal of the American College of Sports Medicine 29,* S5-S9, S36- S38.

Lindquist, C.H., Gower, B.A., & Goran, M.I. (2000). Role of dietary factors in ethnic differences in early risk of cardiovascular disease and type 2 diabetes. *American Journal of Clinical Nutrition, 71,* 725-732.

Ludwig, D.S., Pereira, M.A., Kroenke, C.H., Hilner, J.E., Van Horn, L., Slattery, M.L., et al. (1999). Dietary fiber, weight gain, and cardiovascular disease risk factors in young adults. *The Journal of the American Medical Association, 282,* 1539-1546.

Mayer-Davis, E.J., Monaco, J.H., Hoesn, H.M., Carmichael, S., Vitolins, M.Z., & Rewers, M.J. (1997). Dietary fat and insulin sensitivity in a triethnic population: The role of obesity. The Insulin Resistance Atherosclerosis Study (IRAS). *American Journal of Clinical Nutrition, 65,* 79-87.

Molnar, K. (2004). The prevalence of the metabolic syndrome and type 2 diabetes in children and adolescents. *International Journal of Obesity, 28,* S70-S74.

National Academy of Sciences. (2002). Unequal treatment: Confronting racial and ethnic disparities in health care. Retrieved from http://www.nap.eduopenbook/030908265X.html.

National Heart, Lung, and Blood Institute. (2004). Fourth report on the diagnosis, evaluation and treatment of high blood pressure in children and adolescents. Retrieved from http://www.nhlbi.gov/guidelines/hypertension/child_tbl.htm.

National Institutes of Health. (2001). Third report of the National Cholesterol Education Program Expert Panel on detection, evaluation and treatment of high blood cholesterol in adults. Bethesda, MD: National Institutes of Health [NIH Publication 01-3670].

Neufeld, N.D., Raffel, L.J., Landon, C., Dhen, Y.D., & Vadheim, C.M. (1998). Early presentation of type 2 diabetes in Mexican–American youth. *Diabetes Care, 21,* 80-86.

Ogden, C.L., Flegal, K.M., Carroll, M.D., & Johnson, C.L. (2002). Prevalence and trends in overweight among US children and adolescents. *The Journal of the American Medical Association, 288,* 1728-1732.

Raitakari, O.T., Porkka, K.V.K., Ronnemaa, T., Knip, M., Uhari, M., Akerblom, H.K., et al. (1995). The role of insulin in clustering of serum lipids and blood pressure in children and adolescents: The Cardiovascular Risk in Young Finns Study. *Diabetologia, 38,* 1042-1050.

Roberts, K., Dunn, K., Jean, S.K., & Lardinois, C.K. (2000). Syndrome X: Medical nutrition therapy. *Nutrition Reviews, 58,* 154-160.

Rockett, H.R.H., Breitenbach, M., Frazier, A.L., Witschi, J., Wolf, A.M., Field, A.E., et al. (1997). Validation of a youth/adolescent food frequency questionnaire. *Preventive Medicine, 26,* 808-816.

Rockett, H.R.H., & Colditz, G.A. (1997). Assessing diets of children and adolescents. American *Journal of Clinical Nutrition Supplement, 65,* 1116S-1122S.

Shaibi, G.Q., Cruz, M.L., Ball, G.D., Weigensberg, M.J., Kobaissi, H.A., Salem, G.J., et al. (2005). Cardiovascular fitness and the metabolic syndrome in overweight Latino youths. *Medicine and Science in Sports and Exercise, 37,* 922-928.

Sorof, J.M., Lai, D., Turner, J., Poffenbarger, T., & Portman, R.J. (2004). Overweight, ethnicity, and the prevalence of hypertension in school-aged children. *Pediatrics, 113,* 475-482.

Srinivasan, S.R., Myers, L., & Berenson, G.S. (1999). Temporal association between obesity and hyperinsulinemia in children, adolescents and young adults: The Bogalusa Heart Study. *Metabolism, 48,* 928- 934.

Steinberger, J. (2003). Diagnosis of the metabolic syndrome in children. *Current Opinion in Lipidology, 14,* 555-559.

Steinberger, J., & Daniels, S.R. (2003). Obesity, insulin resistance, diabetes, and cardiovascular risk in children. An American Heart Association Scientific Statement from the Atherosclerosis, Hypertension, and Obesity in the Young Committee (Council on Cardiovascular Disease in the Young) and the Diabetes Committee (Council on Nutrition, Physical Activity, and Metabolism). *Circulation, 107,* 1448-1453.

Stroehla, B.C., Malcoe, L.H., & Velie, E.M. (2005). Dietary sources of nutrients among rural Native American and white children. *Journal of the American Dietetic Association, 105,* 1908-1916.

Sullivan, C.S., Beste, J., Cummings, D.M., Hester, V.H., Holbrook, T., Kolasa, K.M., et al. (2004). Prevalence of hyperinsulinemia and clinical correlates in overweight children referred for lifestyle intervention. *Journal of the American Dietetic Association, 104,* 433-436.

Suminski, R.R., Poston, W.S., & Foreyt, J.P. (1999). Early identification of Mexican American children who are at risk for becoming obese. *International Journal of Obesity, 23,* 823-829.

Valdez, R. (2000). Epidemiology. *Nutrition Reviews, 58,* S4- S6.

Valle, M., Gascon, F., Martos, R., Ruz, F.J., Bermudo, F., Morales, R., et al. (2002). Metabolic cardiovascular syndrome in obese prepubertal children: The role of high fasting insulin levels. *Metabolism, 51,* 423-428.

Van Horn, L. (1997). Fiber, lipids, and coronary heart disease. *Circulation, 95,* 2701-2704.

Variyam, J.B., Smallwood, C., & Basiotis, P.P. (1998). USDA's healthy eating index and nutrition information. Washington, DC: USDA Center for Nutrition Policy and Promotion [Technical Bulletin No. 1866].

Weigensberg, M.J., Ball, G.D., Shaibi, G.Q., Cruz, M.L., Gower, B.A., & Goran, M.I. (2005). Dietary fat intake and insulin resistance in black and white children. *Obesity Research, 13,* 1630-1637.

Weiss, R., Dziura, J., Burgert, T.S., Tamborlane, W.V., Taksali, S.E., Yeckel, C.W., et al. (2004). Obesity and the metabolic syndrome in children and adolescents. *New England Journal of Medicine, 350,* 2362-2374.

Weitzman, M., Cook, S., Auinger, P., Florin, T.A., Daniels, S., Nguyen, M., et al. (2006). Tobacco smoke exposure is associated with the metabolic syndrome in adolescents. *Circulation, 112,* 862-869.

Williams, C.L., Hayman, L.L., Daniels, S.R., Robinson, T.N., Steinberger, J., Paridon, S., et al. (2002). Cardiovascular health in childhood: A statement for health professional from the Committee on Atherosclerosis, Hypertension, and Obesity in the Young (AHOY) of the Council on Cardiovascular Disease in the Young, American Heart Association. *Circulation, 106,* 143-160.

Yensel, C.S., Preud'Homme, D., & Curry, D.M. (2004). Childhood obesity and insulin-resistant syndrome. *Journal of Pediatric Nursing, 19,* 238-246.

Young, T.K., Dean, H.J., Flett, B., & Wood-Steinman, P. (2000). Childhood obesity in a population at high risk for type 2 diabetes. *Journal of Pediatrics, 136,* 365-369.

Ziegler, P., Hanson, C., Ponza, M., Novak, T., & Hendricks, K. (2006). Feeding infants and toddler study: Meal and snack intakes of Hispanic and non-Hispanic infants and toddlers. *Journal of the American Dietetic Association, 106,* 107-123.

Zimmet, P., Magliano, D., Matsuzawa, Y., Alberti, G., & Shaw, J. (2005). The metabolic syndrome: A global public health problem and a new definition. *Journal of Atherosclerosis and Thrombosis, 12,* 295-300.